KV-351-634

The New Medicine

OTORHINOLARYNGOLOGY

The New Medicine

An Integrated System of Study

The New Medicine

An Integrated System of Study

Series Editors R. Harden and A. Marcus

Volume 4

OTORHINOLARYNGOLOGY
including oral medicine and surgery

Edited by A. G. D. Maran

The New Medicine Series has been produced in collaboration with Update Publications Limited

1983 **MTP PRESS LIMITED**
a member of the KLUWER ACADEMIC PUBLISHERS GROUP
BOSTON / THE HAGUE / DORDRECHT / LANCASTER

Published by
MTP Press Limited
Falcon House
Lancaster, England

British Library Cataloguing in Publication Data

Maran, A.G.D.
   Otorhinolaryngology.—(New medicine; 4)
   1. Otorhinolaryngology
   I. Title 11. Series
   616.2′2   RF46

ISBN 0-85200-402-8

Copyright © 1983 MTP Press Limited

All rights reserved. No part of this publication may be
reproduced, stored in a retrieval system, or transmitted in any
form or by any means, electronic, mechanical, photocopying,
recording or otherwise, without prior permission from the
publishers.

Typeset by Servis Filmsetting Ltd., Manchester
Colour origination by Speedlith Photo Litho Ltd., Manchester
Printed and bound by Redwood Burn Ltd., Trowbridge

CONTENTS

LIST OF CONTRIBUTORS

EDITOR

A.G.D. Maran, MD, FRCS, FACS
Consultant Otolaryngologist
The Royal Infirmary
Edinburgh, Scotland

CONTRIBUTORS

Andrew Baxter, FRCS
Department of Otolaryngology
Stobhill Hospital
Glasgow, Scotland

D. Chisholm, BDS, PhD, FDS
Professor of Oral Medicine
Dundee Dental School
Dundee, Scotland

D.L. Cowan, MB, ChB, FRCS(Ed)
Consultant Otolaryngologist
City Hospital and Royal Hospital for Sick Children
Edinburgh, Scotland

B.A.B. Dale, FRCS(Ed)
Consultant ENT Surgeon
The Royal Infirmary
Edinburgh, Scotland

P.R. Geissler, DDS, FDSRCS(Ed)
Senior Lecturer
Department of Prosthetic Dentistry
University of Edinburgh
Scotland

A.I.G. Kerr, MB, FRCS
Consultant Otolaryngologist
The Royal Infirmary
Edinburgh, Scotland

A.G.D. Maran, MD, FRCS, FACS
The Royal Infirmary
Edinburgh, Scotland

D. Mason, BDS, MD, FRCS, FDS, FRCPath
Professor of Oral Medicine
Glasgow Dental School
Glasgow, Scotland

D.S. Murray, FRCS
Consultant in Plastic and Reconstructive Surgery
West Midlands Regional Plastic and Jaw Surgery Unit
Wordsley Hospital
Wordsley, Stourbridge, West Midlands

SERIES EDITORS

R. McG. Harden, MD, FRCP(GLAS)
Centre for Medical Education
Ninewells Hospital and Medical School
University of Dundee
Scotland

A. Marcus, MB, B CH
Chairman
Update Publications Ltd
London
England

CO-ORDINATING EDITOR

R. Cairncross
Centre for Medical Education
Ninewells Hospital and Medical School
University of Dundee
Scotland

INTRODUCTION

The need for a new approach to textbooks

Many books have been written for students of medicine. The conventional textbook, however, imposes many constraints upon the reader and the author. While a considerable effort has been put into developing newer, more sophisticated methods of learning such as television, audio-tape and slides, and computers, few attempts have been made to improve the more traditional approach – the book. The aim of this series of textbooks is to minimize the limitations of the standard text and to maximize the usefulness of the book as an aid to learning.

We believe that in a number of ways this series is unique. It is the first textbook to be produced as a collaborative project between a publisher and a University Department of Medical Education. The intenton has been to produce a series of textbooks which take into account three significant trends in medical education: a move towards a more integrated approach to teaching, an increased emphasis on student-centred learning, and greater use of problem-based learning.

A more integrated text

Firstly, there is a general move to a more integrated approach to learning, a trend reflected in the curricula of many schools. This involves a shift from subject- or discipline-based teaching where the emphasis is on the individual subjects or disciplines such as medicine, surgery and therapeutics, to a multi-disciplinary or integrated approach where the student is encouraged to take a more holistic view of medicine and to learn the appropriate medicine, surgery or therapeutics in relation to each system such as the cardiovascular system, respiratory system, etc. Unfortunately, textbooks, in general, have not kept pace with these developments and many textbooks still look at medicine from the point of view of each separate discipline. Patients, however, present to the doctor with symp-

toms such as abdominal pain, or swellings in the neck, and don't come neatly labelled as a surgical case or a medical case. The examination of the patient, and his further investigation and management, must take into account both 'medical' and 'surgical' pathologies. The advantages and indications for medical treatment must be reviewed alongside those of surgical intervention. This series of medical textbooks presents such an integrated view of medicine and has been written by a multi-disciplinary team.

One approach to the production of an integrated textbook is to ask a series of specialists from different backgrounds each to prepare a chapter or section looking at the subject from his own view point. Unfortunately, such a strategy frequently results in a disjointed look at the subject and the juxtaposition of sections written by a surgeon, a physician and a general practitioner is a poor substitute for a truly integrated book.

In this book the contributors have worked together as a team, planning and writing the book under the direction of an editor. As a group they have taken overall responsibility for its contents. It is hoped that the result will be a more meaningful integration of the subjects.

A useful aid to the student

A second trend in medical education is the move towards more student-centred learning where the emphasis is on the student and what he learns rather than what he is taught. This is a move away from a more teacher-centred approach when the emphasis is on the teacher and what he teaches.

A student-centred approach results in more effective learning and prepares the student better for his continuing education or life-long learning. This series of books has been designed to provide the teacher and the student with an effective resource for learning. It can be used as a basis for a course where the emphasis is on independent learning, as a resource to provide background information for small group work and as a text for use in relation to a lecture course.

Each volume contains questions relating to the content of the volume. The reader can use these to assess his knowledge of the subject. They can be used either before or after he reads the relevant sections of the book. The reader by trying to answer the questions can obtain an indication as to the extent to which he has mastered the subject and to which further reading is necessary.

A more problem-based approach to medicine

A third trend in medical education is the move towards a more problem-based approach to learning. In the past the emphasis in medical education has been placed on the teaching of facts about patients and their diseases rather than on the application of the facts and the use of the information to solve problems relating to patients. To take account of this trend, each volume in the series contains a section which looks at how patients present with problems relating to the system under consideration. It is hoped that this will encourage a more problem-based approach to medicine and provide a resource which can be used in more problem-based curricula.

Format of books

The volumes in the series have a standard format. Each volume has five sections and each section tackles the subject from a different direction. Section one presents appropriate background information and briefly reviews the relevant general anatomy, biochemistry, pathology and epidemiology. Section two considers how to take a history from a patient and

conduct a physical examination in relation to the system under consideration. Section three discusses the investigation and management of the common clinical presentations and leads to a series of differential diagnoses. Section four considers the diseases relating to the system and discusses their management. Section five covers in more detail some aspects of the surgery, pharmacology and therapeutics.

For whom is the text intended?

Undergraduate students can use the books in this series as they work their way through the curriculum. The series will be of value not only in schools with integrated curricula but in more traditional schools. The texts will provide the necessary information on each subject while at the same time encouraging the student to relate the various subjects he is studying one to another. While the books will be of particular value in the later years of the cirriculum, they can also serve to introduce students to medicine in the earlier years. Many teachers have attempted in recent years to introduce a more clinical approach in the early phases of the medical school curriculum and to relate the basic and paramedical sciences to clinical medicine. This series has been designed to encourage the student to relate the medical sciences to the practice of medicine.

The series also has a place in postgraduate and continuing education. For postgraduate students the series can serve as introductory texts in each area. For doctors who have completed their vocational training, it can provide a useful and up-to-date review of medicine. While participation in courses, attendance at meetings, reading of journals and interaction with colleagues are all useful in continuing medical education, a readily available reference source is also necessary. This series of books can be used for this purpose.

PART 1

THE EAR

SECTION I

Background to disease of the ear

BACKGROUND

Some background information is essential if you are to understand the ear. A summary of the relevant points is contained in this section. More detailed information can be obtained from standard reference books.

ANATOMY

The external auditory canal

The ear develops in the first trimester from the first and second branchial arches and the first branchial groove (LD-1, LD-2). The auricle (LD-3) arises from six surface tubercles and is comprised of cartilage covered with closely adherent skin.

Failure of development will lead to malformations:

- anomalies of the auricle from failure of fusion of the tubercles
- complete or partial atresia of the ear canal
  This may be associated with deformities of the auricle and middle ear.
- deformities of middle ear
- inner ear anomalies

The external auditory canal is about 2.5 cm (1 inch) in length and comprises an outer cartilaginous portion and an inner bony portion. Hair follicles and glands lie within the skin of the cartilaginous portion. In the bony canal the skin is applied directly to the periosteum. The glands of the canal are pilosebaceous (related to the hair follicles) and ceruminous (wax producing). The deep anteroinferior portion of the

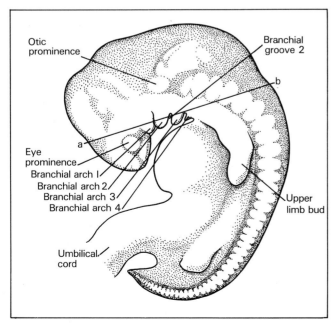

LD-1. *External features of a 5 mm embryo in the fifth week of life*

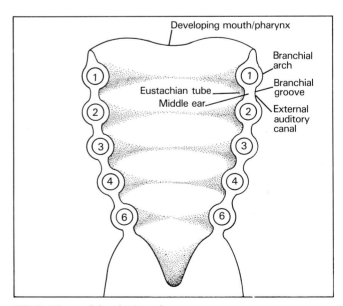

LD-2. *Floor of developing pharynx*

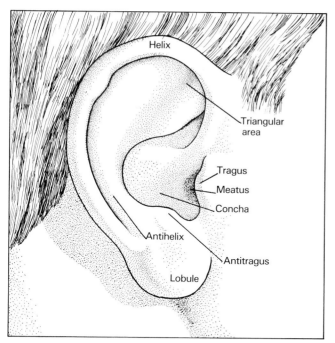

LD-3. *The right pinna*

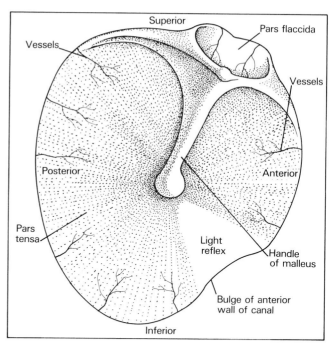

LD-4. *The right tympanic membrane*

canal often bulges into the lumen and a recess is created extending down to the tympanic membrane: in this, wax and debris may collect.

Anterior to the canal are the parotid gland and the temporomandibular joint. The mastoid process lies posterior to the canal.

Lymphatic glands are found pre-, post- and infra-auricularly.

The nerve supply to the ear canal is derived from the trigeminal nerve, the posterior roots of the second and third cervical nerves and a branch of the vagus which innervates the deep canal (this last being known as Arnold's or Alderman's nerve.)

The tympanic membrane

The three layers which compose the tympanic membrane are:

- skin
- fibrous
- mucosal

The upper part of the membrane is known as the 'pars flaccida'. This has no fibrous layer. The 'pars tensa' comprises the remainder and greater portion of the tympanic membrane.

The membrane is set at an angle to the ear canal. The anteroinferior portion is deepest in the canal

such that a light directed on to the membrane appears coned anteroinferiorly (LD-4). The membrane is grey in colour, with blood vessels around the periphery and along the handle of the malleus.

The tympanic cavity

The tympanic cavity is similar to a rectangular box (LD-5), narrower in the mediolateral dimension. The principal contents of the middle ear are:

- three bones (the ossicles):
  malleus
  incus
  stapes

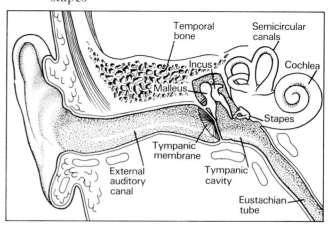

LD-5. *The middle ear*

- two muscles:
  - stapedius
  - tensor tympani

- three nerves:
  - facial nerve
  - tympanic plexus from the ninth cranial (glossopharyngeal) nerve
  - chorda tympani (sensory element of the facial nerve)

The Eustachian tube leads from the nasopharynx to the anterior wall of the tympanic cavity. The posterior wall opens superiorly into the short canal, known as the aditus, which leads to the mastoid antrum.

Respiratory mucosa lines the tympanic cavity. It is continuous with the nasopharynx and passes through the middle ear into the mastoid cells.

The *mastoid antrum* is the first of the mastoid air cells and the mastoid cellularity develops from it.

The *surface marking* of the mastoid antrum is 'Macewen's triangle', which can be outlined on the mastoid process, postero-superior to the bony external canal.

The ossicles

The ossicles (LD-6) are arranged from lateral to medial with the malleus attached to the tympanic membrane and the stapes inserted into the oval window. The stapes communicates through its footplate with the fluid of the inner ear. The incus bridges the gap between the malleus and the stapes. The stapedius muscle is attached to the stapes and the tensor tympani to the malleus.

There are two potential openings in the medial wall of the cavity: (1) the oval window into which the stapes footplate is inserted and (2) the round window which contains a dense fibrous membrane. A bulge in the medial wall known as the promontory separates the two windows.

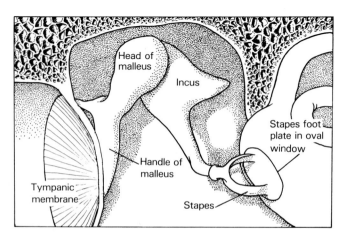

LD-6. *The ossicles*

The nerves

The facial nerve traverses the medial and posterior walls of the cavity to enter the neck below the external canal through the stylomastoid foramen. In the child under the age of 2 it comes to the surface more superficially behind the auricle. As it traverses the cavity within its bony covering known as the Fallopian canal, the nerve is liable to damage through trauma or infection.

The chorda tympani passes backwards across the cavity between the malleus and the incus and joins the seventh nerve in its vertical segment. It carries taste sensation from the anterior two thirds of the tongue (LD-7).

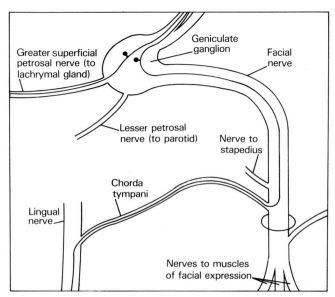

LD-7. *The facial nerve. Although primarily a motor nerve, it contains a few sensory fibres which relay in the cells of its geniculate ganglion. They are predominantly concerned with taste sensations*

The tympanic plexus overlies the medial tympanic wall and is sensory to the tympanic cavity.

The inner ear

The inner ear comprises an outer bony casing, the osseous labyrinth, and an inner membranous labyrinth which is surrounded by fluid known as perilymph. It contains another fluid, endolymph. Two sensory mechanisms are represented within the membranous labyrinth. The sensory end organ of hearing is the cochlea, and that of balance is comprised of the utricle and the semicircular canals of the vestibule (LD-8).

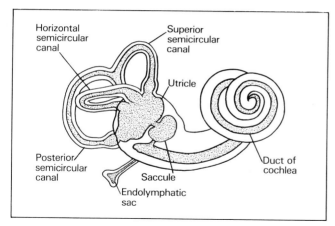

LD-8. *The membranous labyrinth*

The three semicircular canals are the posterior, the superior and the horizontal or lateral.

The eighth cranial or statoacoustic nerve is initially in two parts – the vestibular division and the cochlear division. The two join and pass medially through the internal auditory canal to the brain stem.

A fine sensorineural epithelium lies on the basilar membrane of the cochlea and is also present within the utricle and the semicircular canals. It is this epithelium which on stimulation results in sensory transmission along the nerve (LD-9, LD-10).

THE PHYSIOLOGY OF HEARING

A sound wave must stimulate the cochlea before it may be heard. This may be achieved in two ways.

- by bone conduction directly through the bones of the skull
- by air conduction by traversing the external canal and crossing the tympanic membrane to the stapes footplate

We hear by both routes but principally by air conduction.

The auricle in man has lost its primitive function of moving to locate sound.

Transmission of the sound wave in the middle ear

The sound wave passes through the external canal to strike and cause vibration of the tympanic membrane. This, by means of its physical connection with the

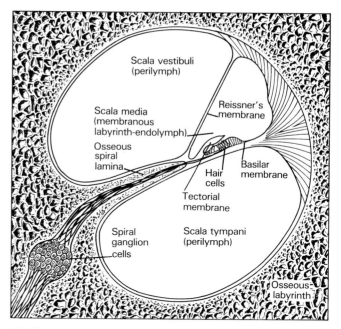

LD-9. *Section of the cochlear duct*

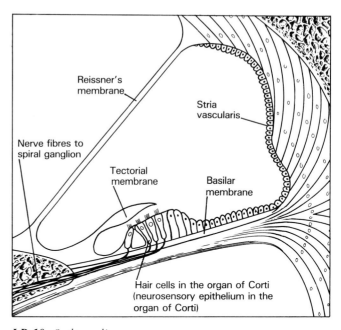

LD-10. *Scala media*

malleus, in turn sets up a vibration in the ossicular chain and results in the stapes footplate moving within the oval window.

The tympanic membrane–ossicular chain system enables the sound wave to be transmitted from the medium of air in the external auditory canal to the medium of fluid within the labyrinth. It reduces the acoustic impedance that occurs when sound passes from one medium to another.

Optimum function of the tympanic mechanism is dependent upon the pressures on either side of the tympanic membrane being equal and upon satisfactory aeration of the round window. This is made possible by the ventilatory function of the Eustachian tube.

The *Eustachian tube* opens at its nasopharyngeal end by the action of the tensor and levator palati muscles. The tube opens on yawning and swallowing.

The *intratympanic muscles* probably have two functions. They protect the inner ear through their potential to firm the ossicular chain under the stimulus of high intensity sound and they also help to suspend the ossicular chain.

Transmission of the sound wave in the inner ear

Vibration of the stapes results in movement of the perilymphatic fluid of the labyrinth. This movement sets up a wave-like motion which travels down the cochlea in the upper scala vestibuli, passing to the apex and then along the lower scala tympani and back to the round window where an equal and opposite movement to that of the stapes occurs (LD-11). Movement of the perilymph causes movement in the membranous labyrinth and particularly in the basilar membrane in which the sensorineural epithelium lies.

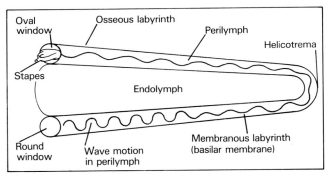

LD-11. Sound conduction in the cochlea

The hair cell is the functional auditory unit of the sensorineural epithelium. Distortion of the so-called hairs on these cells results in an electrical impulse being developed within the cell. This charges the primary auditory neurons.

This impulse is carried through the second and subsequent order neurons and via the cochlear nuclei in the brain stem to the superior temporal gyri, where cortical appreciation of the sound stimulus occurs.

THE PHYSIOLOGY OF BALANCE

Balance is maintained by input from various sources and is coordinated centrally. The vestibular apparatus of the labyrinth is most important but stimuli arise from other sensory sources. These include the eye, receptors in the soles of the feet and the knee joints as well as joint and muscle position sensation in the lower limbs. Maintenance of balance also requires intact extrapyramidal and pyramidal tracts.

The vestibular apparatus

Movement of endolymph within the vestibular apparatus results in stimulation of the fine sensorineural epithelium lying within the ampullae of the semicircular canals and the otolithic membrane of the utricle. This stimulus then triggers the first order neuron.

Nystagmus

The vestibular apparatus of each ear is coordinated with the other and, as such, exerts an equal input to the brain stem. Outflow from the brain stem influences the position of the eyes. An alteration in response on one side as opposed to the other will result in an imbalance in the central response. This affects the control of the eyes and produces the phenomenon of nystagmus, which is an involuntary oscillatory movement of the eyes. If it follows a disturbance in the peripheral labyrinth, it is generally in the horizontal or rotatory plane.

It should be remembered that there are certain non-pathological situations in which the inner ear can be abnormally stimulated. These include rotation, and abnormal visual stimuli such as ascending to unaccustomed heights.

SECTION II
History and physical examination of the ear

HISTORY

The main complaint should be established first, with particular regard to onset, duration and recurrence. In taking an aural history enquire specifically into the six likely presenting symptoms. These are:

- hearing loss
- vertigo and imbalance
- tinnitus
- discharge
- earache
- facial nerve palsy or weakness

These symptoms may be accompanied by both nausea or vomiting and headache.

Hearing loss

Points to elicit are as follows.

- Was the onset sudden or progressive?
- Is the deafness fluctuant?
  This occurs in Ménière's syndrome and Eustachian tube dysfunction.
- Is there a family history of hearing loss?
- Can the patient hear better in a noisy background (paracusis)?
  This is a feature of otosclerosis.
- Is there a history of exposure to noise?
- Has there been trauma to the ears?
- What is the patient's occupational history?
- Does the patient smoke, take drugs or consume alcohol?
- Was the onset associated with a head cold?
  This can follow Eustachian tube obstruction.
- Does the patient suffer from nasal symptoms?

Otorrhoea

The term otorrhoea means discharge from the ear. Points to elicit are as follows.

- How long has the discharge been present?
- Has it been continuous or recurrent?
- What is its colour?
- Is the discharge mucoid, mucopurulent or frankly purulent?
- Has it been blood stained?
- Is it offensive to smell?
- Is there related pain or pruritis?

Vertigo

The term vertigo implies a real or imaginary sensation of imbalance relative to the patient or his surroundings.
Points to elicit are as follows.

- How long has the symptom been present?
- Is it intermittent?
- How long does an individual attack last?
- Can the patient describe an individual attack?
- Is there any element of rotation with regard to the patient himself or his surroundings or is it merely lightheadedness that is the main complaint?
- Is there any associated headache?
  This may suggest an intracranial pathology.
- Does the patient experience nausea or vomiting?
- Is the symptom brought on by a specific provocative action?
  Benign paroxysmal vertigo may be produced by headturning or extending or flexing the cervical spine.

- Was there a history of a head cold prior to the symptom commencing?
  This is a common feature of 'viral' labyrinthitis.
- Does the patient feel that he staggers predominantly to one side or the other?
  This will help to localize the lesion.
- Has the patient ever had a similar occurrence?
  Ménière's syndrome is recurrent.
- Has the patient been taking any medication?
  Ototoxic drugs or hypotensive agents may be a cause.
- Is there a history of emotional or physical stress?

Tinnitus

Noise in the ears or head such as ringing, buzzing, clicking or roaring constitutes tinnitus.

A description of the tinnitus in itself is not helpful, except where the patient describes it as being pulsatile. This would be suggestive of a vascular tumour either in the neck or in the tympanic cavity itself. Always ask about the relationship of the tinnitus to other aural symptoms.

Enquire about:

- general health
- drug history
- evidence of emotional or physical stress

Otalgia

This is pain in the ear.

Points to elicit are as follows.

- Is the pain associated with a head cold?
  This occurs in an acute aural infection.
- Is the ear itself sore to touch or is the pain deep within the ear?
  Localization to canal or middle ear is helpful.
- Is the pain continuous or remittent?
- What is its relationship to other aural symptoms?
- Is there a history of hoarseness or dysphagia?
  Referred otalgia via cranial nerves IX, X can occur.
- Is there any pain in the back of the neck or on opening the mouth?

Referred otalgia can come from the cranial nerves V and central roots 2 and 3.

Facial paralysis

With the exception of the muscles of mastication, the motor nerve to the face is the facial nerve.

Points to elicit are as follows.

- Was the onset sudden or progressive?
- Is there associated pain in the face or around the ears?
  This may be of assistance in the prognosis of Bell's paralysis.
- Is there a history of trauma?
- Is there a history of ear disease?
- Is there any alteration of taste?
  This helps to localize the level of the lesion.
- Is there dryness of eyes?
  This helps to localize the level of the lesion.
- Are there other physical symptoms of weakness or paralysis in the rest of the body?
  This suggests an upper motor neuron paralysis.

Associated symptoms

When a satisfactory history of the presenting symptom is obtained, the patient should be thoroughly questioned about any associated symptoms in the nose and throat. The general health of the patient should also be noted as well as any recent or present medication.

EXAMINATION

On examination of the ear the clinician should resist the temptation of looking straight into the ear with the auriscope. Time should be taken to examine the ear both front and back, looking for any scars, accessory auricles, pedicles or fistulae.

Tenderness may be elicited over the mastoid, and swelling in this region may indicate an abscess or lymphadenopathy which may or may not be secondary to pathology in the ear. Tenderness may also be found on moving the pinna or cartilaginous canal.

Note that the parotid gland lies anterior to the ear and that postauricular nodes may be infected from a scalp lesion.

The external auditory canal and tympanic membrane

These may be inspected using the electric auriscope.

Examination of the ear, as with the nose, throat and larynx, calls for great gentleness and time must be taken to gain the confidence and co-operation of the patient. This is particularly so with children.

Use of the head mirror takes time to perfect. It requires a reflected light source and is generally unsuitable for general practice.

The correct size of speculum must be selected – neither so large as to cause discomfort or pain, nor so small as to inhibit adequate visualization. The auricle should be gently pulled upwards (downwards in the infant) and backwards to straighten the natural curve of the canal. The speculum of the auriscope can then be inserted in the canal carefully and not too deeply. The instrument may be moved to alter the direction of illumination and vision so that the entire canal and tympanic membrane may be studied. An insufflator bulb (LD-12) may be applied to the auriscope and through this the pressure on the tympanic membrane can be altered and mobility observed.

Wax or squames may be present in the canal and these must be removed before the tympanic membrane may be adequately viewed. A probe or cotton carrier with a wisp of cotton rolled on the end can be used (LD-13). If the canal cannot be cleaned, the

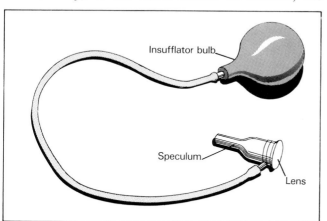

LD-12. *An insufflator bulb altering the pressure on the tympanic membrane*

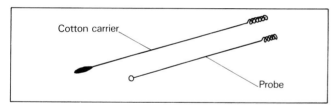

LD-13. *Probe and cotton carrier*

material may be removed by syringing, especially if wax is present. Discharge within the external auditory canal should be swabbed for bacteriological examination. The ear should not be syringed if a dry perforation is present.

A cough reflex may be produced on manipulating the deep external canal due to referral through Arnold's nerve, a branch of the vagus.

Further examination

Following the examination of the ear itself, the nose, nasopharynx, pharynx and larynx must be adequately examined – especially in a case of hearing loss or otalgia. The neck must be palpated, particularly when there is tinnitus.

INVESTIGATIONS

Hearing tests

Free-field speech

The simplest method by which hearing can be assessed is by testing the ability of the patient to respond to the spoken word. From this test it is possible to say whether the patient has or has not a significant degree of hearing loss and to estimate roughly its severity. This is known as 'free-field speech'. It is the basic hearing test and requires no instrumentation.

The non-tested ear should be occluded by the examiner or the patient pressing over the tragus. It should be turned from the examiner. The patient is then required to repeat a list of words spoken in a forced whisper, with the examiner coming closer to the ear until a response is obtained. If this fails the words should be delivered in a conversational voice. Failure to respond indicates a severe level of hearing loss.

The words used for testing are of two types:

- phonetically balanced words such as 'mark', 'bark', 'park' and 'lark'

- spondee words such as 'nightlight', 'blackboard', 'blackbird' and 'daydream'

The former are more difficult to discriminate.

From this test we are able to state whether the patient has a hearing loss and to estimate roughly the severity.

Tuning fork tests

The tuning fork tests help in assessing the type of hearing loss. It should be possible to decide whether the patient is suffering from a conductive deafness or a sensorineural deafness. A disturbance of the conduction system from the external auditory meatus to the stapes footplate will result in conductive deafness. Sensorineural deafness is related to some upset involving the cochlea, the cochlear nerve or more central connections.

Where there is a bilateral deafness it is possible to decide which is the better of the two ears and to estimate the degree of deafness in comparison with the examiner. (It is assumed that the examiner's hearing is normal.) The most commonly used tuning fork is pitched at 512 cycles per second. LD-14 shows a 512 c/s fork and Barany box.

The Barany box is of use in masking the non-tested ear. Masking is a technique for reducing the response of a non-tested ear in order to eliminate crossover of sound from the tested ear if there is hearing loss of greater magnitude than that of the non-tested ear.

Rinne test

The Rinne test compares the air conduction (AC) with the bone conduction (BC) in the one ear (LD-15).

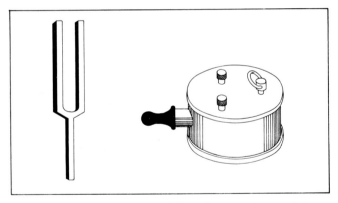

LD-14. A 512 c/s tuning fork (left) and Barany box (right)

To perform the Rinne test, the tuning fork is struck on a dull surface such as the patella or elbow to obtain a tone of moderate intensity. The patient is then asked to compare his ability to hear the fork at the external auditory meatus (AC) with that when the fork is placed over the mastoid antrum (BC). Results are as follows.

Normal
    Rinne Positive
    AC > BC.

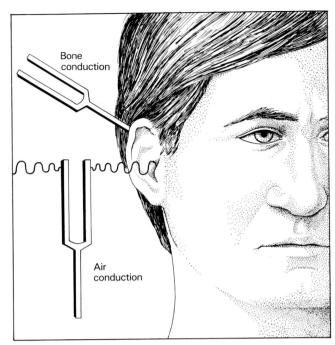

LD-15. Rinne test

Conductive hearing loss
    Rinne Negative
    BC > AC.

Sensorineural hearing loss
    Rinne Positive
    AC > BC
    (But both are reduced when compared with a normal ear).

Total unilateral sensorineural deafness
    False Rinne Negative
    AC not heard
    BC referred to opposite side
    (BC can be eliminated by use of Barany box).

Weber test

The Weber test is purely a bone conduction test and enables the examiner to decide which is the better of the two ears. It is performed by placing the sounded tuning fork on the vertex in the middle of the forehead, on the clenched teeth or on the tip of the chin. The patient is then asked to indicate on which side he hears the sound better (Weber right or left), or if it is central (LD-16–18).

Audiometry

Pure tone audiometry

Pure tone audiometry determines not only the level of the patient's hearing for pure tones but also enables

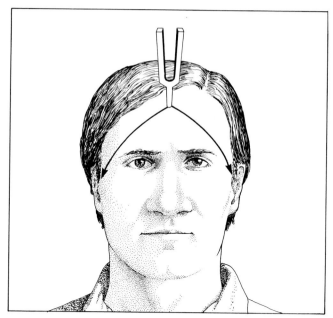

LD-16. *Weber test*

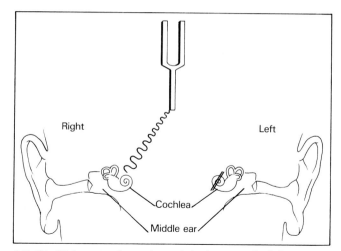

LD-17. *Weber test. Sensorineural deafness on the left – with a Weber test the sound is heard better by the right ear*

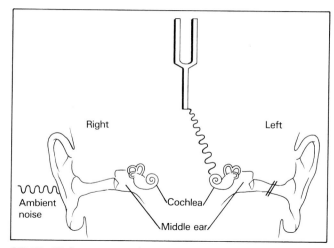

LD-18. *Weber test. Conductive deafness on the left – with a Weber test the sound is heard better on the left. Ambient noise masks the better cochlea*

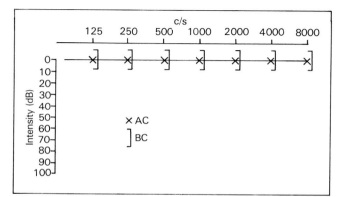

LD-19. *Audiograph – normal hearing. The threshold is < 10 dB. Left ear*

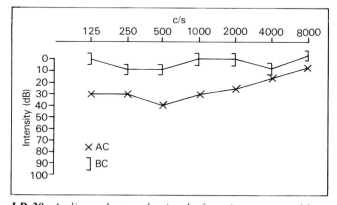

LD-20. *Audiograph – conductive deafness (e.g. serous otitis media). Left ear*

the clinician to say which type of hearing loss the patient is experiencing – whether it is conductive, sensorineural, or a mixture of the two.

In this form of testing the patient's hearing is tested both for air conduction, using earphones, and for bone conduction, using a receiver over the mastoid process. Each ear is tested individually over a range of pure tones varying from 250 to 8 000 c/s (LD-19–21).

Speech audiometry

Speech audiometry is simply a further extension of free-field speech testing in which tape recorded phonetically balanced words are played to the patient through earphones. The ability of the patient to score on repeating the words is marked on a percentage basis.

This is an important test particularly prior to operating for hearing loss. It is necessary to have a

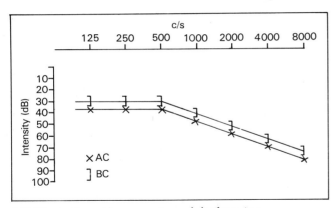

LD-21. *Audiograph – sensorineural deafness (e.g.*
presbycusis). Left ear

baseline of the patient's ability to discriminate speech.
Discrimination is essential for communication.

Special tests

There are a number of other special tests.

Bekesy audiometry. The patient records his own hearing level
in response to a sound which is constantly changing in frequency
and intensity. It is relayed through earphones to the tested ear.

Fowler's loudness balance test for the phenomenon of
recruitment. One ear is tested against the other where there is a
difference of threshold between the two for bone conduction.

Recruitment is a phenomenon thought to be purely related to
cochlear hearing loss. It occurs when the patient experiences an
abnormal sensitivity to an increase of sound intensity, above the
individual threshold for hearing.

Fowler's loudness balance and *loudness discomfort level* are
important tests in helping to determine sensory or cochlear
deafness from neural or nerve deafness.

Acoustic impedance audiometry reflects the ability of the
middle ear structure to overcome the acoustic impedance which
occurs when sound travels from one medium to another. The test
is of great importance in the diagnosis of pure middle ear
conditions such as otosclerosis, Eustachian tube obstruction and
ossicular discontinuity, and in the definition of inner ear hearing
loss. It is also of assistance in localizing a lesion in facial nerve
paralysis by measuring the response of the stapedius muscle to
high intensity sound (stapedius reflex).

Vestibular tests

The labyrinth, unlike the cochlea, tends to be tested in
a rather crude manner.

The fistula test

A fistula may be present on the lateral bony wall of the
labyrinth following a previous fenestration operation,
subluxation of the stapes footplate, an infection of the
middle ear or cholesteatomatous erosion. Compres-

sion of the ear in the external canal wall produces a
sensation of imbalance and a brief nystagmic response
in the direction of the stimulated ear can be observed.

This test can be performed by compressing the tragus into the
external auditory meatus or by using a pneumatic speculum.

Caloric testing

Caloric testing is the main test for the labyrinthine
system. It should be coupled with electronystagmography (ENG).

In electronystagmography, electrodes are applied to the skin at
the outer canthus of each eye. A central electrode is attached in the
midline. The electrodes are placed in these positions to pick up the
corneo-retinal potentials which are produced by rotation of the
eyes from the midline. These potentials can be graphed on an
amplifying recording unit. From the recording, measurements of
the frequency, angle of rotation and duration of nystagmus can be
made (LD-22).

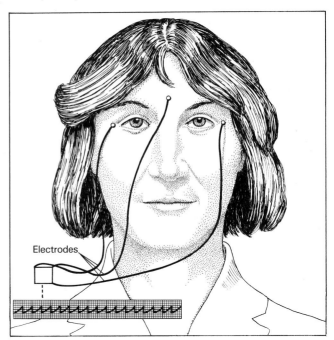

LD-22. *Electronystagmography*

Method of test

Water warmed or cooled 7 °C above or below body
temperature – 44 °C or 30 °C – or a minimal stimulus
using 1 cc of iced water is applied through the external
auditory canal to the tympanic membrane of the ear
under test.

If the patient has a mastoidectomy cavity or a
perforation of the tympanic membrane, water should
not be applied to the ear, because of the risk of
producing an acute infection. A system known as the
Dundas Grant tube should be used to apply cold air to
the middle ear.

The purpose of the test is to create a convection current in the endolymph. This causes a stimulus of the sensorineural epithelium within the ampulla of the horizontal semicircular canal. This movement of fluid is either towards or away from the sensorineural epithelium, depending upon the temperature of the fluid. Nystagmus is produced and the patient may or may not experience a sensation of imbalance. The direction of the nystagmus produced will depend on whether a hypo (cold) or a hyper (hot) function has been created in the tested ear (LD-23).

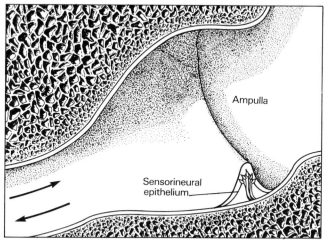

LD-23. *Caloric testing. The illustration shows section of a semicircular canal. Arrows indicate convection currents in the endolymph: the direction of these depends on the stimulating temperature*

In practice, the patient is laid supine on a couch with the head end raised 30° to the horizontal (LD-24). This has the effect of bringing the horizontal semicircular canal into the vertical plane with the ampulla uppermost. The stimulus is then applied to the ear and kept in contact with the tympanic membrane for a period of 30 seconds. The nystagmic response produced in a normal ear will last for approximately $2–2\frac{1}{2}$ minutes. Each ear is tested individually and comparisons made between the two sides.

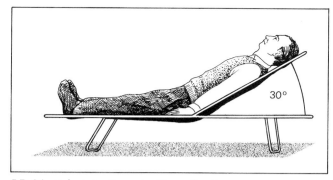

LD-24. *Caloric testing – position of patient*

Positional testing

This is a test of the posterior semicircular canal. It involves moving the patient quickly from the upright position, when sitting, to a fully supine position with the head hanging over the end of the couch and turned

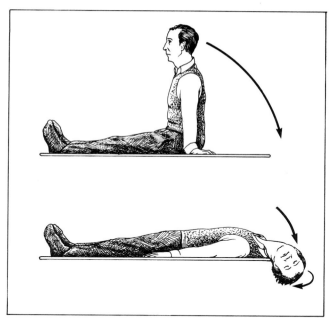

LD-25. *Positional testing*

to one side (LD-25). Nystagmus may be produced in the head down position. By repetition of the manoeuvre, either a benign paroxysmal positional vertigo or a central lesion may be diagnosed.

Other tests

These include:

- Rhomberg's test
- observation of gait for staggering to one side
- past pointing with the eyes open and closed
- dysdiadochokinesis

Tests for facial nerve function

Determining the level of lower motor neuron paralysis

An attempt should be made to determine the level of the lesion when considering lower motor neuron paralysis. The methods used include acoustic impedance audiometry, assessment of lachrymation and electrogustometry.

Acoustic impedance audiometry

Hyperacusis – an abnormal sensitivity to sound intensity – indicates a lesion above the stapedius nerve. The stapedius nerve reflex can be tested using acoustic impedance audiometry.

Assessment of lachrymation

Absence of lachrymation as assessed by Schrimer's tear test will establish a lesion at the level of the geniculate ganglion. Here the parasympathetic fibres leave the nerve.

Electrogustometry

This is a test of taste sensation. It assists in establishing the level of the lesion in relation to the point at which the chorda tympani nerve joins the facial nerve.

Determining prognosis in lower motor neuron paralysis

Electrodiagnostic tests

These are used to determine function and prognosis and include:

- nerve conduction time to assess nerve conductivity
- strength duration tests
  Assess the degree of degeneration or neuropraxia within the nerve. Sequential strength duration curves are taken for comparison and assistance in the management and prognosis of a case.

RADIOLOGY

Straight radiology, tomography and contrast studies are the three methods of investigation in common use.

Straight radiology

Table 1 summarizes the standard views for straight radiology.

TABLE 1

View	Structure(s) visualized
Lateral oblique	Lateral sinus
	Air cells
Stenver's (X-1)	Petrous bone
	Antrum
Towne's (X-2)	Internal auditory canal
Transorbital (X-3)	Internal auditory canal
Submento-vertical (X-4)	Middle ear
	Eustachian tube
	Petrous apex
	Antrum

The pathological appearances which may be visualized on X-ray are summarized in Table 2.

TABLE 2

Pathology	Appearance
Infection	
Acute	Clouding of cells (X-5)
	Destruction of individual cell boundaries
Chronic	Sclerosis (X-6)
Cholesteatoma	Evidence of bony erosion within the attic and mastoid (X-7)
Fracture (X-8)	
Acoustic neroma	Expansion of internal auditory canal (X-9)
Tumour	A simple bony osteoma can be visualized in the external auditory canal
	Malignant appearances may be identified by erosion of the mastoid, external auditory canal, tegmen or petrous bone

Tomography/polytomography

This is principally used to elucidate abnormalities or pathology demonstrated on straight radiographs. The structures visualized include:

- the content of the middle ear – ossicles
- the labyrinth
- the internal auditory canal (X-9)
- fractures

CAT scan (computerized axial tomography)

This technique is of use in the delineation of space-occupying lesions in the region of the temporal bone.

Contrast

Carotid angiography and retrograde venography may reveal a chemodectoma, glomus tumour, of the middle ear.

Pantopaque studies may demonstrate a filling defect in the internal auditory canal, due to an acoustic neuroma.

SECTION III

The presentation of disease of the ear and the diagnostic possibilities

INTRODUCTION

The patient, through his appearance, behaviour and background, supplies diagnostic clues to the physician, who interprets them according to his own experience and training. The doctor then forms a hypothesis which may be accepted or rejected as the result of further investigation. At some stage a diagnostic label may be applied and appropriate management instituted. The response to treatment may itself alter the original hypothesis.

This move from clues to management without a firm 'diagnosis' is a technique used in good general practice – a legitimate short cut adopted to save time. Frequently it is the only rational course in a field where a minority of conditions have been clearly defined.

The student must be aware of this situation and must learn to tolerate a degree of diagnostic uncertainty, if he or she is to avoid self-delusion and spurious diagnostic precision on the one hand and fruitless overinvestigation of his or her patient on the other.

This section considers the approach to patients presenting with complaints referable to the ear. Thus, instead of considering the diseases in turn, each with its catalogue of signs and symptoms, we begin with the symptoms and signs and follow through to the possible diagnosis – a presentation-orientated approach. This more closely approximates the clinical situation faced by the practising doctor. However, it must be appreciated that diagnostic clues are rarely presented singly, and the interrelationships created may themselves be diagnostic. This 'pattern recognition' is a function of experience. Here, for descriptive purposes, the clues have been separated and are considered singly.

DEAFNESS

Hearing loss should be considered in three categories:

- conductive
- sensorineural
- non-organic or psychogenic

Conductive deafness arises from any pathology or physical obstruction of the sound wave from the point at which it enters the external auditory meatus to the stapes footplate.

Sensorineural deafness – also referred to as 'perceptive', 'nerve', 'cochlear' and 'inner ear' deafness – results from pathology involving the cochlear labyrinth, the pathway of the nerve from the hair cells to the brainstem ganglia or the central connections from the brainstem.

Clinical approach

The clinician's approach to the problem presented by a deaf patient should cover:

- obtaining a history
- examination of the external ear for scars and other abnormalities
- speculum examination of the ear canal and visualization of the tympanic membrane
  Swelling, perforation and any wax or discharge should be noted.
- speech and tuning fork tests
- examination of the nose, paranasal sinuses, and postnasal space
- examination of the pharynx and larynx
- audiometry

Conductive deafness in the adult

There are many causes for this:

- wax
- chronic otitis media, either active or resolved
  The latter can be associated with perforation, fibrosis or discontinuity of the ossicular chain.
- external otitis
- chronic stenosing external otitis
- acute bacterial infections of the middle ear
- acute viral conditions
  Acute myringitis bullosa haemorrhagica involves the tympanic membrane.
- otosclerosis
- trauma of the tympanic membrane or ossicular chain
- osteoma of external canal
- Eustachian tube blockage
  This may be associated with a head cold, chronic rhinitis, sinusitis, barotrauma or nasopharyngeal tumours. In the adult carcinoma should be considered – in the adolescent a juvenile angiofibroma.

Conductive deafness in the child

The following may result in conductive deafness:

- serous otitis media
- acute otitis media
- acute suppurative otitis media
- chronic otitis media
- wax
- trauma
  This usually follows a foreign body in the external auditory canal.
- congenital causes
  Failure of the external auditory canal to canalize is a rare cause of conductive deafness and can be associated with malformations of the ossicular chain. It is usually easily recognized, as there is generally an associated deformity of the auricle.

Sensorineural deafness in the adult

The following are causes of sensorineural deafness:

- presbycusis – deafness associated with ageing
- noise induced deafness or acoustic trauma
- Ménière's disease
- hereditary disease
- fracture of the skull
- ototoxic drugs
- inflammatory conditions of the labyrinth
  These are commonly viral. Bacterial infection may be associated with bacterial meningitis or acute otitis media or chronic otitis media in the presence of cholesteatoma.
- acoustic neuroma
- unilateral deafness in the younger adult
  If no aetiological factor can be established, it is possible that vascular occlusion of the blood supply to the cochlea may be the cause.

Sensorineural deafness in the child

This is much less common than conductive deafness. When present it is most commonly related to prenatal, perinatal or neonatal circumstances. The result is generally bilateral deafness. It is vitally important to recognize the deficit as early as possible in order that corrective measures may be taken in the prelingual stage.

Causes include:

- viral labyrinthitis – most commonly mumps
- maternal rubella within the first trimester
- birth trauma
- prematurity
- hereditary disease
- rhesus incompatability
- congenital syphilis

Non-organic deafness

There are two principal causes for this:

- malingering
- psychological

If such a reason for deafness is suspected, the diagnosis may be extremely difficult. However, with the assistance of sophisticated audiometric tests the condition can be revealed. In the case of malingering – when confronted, the patient will generally confess.

OTORRHOEA

Discharge from the ear commonly arises after infection of the middle or external ear. Certain cases of otitis externa are related to generalized dermatological disorders – contact dermatitis, eczema, seborrhoeic dermatitis, or psoriasis.

Clinical approach

The clinician's approach to otorrhoea should include:

- obtaining a detailed history
- inspection of the discharge
- sending a specimen for culture
- examination of the canal and tympanic membrane
  After mopping a speculum may be used to assess the integrity of the tympanic membrane.
- speech and tuning fork tests
- audiometry
- radiological examination

The nature of the discharge

The character of the discharge can be helpful, as shown in Table 3.

TABLE 3

Appearance	Clinical association
Offensive	Osteitis, cholesteatoma
Mucoid	Anterior perforation of the tympanic membrane with disease restricted to the tympanic cavity and associated with Eustachian tube malfunction
Purulent	Frank infection
Bloody	Acute otitis media, acute myringitis bullosa haemorrhagica, trauma, granulation tissue, glomus jugulare tumour or carcinoma – the latter two are rare
Watery	Eczema, contact dermatitis, cerebrospinal fluid leak may follow trauma and can be confirmed with Clinistix
Black and seed like or white and powdery	Mycotic infection
Cheese-like	Cholesteatoma

OTALGIA

Earache is generally associated with infective conditions of the external and middle ear. It may however be associated with non-infective conditions related to the ear and can also be the result of referred pain from other regions within the head and neck.

Clinical approach

The clinician's approach should include:

- obtaining a detailed history
- examination of the external ear
  Swelling may be apparent behind or around the auricle and tenderness may be present on moving the pinna and cartilaginous canal.
- speculum examination
- speech and tuning fork tests
- examination of nose, paranasal sinuses, post-nasal space, pharynx and larynx
- a radiological examination if indicated

Otalgia of aural origin in the child

Middle ear disease tends to be a common source of earache in the child. The causes include:

- acute otitis media
- serous otitis media
- external otitis
- furunculosis
- a foreign body
- myringitis bullosa haemorrhagica

Otalgia of aural origin in the adult

The causes here include:

- external otitis
- furunculosis
- wax
  Wax impinges on the tympanic membrane or is impacted in the external auditory canal.
- myringitis bullosa haemorrhagica

- chronic otitis media
    Here otalgia often heralds complication.
- acute otitis media
- trauma to the pinna, the canal or the tympanic membrane
- malignant disease

Referred otalgia

Referred otalgia is possible because of the multiple nerve supply to the auricle, external canal and the middle ear. The nerves involved are the:

- trigeminal (V)
- facial (VII)
- glossopharyngeal (IX)
- vagus (X)
- posterior roots of C2,3

Pathology arising in other branches of these nerves may result in earache due to the phenomenon of referred pain. It is summarized in Table 4.

TABLE 4

Nerve	Stimulus for referred pain
The trigeminal nerve	Malocclusion Impacted molars in the lower jaw Dental caries Dental abscess Lesions of the temperomandibular joint, e.g. osteoarthritis, recurrent dislocation Sinusitis
The facial nerve	Herpes zoster of the geniculate ganglion (Ramsay Hunt syndrome)
Glossopharyngeal/vagus	Post-tonsillectomy earache – it should be remembered, however, that all post-tonsillectomy earache is not referred and the pain may actually be due to an acute otitis media Neoplastic lesions of the tonsil, posterior third of tongue, vallecula, larynx, pyriform fossae and hypopharynx
C2,3	Cervical disc lesions Osteoarthritis

FACIAL PARALYSIS

Facial nerve paralysis may be either partial or total. The lesion may be nuclear or supranuclear, or infranuclear, within the distribution of the nerve from its nucleus in the brain stem.

Clinical approach

The clinician's approach should include:

- obtaining a detailed history
- establishing if the paralysis is partial or complete
- excluding trauma and local swelling especially of the parotid gland (CP-1)
- a routine examination of the ear
- a neurological examination
- radiological investigation if indicated
- an ophthalmological assessment
- tests to assist in determining the level of a lower motor neuron lesion
- an electrodiagnostic assessment

Disturbances of facial movement are described according to the facial nerve distribution – i.e. to the forehead, the eye and the mouth.

Supranuclear lesions

It should be remembered that there is bilateral cortical representation of the forehead muscles, and so the upper part of the face is unlikely to be affected and involuntary movements of an emotional nature may be retained even in the lower half of the face.

Infranuclear lesions

Arising within the temporal bone

These are listed in Table 5.

Arising outwith the temporal bone

These include:

- direct trauma
- carcinoma of parotid gland
- perinatal trauma

TABLE 5

Cause	Specific disorder
Unknown	Idiopathic (Bell's palsy)
Infection	Chronic otitis media with cholesteatoma
Trauma	Fracture of the temporal bone
Iatrogenic	From surgery of the middle ear and mastoid

Tumour	Benign
	   acoustic neuroma
	   glomus jugulare
	Malignant
	   carcinoma of the middle ear

Where division of the facial nerve is noted immediately after surgery or in relation to skull trauma and if there is deafness and bleeding from the ear, then surgical intervention should be considered. Nerve grafting may be necessary. If the paralysis following surgery develops 24 or 48 hours later, this is generally due to oedema of the nerve in its sheath or pressure from the packing within the ear. Removal of the packing will generally suffice to promote complete recovery.

VERTIGO

Clinical approach

The clinician's approach to vertigo should include:
- obtaining a detailed history
- an assessment of nystagmus when present
- a full otological examination
  This should include testing for the presence of the fistula sign.
- general assessment of balance
- a full physical examination – including blood pressure, full blood examination serology
- an audiological assessment
- caloric testing
- radiological examination if indicated
- neurological assessment

Labyrinthine causes of vertigo

These are listed in Table 6.

Non-labyrinthine causes of vertigo

These are listed in Table 7.

TABLE 6

Cause	Clinical association
Ménière's syndrome	Tinnitus Episodic vertigo Progressive sensorineural deafness (usually unilateral)
Bacterial	Chronic otitis media with cholesteatoma Acute meningitis
Viral labyrinthitis	This is often related to a recent upper respiratory tract infection
Ototoxicity	
Trauma	Fracture of the petrous temporal bone Concussion with no fracture
Postoperative	Stapedectomy
Benign positional paroxysmal vertigo	
Glomus jugulare	From labyrinthine invasion

TABLE 7

Cause	Association
Wax	If swollen with water this can cause pressure on the tympanic membrane
Eustachian tube obstruction	Respiratory tract infection
Acoustic neuroma	
Ramsay Hunt syndrome	Herpes zoster (oticus) involving the geniculate ganglion
Vertebrobasilar insufficiency	Atherosclerosis Osteophytic compression of vascular system in the cervical spine
Vestibular neuronitis	

TINNITUS

Tinnitus is the term used for the sensation of noise in the ear or noise in the head.

All head noises are not necessarily of aural origin. Many may be of a psychological cause or a symptom of a more generalized condition. Rarely, vascular tumours in the neck – such as carotid body tumours – may cause tinnitus.

Clinical approach

The clinician's approach should include:

- obtaining a history
- full aural examination
- palpation of the neck
- audiometry
- radiology of head and neck if indicated
- full physical examination
- neurological assessment

Tinnitus of aural origin may be related to:

- sensorineural deafness
- middle ear disease, including Eustachian tube obstruction
- external canal disorders

Tinnitus of non-aural origin may be related to:

- vertebrobasilar insufficiency
- dental pathology
- anaemia
- hyper- or hypotension
- vascular tumours
- psychogenic causes

In relation to sensorineural deafness, tinnitus may persist for some considerable time. The patient should be reassured that there is nothing seriously wrong and that the condition will settle of its own accord.

In these cases, a mild sedative may be required at night when the patient is in quietened surroundings, the symptom then becoming most disturbing.

SECTION IV

Description of specific diseases of the ear

BAT EARS

Here there is an abnormality of the auricle, which appears to be pushed forward and out. It may be unilateral but is more often bilateral (CP-2). In some children it corrects itself with the development of the mastoid process by the second year. It can be particularly noticeable in boys if the hair is worn short, and the child may be subjected to ridicule at school.

Management

The definitive treatment is pinnaplasty. This is described in Section V, p. 37.

IMPACTED WAX

Wax is produced naturally within the external auditory canal as a normal secretion of the ceruminous glands. The amount of secretion from these glands varies with the individual. The majority of people have no trouble from wax, as it naturally travels outward from the canal. In some cases wax tends to collect within the canal and may build up to such an extent that the canal becomes occluded. Wax in such cases may remain soft, or it may become quite solid and impacted.

Clinical features

The effects of wax are seen in Table 8.

TABLE 8

Effect	Mechanism
Conductive deafness	Obstruction
External otitis	Irritation of the skin Increased susceptibility to infection
Otalgia ⎫ Vertigo ⎬	Pressure on the tympanic membrane
Keratosis obturans ⎭	

Keratosis obturans

Here impacted hard wax, combined with desquamation of the surface skin layer, results in a waxy mass which is difficult to remove. Pressure may cause the underlying bone to be eroded, and it may be necessary to remove the mass under a general anaesthetic.

Management

Usually wax can be removed under direct vision, using a cerumen hook. If this fails the ear must be syringed. Prior to syringing, the patient should be questioned about previous aural trouble. A perforation of the tympanic membrane should be excluded, for if this is present, it is unwise to syringe the ear as there is a risk of producing an acute suppurative otitis media. The wax should therefore be removed either with the cerumen hook or, if necessary, under general anaesthetic.

Syringing

Wax should be softened using a solution of sodium bicarbonate and glycerine in drop form for 1 week.

A solution of 1% sodium bicarbonate as near body temperature as possible should be used. If the water is either too warm or too cold a caloric effect will be produced, and the patient may complain of vertigo.

The tip of the syringe should not be passed deep into the canal and the direction of the jet should be upwards and along the roof.

After the wax has been removed the canal should be examined to ensure that it is entirely clean and free from wax and that the tympanic membrane is intact. It should be dry-mopped, as water left may predispose to an external otitis if the skin has previously been irritated by the wax.

If the ear cannot be completely cleared of wax, then this should be removed under a general anaesthetic.

FOREIGN BODIES

Children are prone to put foreign material into various orifices in their bodies and very commonly into the nose and the ears. In the ear, the presence of a foreign body does not raise the same need for urgency as in the case of nasal foreign bodies. Where bleeding occurs, however, the ear must be adequately inspected as soon as possible. Foreign bodies can generally be removed in the clinic, but, of course, this depends on the age and co-operation of the child. The presence of a foreign body in the ear may not be recognized until infection has occurred in the external canal, or it may only be a coincidental finding on examination.

Management

Paper or cotton wool can be removed with crocodile jaw forceps. Stones, beads and solid materials can often be syringed from the ears.

Vegetable material such as a pea should never be syringed, as such material absorbs fluid and will cause complete blockage and severe tension within the ear canal.

If the patient is unco-operative, removal of the foreign body under a general anaesthetic may be necessary to reduce the risk of iatrogenic perforation of the tympanic membrane. If the membrane has been traumatized, removal of the foreign body under anaesthesia, utilizing the operating microscope, is the best approach.

If the foreign body has pushed through the tympanic membrane into the middle ear, removal through the canal may be extremely difficult and in rare cases the middle ear may have to be approached through the mastoid.

OTITIS EXTERNA

In otitis externa the skin of the external auditory canal becomes oedematous and/or infected. There are general skin conditions which may have local manifestations within the external canal and around the meatus and pinna (CP-3). These include eczema and – in relation to seborrhoea – seborrhoeic otitis externa (CP-4).

Seborrhoeic otitis externa

In this condition the canal is inflamed, and may be oedematous. The common complaint is pruritus.

There may be a watery discharge and crusting around the external meatus. Secondary infection can follow but bacteriological examination is usually negative.

Management

Adequate aural toilet should precede the application of any local treatment. The ears must be kept absolutely dry for as long as 6 months after the episode to prevent recurrence.

In the acute phase, half-inch (13 mm) ribbon gauze wicks with hydrocortisone ointment or the more bland aluminium acetate or ichthyol and glycerine are used. Hydrocortisone cream may be applied around the pinna if this area is affected. Treatment should be aimed at overcoming any seborrhoeic condition of the scalp (see Section V, p. 37).

Infective otitis externa

More commonly, otitis externa is associated with infection of the skin of the canal. It may be an associated feature of otitis media. The principal symptoms are:

- pruritus
- discharge
- deafness
  This varies with the amount of discharge and oedema in the canal.
- tinnitus
  This follows the build-up of debris in the tympanic membrane.

Investigations

Bacteriological examination will reveal the infecting organism to be either bacterial or fungal or a combination of both.

Fungal conditions are often associated with a previous otitis externa which has been overtreated with antibiotic aural drops. It may, however, arise from swimming in infected pools and is not uncommon in patients who have been living in warmer climates. The discharge may be black – *Aspergillus niger* – or powdery white in appearance – *Candida albicans*, pathognomonic of mycotic infection.

Bacterial infection causes the canal to appear red and swollen and there may be an associated lymphadenitis. The pinna is tender to move.

Management

In bacterial infections the organisms are generally streptococcal or staphylococcal but pseudomonous pyocyanea, proteus and coliform organisms may be present. The local treatment is as for non-infective otitis externa.

If an antibiotic is to be used in combination with a hydrocortisone preparation, the sensitivity should have first been obtained. In severe cases systemic antibiotics may be required (see Section V, p. 37).

In treating mycotic conditions antifungal preparations – nystatin or mercurochrome paint – should be used.

Differential diagnosis of otitis externa

This includes:
- furunculosis
- otitis media
- acute mastoiditis
- osteomata of the bony canal

Furunculosis

Furunculosis arises from infection of pilosebaceous glands in the external auditory canal. It presents with pain and swelling at the meatus and in the cartilaginous canal. The pinna is tender to touch, lymphadenitis may be present and the postauricular groove may be obliterated.

The differential diagnosis includes:
- otitis externa

- acute mastoiditis
- lymphadenitis associated with scalp infection

Treatment involves:
- systemic antibiotics
- application of bland local wicks
- analgesia

Otitis media

It is often difficult to assess the integrity of the tympanic membrane.

Osteomata of the bony canal

These may also predispose to external otitis, as they can retain desquamated material from the deep canal, producing a culture media for infection.

ACUTE OTITIS MEDIA

Acute otitis media is an infection of the middle ear commoner in children than in adults and generally associated with an upper respiratory tract infection (CP-5).

It may also follow:
- surgery to the nose and throat – tonsillectomy or adenoidectomy
- postnasal packing
- trauma to the tympanic membrane
- trauma or fracture of the temporal bone
- infected haematoma of the tympanic cavity (haemotympanum)

Clinical features

The clinical features are summarized in Table 9.

Discharge is present only when the tympanic membrane has ruptured. It results in relief of pain and is synonymous with rupture of an abscess at any other site in the body. Short-lasting bleeding may follow rupture of the tympanic membrane.

On examination the tympanic membrane appearance may vary from pink with loss of light reflex to a fiery red with obvious bulging. The discharge has a yellow creamy consistency.

Respiratory tract infection may also occur and

TABLE 9

Symptom	Comment
Children	
Pain	This is the main symptom
Pyrexia	
Mastoid tenderness	If elicited mastoiditis should be suspected
Conductive deafness	
Adults	
Fullness in the ear	An early symptom
Conductive deafness	An early symptom
Tinnitus	
Pain	This develops later. It is described as throbbing and is felt deep in the ear

acute otitis media is frequently associated with Eustachian tube obstruction. In childhood, adenoidal hypertrophy with adenoiditis is an important contributory factor. Acute otitis media is particularly common among young children when 'teething'.

The infecting organism may be either haemolytic streptococcus or *Staphylococcus aureus* or, more rarely, *Haemophilus influenzae*.

The condition – while involving principally the lining of the middle ear – extends down the Eustachian tube and backwards to the lining of the mastoid antrum. Acute mastoiditis may develop if it is not treated quickly and efficiently.

Management

This is summarized in Table 10.

TABLE 10

Treatment	Comment
Bed rest	
Systemic antibiotic	Penicillin is given intramuscularly for the first 48 hours. The organism sensitivity should be identified
Analgesia	
Vasoconstrictor nose drops or menthol inhalations	
Myringotomy (LD-26)	This requires a general anaesthetic and is carried out if the tympanic membrane is bulging
Aural toilet	This is necessary if the ear is discharging. Instillation 10% alcohol drops, boric powder

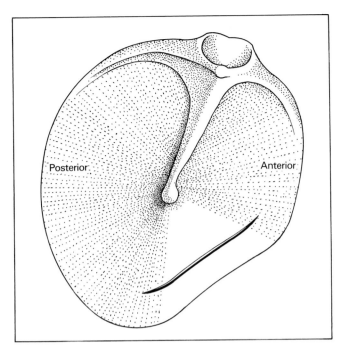

LD-26. *Myringotomy*

ACUTE MASTOIDITIS

Infection may spread to the mastoid and result in acute mastoiditis with the risk of intracranial complications. Mastoiditis is heralded by the presence of pain, tenderness and swelling over the mastoid antrum.

The radiological appearance may be helpful (X-5, X-6).

Failure to eradicate the initial infection in acute otitis media may lead to a subacute condition with residual infection in the middle ear and mastoid. This in turn may progress to a chronic state with thickening of the mucosal lining and osteitis, particularly of the attic and mastoid.

Management

Surgery should be undertaken to open the mastoid and institute drainage. This operation is known as cortical mastoidectomy (see Section V, p. 37).

Systemic antibiotic therapy must also be commenced.

EUSTACHIAN TUBE OBSTRUCTION

The Eustachian tube (pharyngotympanic) is the ventilator of the middle ear cavity.

Causes

The causes of Eustachian tube obstruction are summarized in Table 11.

TABLE 11

Cause	Comment
Nasal obstruction	Acute obstruction from upper respiratory tract infection Chronic obstruction from polypi, septum deflections and chronic discharge from sinuses
Incompetent muscle control	A cleft palate will result in incompetence or incoordination in the muscle controlling the opening of the Eustachian tube
Mass in the nasopharynx	Adenoidal hypertrophy, juvenile angiofibroma or neoplasm in the adult may block the nasopharyngeal orifice
Allergy	Here the associated oedema in the tube results in middle ear problems
Chronic conditions of the middle ear	The narrowest point of the Eustachian tube – the bony isthmus – is especially vulnerable

When the tube is obstructed, ventilation of the middle ear is impaired and a negative pressure develops in the tympanic cavity. The tympanic membrane becomes indrawn and the light reflex is lost or broken. As the obstruction persists fluid collects within the middle ear, arising either from transudation or exudation. This results in a serous otitis media. The effect is to produce a conductive deafness and in some cases otalgia and a sensation of imbalance.

Clinical features

Serous otitis media

This is described below on this page.

Acute barotrauma

Where there is a very rapid alteration from high to low atmospheric pressure, as in flying, the Eustachian tube may fail to adjust to the sudden change in pressure. This can cause acute barotrauma. If there is a nasal obstruction or an upper respiratory tract infection, the risk of obstruction is further increased. Intense otalgia may be experienced and bleeding may take place into the middle ear, producing a haemotympanum.

Management

Treatment of Eustachian tube obstruction is largely treatment of the underlying cause.

In barotrauma, where deafness persists after the resolution of upper respiratory tract infection, auto-inflation can be a therapeutic as well as a preventive measure. Auto-inflation means blowing against a closed mouth and pinched nose and in so doing attempting to force open the tube with the increased nasopharyngeal pressure. This method, while being unphysiological, often suffices temporarily in opening the tube and overcoming the negative pressure. It requires to be repeated regularly. It should not be used when infection exists in nose or nasopharynx.

SEROUS OTITIS MEDIA

Serous otitis media – also referred to as secretory or catarrhal otitis media, glue-ear or otosalpingitis – is a non-infective condition of the middle ear and mastoid and results from Eustachian tube obstruction. It is the commonest cause of deafness in the young child, where it is usually bilateral.

While adenoidal hypertrophy, postnasal discharge and nasal allergy may play a part in serous otitis media in the child, the underlying cause appears to be principally a dysfunction of the opening mechanism of the Eustachian tube. The condition appears to show resolution with age and its incidence is lower in children over 10 years of age.

In the adult, serous otitis media is usually unilateral and is commonly related to an upper respiratory tract infection.

The condition is characterized by fluid within the middle ear. The fluid may range from a thin serous to a thick mucoid material which has a glue-like consistency. It is sterile.

If a cleft palate exists, the condition is present from birth due to the failure of apposition of the muscles which open the tubes. Such infants have a conductive deafness, the severity of which is difficult to estimate in infancy.

Clinical features

The features to note are:
- deafness
- otalgia

In the otherwise healthy child the condition is not

recognized until around the age of 5 years, when a referral to the ENT clinic usually follows failure in the school hearing test. The parents, however, may suspect that the child is deaf prior to this. Confusion may arise as to whether the child is not hearing or is just inattentive and in such cases the parents may delay seeking advice. It should be emphasized that whenever there is any question of a child having hearing difficulties, referral to an audiometric clinic is essential.

Otalgia may be a feature and, when present, is usually short-lasting and nocturnal in character.

Examination

The tympanic membrane lacks lustre, the light reflex is broken or absent and mobility is reduced. There may be increased vascularity around the periphery and down the handle of the malleus.

A yellowish tinge may be appreciated through the tympanic membrane and very occasionally hairlines may be seen through the membrane due to air bubbles within the middle ear.

Failure to recognize this condition may result in a progression from what is essentially a temporary form of deafness to a more permanent form with the development of other pathological features in the tympanic membrane and middle ear. These include:

- tympanosclerosis – white patches on the tympanic membrane
- middle ear adhesions
- retraction or collapse of the pars flaccida into the attic
- formation of a cholesteatoma

Management

Minor hearing loss

Local and systemic decongestant preparations incorporating antihistamines may be tried. Any pathology within the nose and paranasal sinuses should be eradicated (see Section V, p. 37).

Where resolution is not obtained by the above approach, then myringotomy should be considered. The fluid should be completely sucked from the ear. This can be difficult when it is glue-like. A small Teflon tube, known as a 'pressure equalizing tube' or 'grommet', may be inserted through the incision (LD-27). These tubes are generally extruded within 6 months. After insertion of pressure equalizing tubes

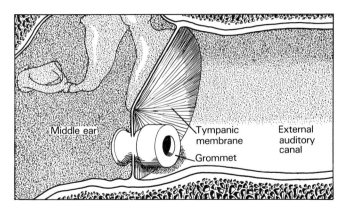

LD-27. *Pressure equalizing tube*

to the tympanic membrane, parents of the patient must be instructed not to permit water to enter the ears as this may lead to an acute suppurative condition (see Section V, p. 37).

The nasopharynx should be examined in all cases – especially in adults, where neoplasm must be excluded. In the child where large adenoids are palpated they should be removed.

After myringotomy the hearing should completely recover. If at subsequent follow-up the hearing is deteriorating, blockage of the tubes should be suspected and the tubes removed. Removal may be carried out in the outpatient department but a general anaesthetic may be required.

MYRINGITIS BULLOSA HAEMORRHAGICA

Myringitis bullosa haemorrhagica is of viral origin associated with upper respiratory tract infection.

Clinical features

These are:

- severe otalgia
  The pain is unrelieved at the onset of discharge – unlike that of otitis media.
- serosanguinous discharge
- haemorrhagic bullous eruptions
  These are found on the tympanic membrane and the skin of the deep canal.
- mastoid tenderness
  This is related to periostitis. Radiology of the mastoid is clear.
- conductive deafness
  This is transient.

Management

Secondary infection should be avoided by non-interference. The ear should be kept dry. The condition will settle spontaneously.

Analgesics are required for the relief of pain.

CHRONIC OTITIS MEDIA

Chronic suppurative otitis media (CSOM) results from failure to achieve resolution in the acute suppurative state. However, where a cholesteatoma is present, the patient may recall no previous history of aural disease. CSOM may be broadly considered to be of two types:

- tubotympanic
- attic or bony

Tubotympanic disease

The tympanic membrane has a central or non-marginal perforation (LD-28) and the discharge is of a mucoid or mucopurulent consistency. The condition may resolve on treatment and recur with each upper respiratory tract infection or with general illhealth. This condition is considered 'safe'. The degree of destruction is usually limited to the tympanic membrane although fibrosis around the ossicles and disruption of the incudostapedial joint may result.

Clinical features

Chronic suppurative otitis media presents with:

- discharge
- deafness
- pain
- nausea and vertigo

These symptoms vary with the degree of destruction of the tympanic membrane and ossicles and with the extent of fibrosis and granulation tissue within the middle ear cavity. Thickening of the middle ear mucosa may actually reach the proportion of polyp formation.

Pain and vertigo herald potential intracranial or labyrinthine involvement and are generally related to an acute or chronic state. They may also occur when a chronically discharging ear suddenly dries up spontaneously.

Investigations

A bacterial swab is taken and past antibiotic therapy noted.

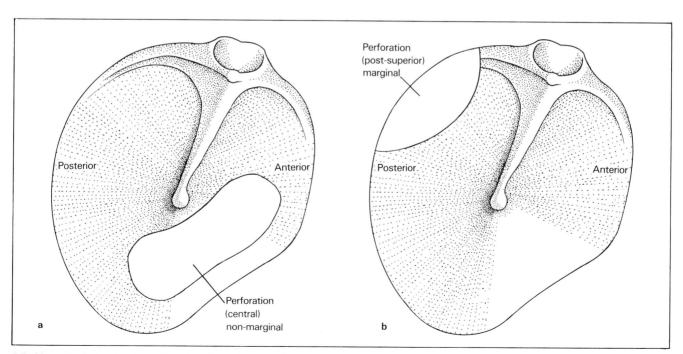

LD-28. **a**, *Tubotympanic perforation.* **b**, *Attic retraction*

Attic or bony disease

This is characterized by posterior or posterosuperior perforation of the tympanic membrane. Being on the margin of the membrane it involves the annulus and leads to an ingrowth of squamous epithelium from the deep canal to the middle ear cavity (LD-28). This results in squamous epithelialization of the mucosal lining of the cavity posteriorly and posterosuperiorly. In the latter instance, the new epithelium may track into the attic region and give rise to a cholesteatoma (CP-6).

The presence of squames or epithelial debris in the discharge may indicate the presence of a cholesteatoma.

Bacteriological examination may reveal a variety of apparently unlikely organisms for the upper respiratory tract – from *Staphylococcus aureus* to *Escherichia coli*, *Pseudomonas pyocyaneus* and *Bacillus proteus*.

Cholesteatoma formation

The condition follows loculation in the middle ear or mastoid of squamous epithelium, and the subsequent failure to achieve natural removal of surface desquamation. Such loculation can either result from ingrowth and epithelialization, or be due to collapse and retraction of the pars flaccida into the attic forming the so-called retraction pocket.

Wherever a cholesteatoma is present within the middle ear, attic or mastoid, it has an erosive potential which can result in the destruction of underlying bone and an osteitis. It may cause destruction of ossicles, particularly the incus and stapes superstructure. The osseous labyrinth and the boundaries of the attic and mastoid may be eroded. There is therefore a risk of bacterial labyrinthitis and intracranial infection. The integrity of the facial nerve is also at risk.

In some cases the cholesteatoma is thought to be of congenital origin arising from an epithelial deposit of ectodermal origin within the temporal bone.

If the membrane cannot be adequately visualized, then examination should be made under the operating microscope with or without general anaesthesia.

Audiometry should be performed.

Radiology may reveal cholesteatomatous erosion in the attic or mastoid (X-7).

Management

For tubotympanic disease, a thorough aural toilet twice daily using sterile cotton wool, the installation of spirit drops or 2 % boric and iodine powder and the limited use of antibiotic preparations with or without steroids is required.

An attic cholesteatoma can be controlled by repeated suction clearance using the operating microscope. Where there is evidence of erosion of bone or failure to control the condition by suction clearance, mastoid surgery must be considered in order to eliminate the disease and prevent the risk of serious complications. A number of operative procedures have been devised to eliminate disease with or without the preservation of hearing. These range from radical mastoidectomy to the combined approach tympanoplasty.

The general health of the patient should be assessed and any chronic focus of infection in paranasal sinuses or tonsils eradicated. Following resolution of the condition tympanoplasty should be considered, if only to produce a sealed membrane and obviate the risk of further infection from injudicious douching of the ear.

Complications of chronic middle ear disease

These include:

- bacterial labyrinthitis
- intracranial complications:
  meningitis
  extradural, subdural or cerebral/cerebellar abscesses
  lateral sinus thrombosis

Complications are generally heralded by the persistence of pain, headache, and vertigo together with nausea, vomiting and pyrexia. While each complication has its own diagnostic criteria, brain abscesses may be insidious and difficult to localize – especially if the patient has been previously treated with systemic antibiotics: these can mask underlying pathology. A neurological assessment should be undertaken.

In meningitis, treatment should be aimed at control of the infection followed by surgery to the temporal bone. In bacterial labyrinthitis and other intracranial complications the focus of infection within the temporal bone should be eliminated by mastoid exploration. Abscess drainage is best achieved through separate burr holes. Systemic antibiotic therapy should be instituted, using penicillin and sulphonamides.

Facial paralysis may be a complication of chronic otitis media following erosion of the Fallopian canal. Mastoid exploration is necessary to relieve pressure on the nerve.

Resolved chronic otitis media

Tubotympanic and limited attic disease may spontaneously resolve on conservative treatment. The principal problems that arise then are:

- perforation
  The tympanic membrane may however heal spontaneously.
- conductive deafness following:
  perforation
  middle ear fibrosis
  ossicular chain disruption

Management

The surgical treatment is by tympanoplasty with or without attic exploration. Selection for an elective procedure depends upon the age and physical condition of the patient. The initial aim of surgery should be the attainment of a sealed tympanic membrane. Satisfactory improvement of hearing may follow this or require a subsequent ossiculoplasty (see Section V, p. 37).

GLOMUS TUMOUR

The chemodectomata are a collection of tumours arising from paraganglionic tissue found around the carotid body, aortic arch and pulmonary artery. They are also found in the temporal bone, where they are known as 'glomus tumours'. They occur in relation to the dome of the jugular bulb or in relation to the tympanic plexus.

The tumour is vascular in nature, comprising vascular channels amid typical polyhedral cells and fibrous tissue. It is slow growing, causing symptoms through expansion. It rarely, if ever, metastasizes.

Clinical features

A glomus tumour can present with:

- conductive deafness
- tinnitus
- a red blush observed through the tympanic membrane

- bleeding from polypoidal formation in the external auditory canal
  This is rare.
- vertigo
  This is slight and indicates a deep expansion of the tumour into the osseous labyrinth.
- hoarseness from involvement of the tenth cranial nerve
  The tumour may reach considerable size and involve a number of the cranial nerves before it presents. On examination a bruit over the mastoid or a pulsatile mass may be felt.

Investigations

The diagnosis is established by biopsy either of a presenting polyp or after tympanotomy. It must be remembered that vigorous bleeding may be encountered. Radiology may be of great assistance in delineating the extent of the tumour. Tomography may show erosion of the temporal bone. Arteriography may reveal a tumour blush, while retrograde venography may demonstrate a filling defect (X-10, X-11).

Management

Where the tumour is small, surgical removal may suffice. Where the tumour has spread extensively within the temporal bone, radiotherapy may reduce the size and vascularity by fibrosis.

The risk of radionecrosis of the temporal bone must be borne in mind when radiotherapy is considered and drainage of the temporal bone by mastoid surgery is required. It should be remembered that the tumour is slow growing and even where neurological involvement is demonstrated the patient may survive and die from unconnected pathology.

LABYRINTHITIS

Causes

Irritation of the labyrinth may result from both infective and non-infective causes. When the labyrinth is irritated, the patient may experience symptoms of imbalance, tinnitus and deafness.

Non-infective labyrinthitis

Post-stapedectomy

The disturbance is thought to be due to the leak of perilymph at operation and to manipulation at the oval window. It should resolve within a few days. Failure to settle will suggest:

- a leak of perilymph around the prosthesis
- that the prosthesis is too long
- the development of an infective labyrinthitis

Traumatic labyrinthitis

A fracture involving the temporal bone may cause disruption of the labyrinth to the extent that both hearing and vestibular apparatus are destroyed. Concussional labyrinthitis may occur in the absence of fracture with the symptoms of vertigo, tinnitus and hearing loss. The hearing usually recovers leaving only a residual degree of deafness.

Infective labyrinthitis

Infective labyrinthitis may be considered under two headings – those of viral and those of bacterial origin.

Viral labyrinthitis

Mumps virus may produce a severe labyrinthitis in which the hearing becomes completely destroyed. The vestibular apparatus may, however, recover. It has generally a unilateral effect.

There are usually a number of cases during a 'flu' epidemic in which vertigo and tinnitus develop as the general symptoms are settling. This may be an example of viral labyrinthitis. An abnormal vestibular response to caloric stimulation may be demonstrated and a residual hearing loss may be evident.

Bacterial labyrinthitis

This may develop as a complication of either meningitis or chronic middle ear disease. The presenting symptoms are vertigo with nausea and vomiting. The 'fistula test' (p. 12) may be positive if the middle ear is the source of infection.

Management

All cases of labyrinthitis should be treated symptomatically, using antivertiginous preparations.

Bed rest is required with light diet in the acute phase, and driving and operating of machinery should be banned until recovery is complete. Graded physiotherapy exercises may be necessary and reassurance and encouragement from the clinician is helpful. Treatment of bacterial labyrinthitis must be aimed at eradication of the source of infection with vigorous antibiotic therapy. In the case of otogenic infection, mastoidectomy and labyrinthine drainage is required (see Section V, p. 37).

Following an episode of infection when both functions are destroyed, the term 'dead ear' is used. Recovery of balance may take some months.

VESTIBULAR NEURONITIS

This is a term used for episodic attacks of sudden vertigo with nausea and vomiting, usually associated with a viral infection of the upper respiratory tract. The hearing is spared and there is no tinnitus.

It has been postulated that as the cochlea is spared the pathology must be central to the peripheral sensory epithelium and may involve Scarpa's ganglion of the vestibular division of the eighth cranial nerve.

Clinical features

There is a spectrum of presentation through vertiginous attacks of varying severity to a feeling of imbalance and unsteadiness of gait.

- There is no nystagmus
- Examination of the ear is normal
- Audiometric testing reveals no abnormality
- There are no other neurological symptoms.

Vestibular testing using caloric stimuli reveals a reduction in response on the affected side. This persists even after recovery. The condition runs a benign course and, although distressing to the individual, generally settles within a month of onset.

Management

The treatment is symptomatic in the acute phase. Antivertiginous preparations such as antihistamines may be given intramuscularly, especially if nausea and vomiting are present. Bed rest and a light diet may be required. The patient must be constantly reassured, should be counselled against driving and should avoid handling machinery until recovery is complete.

MÉNIÈRE'S DISEASE

Ménière's disease is a condition characterized by vertigo, tinnitus and fluctuating sensorineural deafness.

The aetiology is unknown.

The pathology lies within the labyrinth where there is an excess of endolymphatic fluid, due to either overproduction or underabsorption of endolymph. This is produced and absorbed within a closed system.

Clinical features

Many cases are considered to be Ménière's disease without adequately satisfying the diagnostic criteria. It is commoner in males within the 55–65 age group. It is bilateral in 7% of cases.

Vertigo is the feature which draws attention to the condition. It is paroxysmal, varying in severity and duration with individual attacks. Typically the patient will experience a number of attacks over a period of days to weeks followed by a spell of complete freedom from the condition. There is often a record of an attack of vertigo of limited severity which occurred several years previously.

Nausea and vomiting may accompany an attack. Headache is not a feature, but 10% of migraine sufferers may develop Ménière's disease.

A prodromal symptom of fullness in the ear may be described. The attacks, however, may occur suddenly and without warning. At the time of an attack, tinnitus becomes more severe and the deafness is increased. Both are relieved by the onset of vertigo.

The appearance of the ear is normal and no other neurological symptoms or signs are present.

Nystagmus will be present during an attack, with the quick component moving towards the good ear.

Audiometric examination is helpful in defining the cochlear deafness and vestibular testing may reveal a diminished caloric response on the affected side. Radiology is of no assistance.

The differential diagnosis is from other peripheral causes of vertigo but most importantly from an acoustic neuroma.

Management

The treatment of Ménière's disease is both medical and surgical.

Medical treatment

Medical treatment is difficult to assess because of the episodic nature of the condition. However, salt and fluid restriction may be helpful.

Medical treatment is best reserved for symptomatic relief of an individual attack of vertigo using anti-vertiginous preparations such as the antihistamines. These may be given intramuscularly if vomiting is present, and in the acute phase bed rest and a light diet may be required.

Surgical management

Surgery of the labyrinth, unless conservative, will lead to destruction of both the vestibular and the cochlear apparatus (Section V, p. 37).

Membranous labyrinthectomy should be reserved for those cases where there is no longer any usable hearing or where the patient's life is threatened by the condition. Following labyrinthectomy there is always a degree of persisting vertigo. This may take several months to settle.

Conservative surgery

This includes:

- ultrasonic destruction of the vestibular labyrinth
- decompression of the endolymphatic sac
- endolymphatic shunt

Conservative surgery has varied success.

Bilateral Ménière's disease is extremely difficult to treat, and a combination of ablative and conservative surgery matched to the severity of the condition in each ear may be the only answer. Streptomycin sulphate has been used to destroy the vestibular response with hearing preservation.

ACOUSTIC NEUROMA

An acoustic neuroma is a benign tumour arising from the vestibular division of the eighth cranial nerve. It arises from the sheath of the nerve and as such it is neither acoustic nor a neuroma but, rather, a vestibular neurilemoma. However, tradition calls for the retention of inaccurate terminology.

The tumour arises within the internal auditory

canal. Its presentation is due to local expansion and pressure necrosis of the walls of the canal. It eventually expands into the intracranial cavity and behaves like a true cerebellopontine angle tumour. As it expands within the canal the vestibular division of the eighth nerve becomes replaced by tumour, and the blood vessels supplying the cochlea are compressed in addition to compression of the cochlear division of the nerve itself.

The facial nerve becomes compressed, producing a facial paralysis of a lower motor neuron type.

Clinical features

The tumour generally presents between the ages of 30 and 60, but may occur at an earlier age. Bilateral cases are rare and are associated with multiple neurofibromatosis.

Unilateral deafness is the main presenting feature.

Symptoms are progressive, although sudden unilateral deafness of a sensorineural type can occur.

Tinnitus may be present, and vertigo in the early stages may be transient and almost disregarded by the patient.

With expansion of the tumour, facial paralysis develops. Early signs of trigeminal involvement should be sought and may be demonstrated before facial paralysis develops. Tingling and numbness of the face and loss of the corneal reflex all point to pressure on the trigeminal nerve. As intracranial expansion occurs, headache develops with nausea and vomiting. At this stage papilloedema will be present.

Cerebellar involvement may be heralded by staggering to the affected side and clumsiness, and the development of a coarse type of nystagmus.

Investigations

A high index of suspicion is required.

Specialized audiometry will enable a diagnosis of cochlear or neural deafness to be made. Vestibular testing should reveal a complete loss of function on the affected side. Tomography and the use of contrast media will reveal erosion of the bony canal walls and/or a filling defect (X-9, X-12, X-13). The cerebrospinal fluid (CSF) will have increased protein. Lumbar puncture can be a dangerous examination if a large tumour is suspected, because of the risk of coning.

Differential diagnosis

The condition must be differentiated from:
- Ménière's disease
- intracranial tumours involving cerebellopontine angle and posterior fossa
- multiple sclerosis

Management

The tumour is slow growing, and although surgical removal is indicated in the younger patient, in the older individual a conservative approach may be employed, as the patient may well die from a coincidental cause.

A small tumour may be removed by entering the canal through the labyrinth and sparing the facial nerve. Where the tumour has expanded intracranially, neurosurgical assistance will be required for removal. (Section V, p. 37).

VERTEBROBASILAR INSUFFICIENCY

The labyrinth receives its blood supply from the vertebrobasilar system. Atherosclerosis or intermittent nipping from cervical spondylosis will result in ischaemia of the labyrinth. Symptoms of sensorineural deafness, tinnitus and vertigo may develop. The vertigo is precipitated by head movement.

Atherosclerotic disease

In the older age group, atherosclerosis is a commoner cause of vertebrobasilar insufficiency than is cervical spondylosis. The patient may complain of unsteadiness on rising in the morning or on coming up quickly from a stooped position. There may be a constant tinnitus which is often very troublesome to the patient. Reassurance is required and sedation may be prescribed to allow sleep.

Cervical spondylosis

In cervical spondylosis the vertebral arteries become compressed by osteophytic growths.

The typical history is one of imbalance provoked by the patient having his neck in an abnormal position. An attack of vertigo which is usually short-lasting is experienced. Nystagmus may be present. Attacks may also result from turning, extending, or flexing the neck.

Deafness and tinnitus are not constant features and may be unrelated to the pathology. The patient may also complain of pain radiating down the arms due to pressure on the cervical nerves.

The diagnosis is confirmed by radiology of the cervical spine. Vestibular testing is usually of little assistance.

Management

Treatment is aimed at relieving pressure from the osteophytes through the use of an orthopaedic collar. The patient should also be cautioned to avoid the provocative positions.

DRUG TOXICITY

Ototoxic drugs produce labyrinthine symptoms by irritating and destroying the fine sensorineural epithelium within the cochlea and the vestibule. The fetal labyrinth is at risk in the first trimester of pregnancy.

The best-known of ototoxic drugs is streptomycin. Initially dihydrostreptomycin sulphate was used in the treatment of tuberculosis. This drug had a specific predilection for the hair cells within the organ of Corti as well as affecting the vestibule. A number of the first patients treated with the drug developed a total bilateral deafness which was irreversible.

The aminoglycoside drugs dihydrostreptomycin, streptomycin, neomycin, kanamycin, viomycin and gentamicin are all ototoxic and can produce an irreversible effect when taken systemically. Quinine, alcohol and salicylates also produce an effect on the cochlea. This is, however, reversible.

It is thought that aural drops containing framycetin or neomycin may produce an ototoxicity by penetrating the round window membrane.

Clinical features

The symptoms produced by ototoxic drugs are:
- tinnitus
- vertigo
- sensorineural deafness

When an ototoxic drug has been used the development of tinnitus should be taken as an early warning sign of imminent toxicity.

BENIGN POSITIONAL VERTIGO

This is a condition usually occurring in females in which vertigo is experienced on turning the head into a specific position. The attack is always brought on when the head is put into the provocative position and the vertigo is also experienced fleetingly when the head is returned from the provocative position. The attacks are short-lasting and are usually present when turning in bed from one side to the other, or induced by lying down with the head turned to one side. It is thought that a disturbance within the utricle is responsible.

It may also be found in patients who have had previous surgery involving the labyrinth or who have sustained a head injury.

Investigations

Audiometry and caloric testing are normal. Positional testing produces a subjective response and nystagmus can be demonstrated in the direction of the undermost ear. This diminishes on repeated testing.

Management

The patient should be advised to avoid the provocative position. Rarely, vestibular nerve section is necessary.

NOISE DEAFNESS

There are two causes for deafness which follows exposure to high intensity noise:
- acute acoustic trauma
- chronic noise exposure

Acute acoustic trauma

Hearing loss follows exposure to blast or explosion,

the effect on the cochlea producing a sensorineural deafness. There may also be a conductive element if the tympanic membrane is blown in and discontinuity of the ossicular chain produced.

The blast effect is the result of positive and negative compression waves. The intratympanic muscles react to the stimulus, but if the intensity is very great they offer little protection.

Clinical features

The patient experiences deafness which may subsequently improve.

Tinnitus accompanies the deafness and may settle in time.

Vertigo may also be a feature but settles in a matter of weeks. The patient may initially complain of pain, particularly if the tympanic membrane is ruptured.

The trauma is principally to the basal turn of the cochlea and is most severe in the higher frequencies. It should be remembered that the consonants of speech on which discrimination depends are contained in the high frequencies. Therefore such damage will result not only in deafness but also in a difficulty in discrimination or understanding speech.

Management

There is no treatment for the sensorineural element of the deafness. For the conductive element tympanoplastic procedures should correct any defect.

The patient should be cautioned against further noise exposure. The use of ear protectors should be insisted upon if there is continued exposure to noise at work.

Chronic noise-induced deafness

This results from long term exposure to a continued high intensity noise of 90 decibels or over. Those commonly at risk are boilermakers, riveters, sheet metal and loom workers. The duration of exposure is usually in the region of 5 years or more and the damage tends to be bilateral.

The pathology is the same as for acute acoustic trauma. The higher frequencies are first involved but eventually all the frequencies are affected.

Clinical features

The first audiometric sign is a dip at the 4000 cycle/second point on the audiograph. Tinnitus occurs and there may be an individual susceptibility to damage.

Concern has been expressed in recent years over the danger to teenagers at pop concerts or discotheques where high amplification sound is produced. While hearing loss may be experienced, it is due to a temporary shift of the individual's hearing threshold which generally recovers within 24 hours. Tinnitus, however, may persist for longer. The danger is greater to the performers who are constantly being exposed to high level of amplification.

Noise-induced deafness has become recognized for industrial injuries compensation in the United Kingdom.

Management

Treatment should aim at prevention by regularly screening those employed in a noise-producing industry. Employees should be encouraged to use either earplugs or ear protectors and attempts should be made to deaden the noise-producing effect of the machinery. Where damage has occurred there is no hope for the recovery of hearing.

OTOSCLEROSIS

Otosclerosis is a condition in which hearing loss is the presenting symptom. The underlying pathology is of new bone formation initially around the oval window. This arises from vestigial cartilaginous rests, which may also occur in other areas of the temporal bone. The effect is to limit the movement of the stapes footplate. This can progress to complete fixation.

Clinical features

- The condition is commoner in females.
- It is bilateral in 90% of cases.
- It is first noticed in the twenties and is progressive.
- Pregnancy causes acceleration of the condition.
- There is usually a strong familial tendency.
- Tinnitus may also be a feature.
- There is no associated history of otalgia or otorrhoea but vertigo and severe tinnitus indicates further involvement of the osseous labyrinth.
- On examination there is a normal mobile tympanic membrane.

A flushed appearance through the membrane is due to increased vascularity on the promontory mucosa. It is said to indicate active disease.

Investigations

Pure tone audiometry confirms a conductive deafness. Acoustic impedance audiometry is helpful in differentiating it from ossicular chain disruption and serous otitis media.

Speech audiometry should be performed and is of vital importance when considering surgery.

There are no characteristic radiological findings.

Management

There is no medical treatment for otosclerosis.

There are two approaches – surgery or amplification by hearing aid. In the elderly, or where there is severe sensorineural component, a hearing aid should be considered.

Surgery

Stapedectomy

The aim of surgery is to close the air–bone gap of the conductive deafness. If the bone conduction loss is greater than 30–40 dB, closure of the gap will not improve the patient's overall performance but will give greater gain from the use of a hearing aid.

Fenestration of the lateral semicircular canal was the earliest operation for otosclerosis. It has now been discontinued.

PRESBYCUSIS

Deafness due to ageing is termed 'presbycusis'; it generally occurs after the age of 60 years. Such deafness is bilateral, progressive and sensorineural in character. It may be well-developed before the patient appreciates the loss of auditory acuity. It is more often the patient's relatives who are first aware of the problem.

Clinical features

The pathology may occur at two points in the peripheral auditory system.

In the 'younger' group, sensory presbycusis, degeneration occurs in the hair cells. With the loss of hair cells there may be marked recruitment. The characteristic comment of the patient is: 'Don't shout, I am not deaf'.

In the older group, neural presbycusis, probably occurs after 75 years. Atrophy is present in the nerve cells of the spiral ganglion in addition to those of the hair cells. This has the effect of producing a marked reduction in speech discrimination. While the patient may hear speech, the ability to understand is impaired. This is an important point when considering the role of a hearing aid. Tinnitus may be a troublesome accompaniment in both groups.

It should be possible to differentiate sensory from neural presbycusis by the use of advanced audiometry. However, in the aged the ability to concentrate through a series of audiometric tests may be limited.

Management

Where the hearing has fallen below 30dB, the socially acceptable limit for hearing, treatment consists of amplification by the use of a hearing aid. The ability to lip read may be acquired and should be encouraged.

The patient with presbycusis should be spoken to clearly and slowly. Patience is necessary, as in all contact with the deaf.

BELL'S PALSY

Bell's palsy is idiopathic facial paralysis. The aetiology is unknown but the condition is thought to be secondary to oedema within the nerve sheath as it lies in the Fallopian canal.

Clinical features

The patient may often describe an exposure to a draught. Paralysis is sudden in that the patient may awaken with the condition.

The unilateral facial paralysis of lower motor neuron type may be total. It is frequently associated with, or preceded by, pain or discomfort between the mastoid tip and the angle of the mandible.

In making a diagnosis other causes of facial paralysis should be excluded.

Electrodiagnostic tests for both function and progress may be necessary. Ninety per cent of cases recover spontaneously.

Those who do not completely recover are generally older, or are those patients who have had a considerable amount of pain.

Management

Reassurance is essential.

Physiotherapy can give the patient a greater feeling of well-being, but it is doubtful whether physical improvement is accelerated.

An ophthalmological opinion should be sought as there may be a risk of corneal ulceration.

The use of corticosteroids and adrenocorticotrophic hormone (ACTH) is advocated by some. Surgical decompression of the Fallopian canal has also been advocated.

THE RAMSAY HUNT SYNDROME OR HERPES ZOSTER OTICUS

This condition results from a herpes zoster infection of the geniculate ganglion.

Clinical features

Facial paralysis, otalgia and malaise are all features. There is nearly always a herpetic eruption with vesiculation around the external auditory meatus. Sometimes vesiculation on the pharynx and palate is seen. Other cranial nerves may be involved – VIII, IX, X.

Management

Analgesia is the main form of treatment but the skin of the ear canal should be kept dry. Antivertiginous preparations may be required.

SECTION V

Principles of general management and treatment of the ear

HEARING AIDS AND ADVICE FOR THE DEAF

The modern hearing aid comprises a microphone, an amplifier and a receiver. These may be incorporated into the earpiece of an air conduction aid. The ideal for any hearing aid is that it should be efficient, inconspicuous and low in cost. It is felt by many users that a body-worn aid is too conspicuous. Hiding the amplifier–microphone unit under clothing diminishes its efficiency.

To meet these difficulties, ear level aids have been produced. These are worn behind the ear for air conduction.

Assessment

The patient should have a full otological examination. There is little purpose in using an insert or earpiece where the ear is filled with wax or where there is a discharge. The insert itself may produce a sensitivity reaction. A non-toxic form is available.

In estimating the value which the patient may derive from the use of a hearing aid, both pure tone and speech audiometry should be performed. It should be remembered that although low frequencies allow speech to be heard, high frequencies are essential for understanding speech patterns. Normal speech is at an intensity of 40–70 dB. Therefore, if a patient's hearing loss is greater than 30 dB, some form of amplification is required.

Type of aid

An air conduction hearing aid should be prescribed when possible. In a mixed deafness, however, the air conduction level can be so low as to offer little hope of usable amplification. In such a case a bone conduction receiver may give a satisfactory response. The bone conduction receiver is held over the mastoid antrum by a head band. It may be either aesthetically unacceptable to some patients or uncomfortable.

As a whole, patients requiring hearing aids have a sensorineural loss, although some with conductive deafness may be aided by amplification where age or the extent of the disease or accompanying sensorineural deafness makes surgery impractical.

There is a percentage of patients with sensorineural deafness for whom a hearing aid gives little improvement. These are:

- those with a high frequency deafness
- those with a poor speech discrimination associated with noise induced deafness
- those with marked recruitment phenomenon
  The increased amplification cannot be tolerated.
- those in whom the threshold of hearing is so low that the aid can offer little gain

Management

When an aid is prescribed, adequate time should be given to the patient for trial and rehabilitation. In the aged, this involves time spent explaining the use of the aid to either the patient or perhaps to the home help who may be the patient's only daily contact. Follow-up and information about recognized centres for repair and advice must be provided.

The patient should also be informed of facilities available to boost personal telephone and television reception.

Where the patient's hearing is either of such severity that he or she is unable to appreciate any advantage from the use of a hearing aid, or where there is a marked recruitment phenomenon, lip-reading should be encouraged.

PRINCIPLES OF SURGERY FOR DEAFNESS

With antibiotic therapy and the introduction and development of the operating microscope, surgery for deafness has been made possible. Previously, surgery of the temporal bone was aimed at drainage of infection and the removal of diseased tissue and cholesteatoma to render the ear 'safe'.

The operating microscope permits the meticulous removal of diseased material, allowing specific attention to be paid to the conservation of the fine ossicular chain mechanism and the tympanic membrane. It also permits investigation of the middle ear in the non-infective and postinfective states. The middle ear and mastoid may be approached by three routes (LD-29):

- postauricular (postaural)
- endaural
- transcanal

Myringotomy

The tympanic membrane is incised in its antero-inferior quadrant. The indications for this are acute otitis media and serous otitis media (LD-26).

Postoperative management

In acute otitis media where pus is drained from the ear, the condition generally settles within a week to ten days and the myringotomy closes.

In serous otitis media the incision may close within 24 hours. A pressure equalizing tube (grommet) may be inserted through the incision to allow equalization of pressure (see LD-27).

In all cases water should be kept from the ear until the tympanic membrane has healed. The pressure equalizing tube generally is extruded within 6 months of insertion.

Dangers of myringotomy

These include:

- continuing perforation
- thin scars and tympanosclerotic patches on the tympanic membrane
- disruption of the ossicular chain
  This is a risk if the incision is in the posterior half of the membrane.
- perforation of a high dehiscent jugular bulb
  This would result in a sudden gush of blood. It is easily controlled by packing.

Stapedectomy

The results of the surgical treatment for otosclerosis should be fully explained to the patient. He or she should be told that some imbalance, nausea and vomiting may occur postoperatively.

The poorer ear is always operated upon if the bone conduction is no worse than 30 dB. Where the bone conduction is as low as 30 dB it should be explained

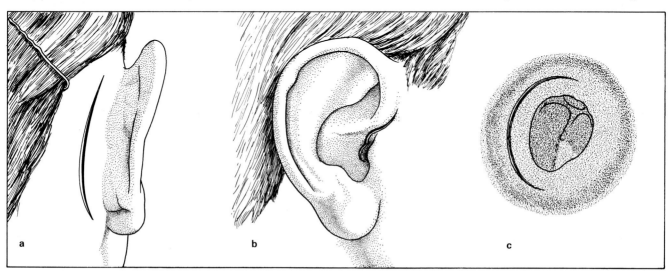

LD-29. *Approaches to the middle ear and mastoid.* **a**, *The postauricular incision.* **b**, *The endaural incision.* **c**, *The transcanal tympanotomy*

that any improvement in hearing will only facilitate use of a hearing aid.

Surgery is performed through an anterior tympanotomy.

The stapes superstructure is removed and the footplate perforated and removed in total or in part. A prosthesis is then inserted onto fat or connective tissue graft in the oval window and attached to the incus (LD-30). An alternative procedure – interposition – involves retaining the stapes superstructure attached to incus and placing it on a fat graft placed in the oval window.

Duration in hospital is 5–7 days.

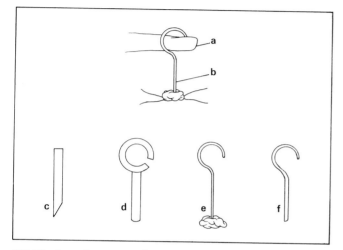

LD-30. *Stapedectomy with a range of prostheses. **a**, Incus. **b**, Wire/fat prosthesis. **c**, Polythene strut. **d**, Teflon piston. **e**, Wire/gelfoam or fat. **f**, Stainless steel*

Postoperative management

The patient should be home within 1 week. Warn against flying, for at least 6 months, and against violent nose blowing.

Complications

Short term complications

These include:

- imbalance, nausea and vomiting
- acute suppurative otitis media
- facial nerve paralysis

Immediately after surgery the patient may experience imbalance with nausea and vomiting for a few days.

Acute suppurative otitis media is an extremely dangerous condition as it may result in acute bacterial labyrinthitis.

Facial nerve paralysis is usually a temporary complication.

Midterm complications

Midterm complications include continuing vertigo. This may result from too long a prosthesis or from a perilymphatic leak around the prosthesis.

Long term complications

Long term complications include sudden sensorineural deafness related to injury or a head cold.

Conductive deafness may occur if the prosthesis slips or if fibrosis develops within the middle ear around the prosthesis. In secondary conductive deafness, re-exploration may be indicated.

The prognosis is reported as 90% success in closure of the conductive gap. Eight per cent remain unimproved and 2% become worse with sensorineural depression.

Pinnaplasty

Pinnaplasty is the operative procedure for bat ears.

Prior to any plastic procedure for correction of a cosmetic defect, photography from the front, the back and the side of the patient should be taken before and after surgery for record and medicolegal purposes (CP-2).

Preoperatively, infection in the area surrounding the pinna and within the external auditory canal must be eradicated to eliminate the risk of perichondritis and destruction of cartilage (CP-7).

The operation involves reconstructing an antihelical fold by removal of the skin on the posterior surface of the auricle and folding back the cartilage with subcuticular sutures. The patient would normally be in hospital for a period of approximately 5–7 days.

Tympanoplasty

Tympanoplasty is the term used for reconstruction of the tympanic membrane and middle ear structures. In its simplest form it is known as myringoplasty.

Myringoplasty

Myringoplasty is a term used for simple reconstruction of a perforation of the tympanic membrane where no middle ear reconstruction is required. Preoperatively two criteria must be met.

The Eustachian tube must be patent.

Infection must be cleared from:
- the middle ear
- the region of the nose
- the throat and paranasal sinuses

While it is hoped that reconstruction of the tympanic membrane will result in improved hearing, the main purpose of the operation is to seal the membrane and thus offer protection to the ear from the risk of recurrent infection. Closure of a perforation permits the patient to live a normal existence without fear if water enters the ear.

Prior to surgery audiometric assessment should be performed.

Procedure

The operation may be undertaken through the external auditory canal or through a postaural incision.

The edges of the perforation are freshened and the graft may be inserted through the drum as an underlay or on top of the drum as an onlay.

In very small perforations a small piece of fat inserted into the perforation may suffice. Material for grafting the larger perforations is either temporalis fascia or preserved dura taken at postmortem.

Complications

Complications are generally associated with infection. This can result in the breakdown of the reconstructed tympanic membrane.

The intact ossicular chain may be traumatized.

Postoperative management

Patients are usually home within 1 week and return to hospital 2 or 3 weeks later for removal of the deep packing laid on the reconstructed tympanic membrane. The ear should be kept dry until the membrane has completely healed.

Tympanoplasty with ossiculoplasty

Reconstruction of middle ear structures as well as repair of the tympanic membrane can be undertaken.

Discontinuity of the ossicular chain generally occurs at the incudostapedial joint. A bone chip may be interposed, to reconstitute the chain. Erosion of the long process of the incus requires reconstruction either by prosthetic material or removal of the incus followed by remodelling and repositioning between the malleus and the stapes (incus interposition). (Homograft incus and malleus may be used in reconstruction.)

The operative approach is similar to myringoplasty.

Postoperative management

The patient will be in hospital for about 1 week and the deep packing is removed from the ear 2 or 3 weeks later.

Complications

Complications are similar to those of myringoplasty. Where there is considerable tympanosclerosis in the tympanic membrane and middle ear, the prognosis for hearing improvement is poor.

Tympanotomy

Anterior tympanotomy involves opening the middle ear and inspecting the middle ear cavity. It is used in cases of conductive deafness where there is an intact tympanic membrane (e.g. otosclerosis). The middle ear is opened by raising a flap from the posterior canal wall, elevating the tympanic annulus.

Complications

Disruption of the ossicular chain at the incudostapedial joint may occur.

Perforation may follow.

Trauma to chorda tympani may occur (patient may complain of altered taste).

Mastoidectomy

This is undertaken for infective conditions of the mastoid cells and cholesteatoma.

There are two forms:
- cortical mastoidectomy
- radical mastoidectomy/modified radical mastoidectomy

Cortical mastoidectomy

The operation is indicated for acute mastoiditis.

The aim of the operation is exenteration and drainage of the mastoid cells. The mastoid is opened through a postauricular incision. The middle ear is untouched. The patient is generally hospitalized for 10 days to 2 weeks.

Radical and modified radical mastoidectomy

Radical and modified radical mastoidectomy procedures are performed for chronic disease of the middle ear and mastoid with or without cholesteatoma. The postauricular or endaural approach is used. Mastoid surgery for chronic ear disease may be combined with tympanoplasty procedures (mastoid-tympanoplasty).

Radical mastoidectomy involves complete mastoid exenteration – removal of all diseased structures within the middle ear itself. Modified procedures stop short of the complete radical procedure.

Combined approach tympanoplasty (CAT)

This may be performed in limited cholesteatoma.

The mastoid is opened postauricularly and the middle ear is entered. The posterior canal wall is thinned but intact. The middle ear can be viewed from behind (posterior tympanotomy) and via the external auditory canal (anterior tympanotomy), allowing greater accessibility for eradication of disease and reconstruction.

The patient is generally hospitalized for 2–3 weeks.

Complications of mastoid surgery

These include:

- damage to the inner ear
- damage to the facial nerve

PRINCIPLES OF NEURO-OTOLOGICAL SURGERY

Intracranial complications of middle ear infection are fortunately seen much less frequently than 20 years ago. This is due mainly to the introduction of antibiotic therapy and improved health education.

Intracranial infection

Bacterial meningitis must be treated by systemic antibiotic therapy in the first instance. Where a suppurative chronic otitis media is the origin of the condition, surgery of the mastoid and middle ear should be contemplated only when the meningitis is controlled. Drainage of the labyrinth may be required.

Intracranial abscesses should be drained through burr holes and mastoidectomy should follow under antibiotic cover.

If venous thrombosis of the lateral sinus is suspected, mastoidectomy, uncapping and exploration of the sinus should be undertaken. If pus is found this must be evacuated.

Surgery of the facial nerve

Surgical exposure of the facial nerve is achieved by approaching from the mastoid. The nerve may be exposed from the stylomastoid foramen to the geniculate ganglion. Opening the Fallopian canal permits the nerve sheath to be slit, giving relief of pressure from oedema.

The nerve may require to be grafted or approximation of the traumatized ends may be sufficient. The lateral cutaneous nerve of the thigh or the great auricular nerve may be used for grafting.

After grafting or reapproximation, residual weakness may occur and incoordination of facial movements may result. Recovery may take from 6 months up to 1 year.

Surgery for acoustic neuroma

Where an acoustic neuroma remains entirely within the internal auditory canal or even when it has expanded into the intracranial cavity, the portion within the internal auditory canal may be removed by a translabyrinthine approach after a preliminary mastoidectomy. In doing this it is hoped to spare the facial nerve, although the result will be a 'dead' ear.

Where the tumour is occupying the cerebellopontine angle, the internal portion must be removed via the posterior cranial fossa.

Surgery for Ménière's disease

Where conservation of hearing is sought, surgical procedures have been devised either to selectively ablate the vestibular apparatus or drain the excess endolymph.

The endolymphatic sac shunt

The endolymphatic sac is approached by a preliminary mastoidectomy followed by extradural entry into the posterior cranial fossa. A drainage tube is inserted into the sac to reduce the excess endolymphatic fluid.

Ultrasonic destruction of the vestibular apparatus

The ultrasonic destruction of the vestibular apparatus involves exposure of the lateral semicircular canal. The endostial bone of the canal is thinned until a grey line is observed and an ultrasonic beam is then directed on to the semicircular canal. The nystagmic response of the patient is monitored until it is abolished.

Membranous labyrinthectomy

Where no usable hearing remains or where the patient's life is threatened due to vertiginous attacks, a membranous labyrinthectomy may be performed. The procedure follows a preliminary anterior tympanotomy. The stapes is removed and the bone between the oval and round windows is drilled out. The membranous labyrinth may then be sucked out and the orifices of the canals probed. The vestibule should be filled with gel-foam and the tympanotomy flap replaced.

PRINCIPLES OF DRUG MANAGEMENT

Aural drops, creams and ointments

Medication can be applied to the ear as cream and ointments or in the form of drops, or insufflated in powder form.

Cream or ointment is best applied on half-inch (13 mm) ribbon gauze wicks, but may also be applied directly into the ear canal or to the pinna.

Drops – 3–4 in number – should be applied into the ear with the head inclined to the opposite side and the position maintained for 5 minutes. A plug of cotton wool should then be placed in the meatus. Drops may also be applied on half-inch (13 mm) ribbon gauze to ensure adequate contact and penetration.

The applications should be as frequent as is necessary, usually twice per day in the early stage of treatment.

Ointments and creams are generally used in the treatment of furunculosis and external otitis, whereas drops are used in middle ear infections.

The medications fall into groups, summarized below.

Bland preparations

These include:

- 1% ichthyol and glycerine

- 8% aluminium acetate cream
- 10% alcohol drops
- sodium bicarbonate 5 g/glycerol 30 ml drops

Steroid preparations

These are used as anti-inflammatory agents.

Steroid antibiotic preparations

Various preparations are available with a steroid base combined with antibiotics.

The antibiotic prescribed should relate to organism sensitivity.

Analgesics

The use of analgesic drops is not encouraged.

Analgesics are more effectively administered systemically.

Antiobiotic preparations

These include:

- framycetin sulphate 0.5% drops
- gentamicin sulphate 0.3% drops
- nitrofurazone 0.2% (ointment)
- framycetin sulphate 0.5%
- tetracycline hydrochloride 1%

Antifungal preparations

These include:

- nystatin powder 100 000 units/g
- amphotericin 3%
- miconazole 2%

} in drop form

Antivertiginous drugs

Antihistamines are used in the symptomatic treatment of vertigo and act at brain stem level.

They include:

- promethazine theoclate
- dimenhydrinate
- prochlorperazine maleate
- thiethylperazine maleate
- cinnarizine

The antihistamines may cause drowsiness and the patient should be cautioned about driving and operating machinery.

Tranquillizers

These are used to allay the apprehension experienced by the vertiginous patient.

Antibiotic policy

Antibiotics may be administered systemically or topically. Their use should be related to organism sensitivity, but in many instances therapy must be begun immediately. The indiscriminate use of antibiotics can, however, play an important part in the development of organism resistance.

All antibiotics have side-effects. Blood levels should therefore be commensurate with the elimination of the bacterial focus.

TEST-YOURSELF QUESTIONS

Part 1 – The Ear

1. The following cranial nerves may be responsible for referred otalgia:
a) Vagus X
b) Abducens VI
c) Glossopharyngeal IX
d) Trigeminal V

2. Post-auricular swelling may arise from:
a) Acute parotitis
b) Pediculosis capitis
c) Acute mastoiditis
d) Furunculosis of the ear canal

3. Cholesteatoma
a) is a benign middle ear tumour
b) may produce an offensive discharge
c) can erode bone
d) may present as otalgia

4. Ménière's disease is characterized by:
a) Conductive hearing loss
b) Tinnitus
c) Episodic vertigo
d) Recurrent otalgia
e) Severe frontal headache

5. Tinnitus
a) is the term used for aural noise
b) may be a presenting symptom of glomus jugulare tumours
c) may be of dental origin
d) is a feature of Bell's paralysis

6. Impacted wax may be associated with:
a) Sensori-neural hearing loss
b) Otalgia
c) Facial paralysis
d) Keratosis obturans

7. In the management of acute otitis media which of the following are of importance?
a) Bed rest
b) Topical antibiotic
c) Myringotomy
d) Systemic decongestants

8. Features of serous otitis media include:
a) Bacterial infection of the middle ear
b) Conductive hearing loss
c) Eustachian tube dysfunction
d) Preceding upper respiratory tract infection
e) Otalgia

9. Myringotomy
a) is the surgical management of serous otitis media
b) involves a post-auricular approach to the tympanic membrane
c) may result in a perforation of the tympanic membrane as a complication
d) is a form of surgical management of vertigo

10. The following are causes of non-labyrinthine vertigo:
a) Acoustic neuroma
b) Ménière's disease
c) Stapedectomy
d) Aminoglycoside therapy

The answers to these questions will be found on p. 191.

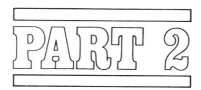

THE NOSE

SECTION I

Background to disease of the nose

BACKGROUND

In lower mammals the sense of smell is all-important. Large areas of the nose are covered by olfactory epithelium on an extensive turbinate structure. This increases the available surface area without taking up too much room.

In man, where the need for olfaction is very much less, the turbinates are small and have largely sequestrated off and developed as sinuses in the rounder skull. Olfactory epithelium exists only in the roof of the nose.

ANATOMY

Maxillary sinus

The maxillary sinus or antrum is bounded by:

- the eye
- the cheek and face
- the nasal cavity
- the teeth and hard palate

Any infective process or trauma to the maxillary sinus can therefore affect these sites.

The bony walls are very thin, especially superiorly and anterolaterally, and so fractures in this area are not uncommon. The maxillary sinus is connected to the nasal cavity by a small ostium in the middle meatus (LD-31).

The ethmoid sinuses

The ethmoid is a separate bone consisting of:

- the crista galli and perpendicular plate of the septum
- the cribriform plate

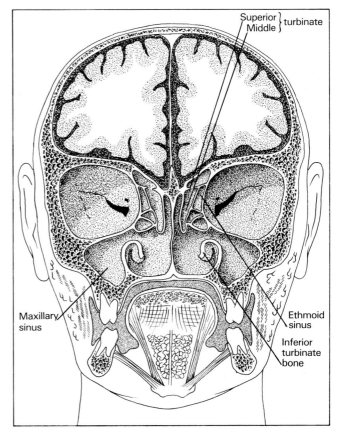

LD-31. Maxillary and ethmoid sinuses and turbinates

- the ethmoid bullae and air cells
- the superior and middle turbinates

It lies medial to the medial canthus of the eye and extends back to the sphenoid sinus which lies below the pituitary fossa. The bone of the ethmoid is paper-thin and infections and tumours spread rapidly from the ethmoid cells to the orbits and adjacent sinuses (LD-32).

The ethmoid cells are contiguous to the maxillary sinus and also to the frontal and sphenoid sinuses.

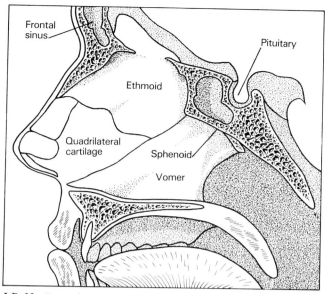

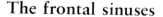

LD-32. Frontal and sphenoid sinuses

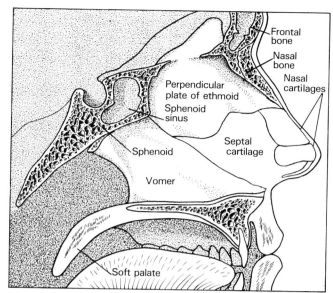

LD-33. Anatomy of the septum and external nose

The frontal sinuses

The frontal sinuses are bound by:

- the forehead
- the orbit
- the anterior cranial fossa (LD-32).

The bone is relatively thick, and so spread of infection and fractures are more rare. The frontonasal duct enters the middle meatus.

The nasal septum

The nasal septum is made up of:

- the quadrilateral cartilage (septal cartilage)
- the perpendicular plates of the ethmoid and the vomer

The cartilage is inserted in a groove in the vomer as it runs along the floor of the nose. After nasal injury it can be dislocated from its groove, causing nasal obstruction and an external nasal deformity (LD-33).

The external nasal skeleton

In the upper third, the external skeleton of the nose is made up of the nasal bones. These articulate with the maxillary and frontal bones. The lower two thirds consist of cartilage, with the upper lateral cartilages in the middle part and the lower lateral cartilages at the tip (LD-34).

Nasal fractures are usually lateral displacements but, if posterior displacement of the nasal bone occurs, then they are pushed into the ethmoid cells.

The lateral walls of the nasal cavity

The lateral wall of the nasal cavity bounds the maxillary and ethmoid sinuses.

The inferior turbinate closes off from the lower part of the maxillary antrum while the middle and superior turbinates form part of the ethmoid complex. The olfactory lining is limited to the superior turbinate and occasionally part of the middle turbinate. The rest of the nose and sinuses are lined by respiratory columnar ciliated epithelium.

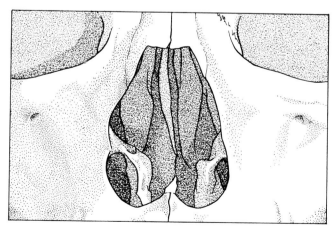

LD-34. Anterior skeleton of nose

The blood supply

The blood supply of the nose is derived from both the internal and external carotid arterial systems. The external carotid through the maxillary artery and its branches – principally the greater palatine and short sphenopalatine arteries – supplies the lateral wall of the nose below the middle turbinate. The internal carotid through the anterior ethmoid arteries supplies the lateral wall above the middle turbinate.

With an epistaxis, the source of bleeding can therefore be deduced by determining whether the blood runs from above or below the middle turbinate (LD-35).

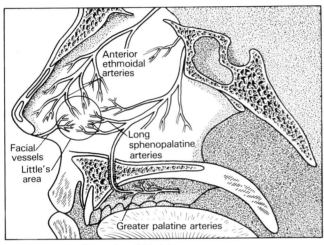

LD-35. *Arterial supply of Little's area*

The blood vessels of the nasal septum all meet at an area 13–25 mm (half-inch to 1 inch) from the mucocutaneous junction known as 'Little's area'. This is the commonest site for an epistaxis from the septum and is easily controlled by cautery.

The arteries involved in the anastomosis are the long spheno-palatine, the superior labial, the greater palatine, and the septal branch of the anterior ethmoidal.

The nerve supply to the nose

Branches of the sphenopalatine ganglion provide the nerve supply to the nose. They are the greater palatine and the long and short sphenopalatine nerves. The anterior ethmoidal nerves also contribute.

The blood vessels and the mucosal glands are therefore under autonomic control. A balance should exist but if the parasympathetic tone is higher the vessels dilate, the turbinates become engorged by venous stasis and the result is nasal obstruction and a watery discharge. If the sympathetic tone is greater then the vessels constrict and the turbinates shrink. Most nose drops produce this effect.

PHYSIOLOGY

The nose has five main functions. They are:
- provision of an airway
- olfaction
- humidification of inspired air
- warming of inspired air
- protection of the lower respiratory tract

The sinuses have no function.

Provision of an airway

The nose primarily provides an airway. On inspiration and expiration the airflow occurs in two streams – one above, and one below, the middle turbinate. In the roof of the nose the air currents form eddies which permit contact with the olfactory epithelium.

Olfaction

This sense is vital in lower animals but not so important in man. Olfactory nerves arise from a specialized mucous membrane situated mainly on the superior turbinate. They pierce the cribriform plate. To make smell possible, air must get to this area and it must be moist. If there is no sense of smell, then it is likely that there will not be a sense of flavour.

Humidification

A patient with a new tracheostomy will get crusting, because the relatively dry atmospheric air directly hits the tracheal mucosa. Normally no crusting occurs in the lower respiratory tract because the air is humidified during its passage through the nose. The nasal mucosa constantly secretes mucus which wets the air. This mucous blanket is moved on by cilia. If the cilia stop functioning the mucous blanket thickens and moves irregularly, and the symptom of 'catarrh' results.

Warming

It is important that air is warmed as well as humidified before it reaches the lungs. This is done quite simply by the air column passing around the vascular turbinates and nasal spaces.

Protection

The nose has hairs at the vestibule which trap particulate matter including allergens such as pollens. Smaller particles, which get past that barrier, stick to the mucus. This is constantly being wafted posteriorly by the cilia and swallowed. The mucus contains lysozymes which have a bacteriocidal function.

SECTION II
History and physical examination of the nose

HISTORY

The main complaint should first be established with regard to onset, duration and recurrence. In taking the nasal history, enquire specifically into the likely presenting symptoms. These are:

- obstruction
- discharge
- bleeding – epistaxis

Obstruction

Nasal obstruction is the commonest symptom of nasal disease. The points that should be elicited are:

- How long has the obstruction been present?
- Is it unilateral or bilateral?
- Has it an allergic aetiology?
- Is it secondary to vasomotor changes?
- Is it due to previous trauma or nasal surgery?
- Is it due to infection?
- Is it due to polypi?
- Is it due to disorders elsewhere?

Has it an allergic aetiology?

Many patients are able to relate the obstruction to contact with a specific precipitating factor such as grass pollen, or an animal dander. Ask therefore about seasonal variations and the environment in which the symptom occurs.

Enquire about a family history of allergy and a personal history of asthma or eczema in childhood.

Is it secondary to vasomotor changes?

Overactive nasal reflexes result in nasal obstruction from venous engorgement of the turbinates. This tends to occur in stressful situations and is stimulated by change in the ambient temperature and posture of the patient.

Ask therefore about nasal blockage on going from a warm to a cold room or on lying down in bed at night.

Is it due to previous trauma or nasal surgery?

Septal dislocation, distortions and collapse of the alar cartilage support are common causes of nasal obstruction.

Ask therefore about previous nasal injury or surgery and determine whether the obstruction is confined to one nostril or not. This is commonly found with a dislocated septum.

Is it due to infection?

The commonest nasal infections are viral in origin. They are the common cold and influenza. A systemic upset and fever may be associated. These infections are of short duration and are self-limiting. Acute sinusitis is a bacterial infection, is more prolonged and is associated with pain over the affected sinuses. Chronic sinusitis gives prolonged symptoms and is associated with purulent catarrh.

Ask therefore about fever, pain around the sinuses and purulent secretions. These would all favour an infective aetiology.

Is it due to polypi?

Nasal polypi are usually bilateral. Before obstructing the nose completely they have an intermittent valve-like effect. They are the commonest cause of loss of sense of smell.

Ask therefore about gradual increase in obstructive symptoms, and about loss of smell.

Is it related to disorders elsewhere?

Spread of infection from the sinuses and the gradual expansion of malignant disease will affect the eye, the teeth, and the soft tissues of the cheek.

Enquire about double vision, proptosis, epiphora, swelling of the cheek, toothache, loosening of the teeth, and ill-fitting dentures.

Discharge

Nasal discharge usually accompanies nasal obstruction. Thin watery discharge is usually blown out the nose – a rhinorrhoea – whereas thick and purulent discharge commonly runs down the nasopharynx and is called catarrh. The following points should be elicited:

- Is it thin and watery?
  This is due to excess mucus production, and suggests a viral infection, allergic or vasomotor rhinitis. Remember also the possibility of CSF rhinorrhoea.

- Is it thick and purulent?
  This suggests a bacterial infection, such as sinusitis.

- Is the discharge foul smelling?
  In the young or the mentally infirm, a foreign body is the commonest cause of offensive nasal discharge. In young and middle-aged patients, consider sinusitis secondary to a dental infection. In the elderly, consider malignant disease.

- Is it related to head position?
  This would suggest a CSF leak, and requires urgent attention – cerebrospinal rhinorrhoea.

Epistaxis

With the exception of menstruation, epistaxis is the commonest cause of spontaneous haemorrhage. It is due to the bursting of an unsupported vessel in the nasal mucosa. In the majority of cases it is an isolated incident, but it can be the presenting symptom of systemic disease. A few simple questions should always be asked to exclude underlying pathology. These are:

- Is it due to trauma?
  This includes major trauma sufficient to cause a fracture of the nasal bones. Minor trauma

such as nose picking, or excessive blowing, is also important. Enquire also about previous nasal surgery.

- Is there evidence of a bleeding disorder?
  Ask about excessive bleeding from minor cuts or excessive bruising from minor knocks. The drug history, especially in the elderly, is important. Excessive aspirin intake, or anticoagulant therapy, can cause epistaxis.

- Is it due to arteriosclerosis or hypertension?
  In the elderly hypertensive patient, epistaxis from bleeding far back in the nose is not uncommon.

- Is it due to infection or neoplasms of the sinuses?
  Enquire about purulent rhinorrhoea and offensive discharge as well as swelling in the region of the sinuses.

Nasal symptoms in childhood

In a child the commonest cause of nasal obstruction is large adenoids. In addition to the obstruction, large adenoids lead to ear infection. Their size increases with local infection. Enquiry should therefore be made about sore ears, deafness and sore throats.

Facial pain

The sensory supply to the face is by the ophthalmic, maxillary and mandibular divisions of the trigeminal nerve. The interior of the nose and sinuses are supplied by the ophthalmic and maxillary nerves.

EXAMINATION

Equipment

Use a headlight and a Thudicum's nasal speculum to examine the anterior nose, and a tongue depressor and a heated postnasal mirror to see the nasopharynx (CP-8).

As an alternative to a headlight, put the biggest aural speculum on an auroscope, take off the magnifier and you will be able to have a reasonable look at the anterior nose (CP-9). It is useful to use a cocaine and adrenaline spray prior to any nasal examination since this will shrink and anaesthetize the nasal mucosa.

Approach

External examination

Look first at the external nose to see if it is straight or bent.

Determine whether it is the bony upper third or the cartilaginous lower two thirds that is twisted.

Finally look at the nose from below and see if the end of the quadrilateral cartilage is in the columella or if it is dislocated.

Internal examination

Examine the nasal septum, determining if it is straight, and the colour of the nasal mucous membrane. The size and colour of the inferior turbinate and, with practice, the middle turbinate should be noted. Where there has been epistaxis, carefully examine Little's area of the septum. Look for polyps around the middle meatus. They are white and translucent. If there is any discharge, note its source and character.

Examining the nasopharynx is difficult but the technique reveals enlarged adenoids, choanal polyps, the large posterior ends of turbinates, tumours beginning around the Eustachian tube (their most usual site) and posterior nasal bleeding.

If a patient has a history suggesting a sinus problem, then palpate the sinus and compare the two sides for evenness of contour and tenderness. If the maxillary sinus is involved, it is necessary to palpate intraorally around the alveolus.

INVESTIGATIONS

Allergy tests

Many patients with nasal symptoms either have an allergy or require to have an allergic cause excluded. No satisfactory method of testing inhalant allergens exists by direct application, and so skin testing is commonly employed.

It is only worth desensitizing patients whose strong reactions to allergens are compatible with their history. For desensitization a vaccine of the allergen is made up in various strengths and a course of 18 weekly injections of increasing strengths is then given.

In skin testing, various allergens are made up in dilute form and applied to the skin of the forearm by a scratch. The allergens are selected using information gained from the patient's history. Common ones are house dust, house dust mite, feathers, cat dander, dog hair, grasses, trees, pollens and various moulds.

The reaction is read at 15 min and is assessed on a scale + to + + +.

RADIOLOGY

A third of the nose and all the paranasal sinuses have bony walls. They are air-containing cavities and therefore present as radiolucent areas. The depth of the mucosal lining and the bony margins are clearly seen.

Radiological views

There are four radiological views in common use. They are:

- occipitomental
  This shows the maxillary antra.
- occipitofrontal
  This shows the ethmoid and frontal sinuses.
- lateral
  This shows the sphenoid sinus.
- an underpenetrated lateral view
  This assesses possible fractures of the nasal bones.

When looking at sinus films (X-14), compare the lucency of one sinus with that of its contralateral partner, and the lucency of both sinuses with that of the orbits. The bony margins should also be carefully traced and compared.

Radiological changes

Fluid level

This is a sign of active infection, and may be acute sinusitis. To be sure that fluid is present a tilted view should be requested (X-15).

Opacity of a sinus

This is due either to the sinus being filled with fluid, mucus or pus, or to gross mucosal thickening (X-16). It is a picture seen in acute or chronic sinusitis, especially when nasal polypi are present.

Mucous membrane thickening

This is the commonest radiological change, but is unfortunately not diagnostic (X-17). Any condition which causes thickening of the nasal lining will give this picture. The degree of radiological thickening may be much more than one would expect when compared with the appearance of the nose. Chronic sinusitis is a likely cause of this.

Expansion of bony sinus walls

This may be associated with opacity of the sinus affected and is seen in mucocoeles of the frontal and ethmoid sinuses, and benign tumours such as transitional cell papillomata (X-18).

Erosion of bony sinus walls

This radiological appearance is diagnostic of malignant tumours, the commonest of which is a squamous carcinoma (X-19).

Tomography of the sinuses

This investigation is important in the preoperative assessment of a patient with malignant disease of the nose or sinus to assess extent and hence operability (X-19).

ANTROSCOPY

The antroscope is a small fibreoptic instrument which can be passed through the nose into the maxillary sinus. It is of particular use in determining the nature and extent of mucosal thickening, especially if there is a possibility that this is due to malignant change.

SECTION III

The presentation of disease of the nose and the diagnostic possibilities

NASAL OBSTRUCTION WITH DISCHARGE

The majority of nasal disease presents with symptoms of nasal obstruction and discharge. The severity of each symptom may vary.

Causes

Colds and influenza

The commonest causes in all age groups are 'colds' and influenza. The obstruction is due to the inflammatory response of the nasal mucosa, and the rhinorrhoea to the irritation of the mucous glands. The lining of the turbinates and septum is equally red and inflamed, and the patient has a systemic upset and fever.

Allergic rhinitis

In this condition the history is of short, sharp episodes of running eyes and with nasal obstruction. It is a response following contact with a specific allergen. The commonest type of allergic rhinitis is hay fever. The mucosa is pale and is oedematous in appearance due to increased extracellular fluid.

Vasomotor rhinitis

In vasomotor rhinitis, the periods of discharge and obstruction result from non-specific stimuli such as a change of ambient temperature or of the posture of the patient. For example the obstruction can be worse on lying down and if the patient lies on one side the undermost nostril will have the greatest obstruction.

Examination of the nose shows the turbinates, particularly the inferior ones, to be engorged. The septum is normal in colour.

NASAL OBSTRUCTION WITH MINIMAL DISCHARGE

Causes

Adenoids

Adenoids are enlarged aggregates of lymphoid tissue in the nasopharynx. Lymphoid tissue undergoes hypertrophy and atrophy relevant to its activity. It is at its largest relative to the size of the patient between the ages of 3 and 6 years. It is rare to find large adenoids beyond the age of 10 years.

Enlarged adenoids obstruct the passage of air through the nose. The muscles of the nasal tip do not develop, the nasal arch remains narrow, and if the condition is not treated the patient may have a poor narrow nasal airway for life.

Polypi

Polypi are aggregates of oedematous mucosa which come down into the nose usually from the ethmoidal sinuses. They initially have a valve-like effect, causing obstruction either on expiration or inspiration, but as they become larger they cause complete obstruction.

As they inhibit the flow of air to the superior meatus, which is the olfactory area, there will be a loss of sense of smell and flavour. Polypi are grey in colour and relatively insensitive to touch, and can be differentiated from turbinates as they do not contain a bony skeleton. They occur in people with a long history of allergic rhinitis or chronic sinusitis.

Deviated nasal septum

A deviated nasal septum is a frequent cause of obstruction. As few nasal septa are completely straight, it is important to ensure that the obstruction is in fact due to the deviation of the septum.

The symptoms are predominantly unilateral, although from time to time patients are seen with bilateral symptoms due to an S-shaped deviation. In addition to the obstructive symptoms, stasis occurs; this leads to catarrh and to infective conditions of the ear, pharynx and larynx.

The causes of a deviated septum are:

- trauma
- birth injury
- unequal growth

Tumours of the nose and sinuses

Tumours of the nose and sinuses are relatively rare but it is important that they are diagnosed early. The symptoms are again predominantly unilateral and are often associated with a foul-smelling serosanguinous discharge.

NASAL DISCHARGE WITH MINIMAL OBSTRUCTION

Causes

Chronic sinusitis

Chronic sinusitis presents with both posterior and anterior catarrh. In the acute exacerbation there is bacterial infection, and the discharge is therefore purulent at these times.

Foreign body

In the young and the feeble-minded, a purulent serosanguinous discharge is presumed to be due to a foreign body until proved otherwise.

The foreign body stimulates a giant cell reaction and granulation tissue forms around it.

Cerebrospinal fluid (CSF) rhinorrhoea

Cerebrospinal fluid (CSF) rhinorrhoea is usually the result of trauma or of an operation on the superior part of the nose or anterior cranial fossa. Occasionally it is spontaneous in the adult. The discharge is clear, is greater when the patient bends, stoops or strains and is commonly unilateral.

As CSF contains sugar, a quick test to lead to a correct diagnosis is to collect some fluid and see if it reacts with Dextrostix. If it does not cease within 2 weeks the leak must be closed surgically, as if left untreated there is a risk of meningitis.

Epistaxis

Epistaxis is common. Whilst its cause is often simple – an exposed dilated vessel on the anterior part of the normal septum – it can also be the presenting symptom of serious disease, such as:

- tumour of the nose, sinuses or nasopharynx
- a bleeding diathesis
- arteriosclerosis with hypertension

When treating a patient with epistaxis, enquiry should always be made about abnormal bleeding and bruising tendencies and symptoms of general ill health. In addition to seeking the source of the bleeding in the nose, it is necessary to exclude abnormal discharge, purulent secretions or foul smell. In the young or feeble-minded these are suggestive of a foreign body, and in the middle-aged and elderly a tumour.

FACIAL PAIN

What is the nature of pain?

It is important to identify the nature of the pain.

A vascular pain occurs when vessels are dilated. This gives a throbbing type of ache which is more marked on raising venous pressure and is exacerbated on stooping and straining. Vascular-type pain occurs in infections – tooth abscess and acute sinusitis – and also in migraine and stress headaches.

Neuralgic pains have a sharp burning or lancinating quality, and occur in trigeminal neuralgia and migrainous neuralgia.

Pain which is associated with altered sensation, such as paraesthesia or numbness in the distribution of the trigeminal nerve, is suggestive of infiltration of the nerve by tumour.

Are there significant features on examination?

In examining a patient with facial pain a specific plan should be followed.

Test for sensation over the trigeminal area to rule out direct neuralgic damage such as could occur from tumour of the sinuses, pterygomaxillary fissure or middle cranial fossa.

If sensation is normal consider the type of pain. If it is a vascular-type pain, exclude infection – boils of the face or vestibule of the nose or sinusitis. Vascular-type pain without infection is often due to migraine.

A dental cause is suggested if the pain is exacerbated by ingestion of hot, cold or sweet sub-stances. The alveolus should be palpated for signs of abscess and the teeth percussed.

Trigeminal neuralgia occurs in sudden self-limiting attacks of lancinating-type pain. There is often a trigger area, and palpation of it can start the pain. In this condition sensation is normal. Carbamazepine may have a fairly specific beneficial effect.

An intraocular cause of pain such as glaucoma should be considered.

If pain occurs during eating, then salivary gland disease could be the cause. The underlying condition will probably be sialectasis with or without calculus formation.

SECTION IV

Description of specific diseases of the nose

EPISTAXIS

Epistaxis is a term used to describe haemorrhage from the nose. It is a common complaint and can occur at any age.

Cause

Eighty per cent of epistaxis arises from blood vessels in Little's area. This is the anterior part of the nasal septum, just behind the mucocutaneous junction where there is a rich anastomosis of blood vessels.

The commonest cause of epistaxis is trauma.

This can be major trauma involving fracture of the nasal bones, minor trauma such as picking the nose or minimal trauma due to damage of the fragile nasal mucosa of Little's area. It can follow a break of the protective mucus blanket. As the latter is wafted posteriorly, the commonest place for deficiency of the mucus is at the anterior part of the septum. The trauma occurs as cold unmoistened air impinges on the delicate mucosa.

Incidence

Epistaxis is common in childhood and adolescence when the actual bleeding from an exposed blood vessel occurs during an upper respiratory tract infection. Virtually all epistaxis in young people originates from Little's area. Bleeding noses are uncommon in middle adult life but become more frequent in the elderly where the proportion of haemorrhages arising from far back or high up in the nasal cavities markedly increases.

Clinical features

Presentation

Patients often claim that they are bleeding from both nostrils. In fact this is very uncommon. Concentrate on the nostril which started bleeding or on the one which is bleeding most.

Examination

Instruct the patient to blow out all the blood clots, and then inspect the nostril carefully, especially Little's area, for evidence of an exposed vessel or a bleeding point.

Management

First aid treatment

Place the patient in a sitting position with the head forward so that blood does not run into the pharynx and cause coughing and spluttering. Get the patient to compress the tip of his nose, thus bringing direct pressure onto the blood vessels of Little's area for 5 minutes. This allows a firm clot to form.

Definitive treatment

Before embarking on definitive treatment, it is necessary to anaesthetize the nostril. The method of choice for treatment is cautery. In areas unsuitable for cautery, packing should be carried out.

Local anaesthesia is best achieved with a pledget of cotton wool soaked in 10% cocaine and then wrung out so that less than 2 ml of cocaine is applied. The safe body dose of cocaine is 200 mg. Cocaine reactions are excessively rare, but overdosage is not uncommon. This pledget of cotton wool is left in place for 10 min. Cocaine is a vasoconstrictor, and itself tends to lessen the bleeding.

Cautery is done by touching the exposed blood vessel with a small fused bead of chromic acid. After cautery the excess acid is removed by mopping. Cautery can only be carried out where a potential bleeding point can be seen and reached and when it is not actively bleeding (see Section V, p. 65).

The nose is packed by inserting double layers of 25 mm (1 inch) ribbon gauze soaked in bismuth iodoform paraffin paste in tiers starting from the floor and building up to the roof. This pack should be left in place for 48 hours, when a firm clot unlikely to be broken down by the fibrinolytic enzymes of nasal bacteria will have formed (see Section V, p. 65).

In addition to stopping the bleeding, general care of the patient is important. The shocked will require admission to hospital and blood transfusion. The anaemic will require iron therapy or blood transfusion. Patients with bleeding disorders will require special care and investigation.

Epistaxis is common and is frequently of little importance. However, a patient can die from epistaxis. It should therefore always be treated enthusiastically. Haemorrhage from the nose is never a safety valve!

Complications

In a very small proportion of cases, cautery and nasal packing will not suffice. This small group includes two quite separate problems.

The first problem is the patient who continues to bleed even after an adequate anterior nasal pack has been inserted. Such a patient should have a postnasal pack inserted.

The second problem is the patient who restarts bleeding once the anterior pack has been removed. He or she should have the feeding blood vessels tied off.

If the bleeding arises from below the middle turbinate, the maxillary artery is tied off in the sphenopalatine fossa. If the bleeding comes from above the level of the middle turbinate, the ethmoidal vessels are tied off as they emerge from the orbit and pass through the fronto-ethmoidal suture line.

ALLERGIC RHINITIS

Allergic rhinitis is a contact mucositis and is the result of an antigen–antibody reaction to an inhaled or ingested allergen.

Clinical features

History

In a true allergic rhinitis the intelligent patient will often know what he is allergic to. If it is seasonal, the allergen is usually a pollen and the condition is known as hay fever. The commonest non-seasonal allergens are the house dust mite, animal dander and feathers.

The patient complains of sneezing and rhinorrhoea and watering eyes, as well as partial nasal obstruc-tion. Although the condition can arise at any age, in many of those patients starting in childhood it is accompanied by asthma and eczema and there is often a strong family history.

A reduced sense of smell is limited to acute attacks.

Examination

The nasal mucosa is pale and swollen due to the increase in extracellular fluid caused by the release of histamine at the site of the antigen–antibody reaction.

If the patient is examined at a time when he or she has no symptoms, the nose will look normal.

Management

There is an enormous variability in the severity of symptoms of allergic rhinitis and it is important that the treatment is tailored to the patient's needs.

Symptomatic therapy

For mild occasional bouts the patient can be adequately managed with instructions to avoid the known allergen and to take decongestant nose drops or oral antihistamines (see Section V, p. 65).

Desensitization

Where there are moderate or severe reactions in either degree or duration, desensitization is the method of choice. Before contemplating this, adequate skin tests must be carried out to identify the causative factors and to make sure that these correlate with the patient's history.

Desensitization is a long and tedious procedure and should only be embarked upon if there is a reasonable chance of success. It has been found to be most effective in patients with pollen allergies (the largest group) and in those with only one or two strong positive skin test reactions.

Sodium cromoglycate

In patients with moderate symptoms and in whom desensitization is less likely to be effective, sodium cromoglycate should be tried as a nasal spray or as an insufflation.

Corticosteroids

Corticosteroids should never be given systemically for allergic rhinitis, because the complications may outweigh the advantages. Local, poorly absorbed steroids, such as beclomethasone dipropionate, are useful, but should be stopped if the patient has an upper respiratory tract infection.

VASOMOTOR RHINITIS

This condition has exactly the same symptoms as allergic rhinitis – sneezing, watery rhinorrhoea and intermittent nasal obstruction. The precipitating factors and nasal signs are, however, completely different.

Causes

The rate of nasal secretion and the vascular supply of the inferior and middle turbinates are under the control of the autonomic nervous system. The parasympathetic nerves stimulate secretion and cause vasodilatation, whereas the sympathetic nerves reduce secretion and cause vasoconstriction. These two systems are normally in balance and should produce sufficient heat and humidification to the inspired air reaching the larynx so that it is 90% humidified and within 1 °C of body temperature.

In vasomotor rhinitis this balance becomes abnormal. The parasympathetic element becomes dominant, resulting in congested turbinates and increased secretions, and the symptoms of nasal obstruction and watery rhinorrhoea.

Recognized underlying causes for this condition are:

- stress
  Vasomotor rhinitis is common in the stress age groups of adolescence, menopausal females and old men.
- change of climate
  Immigrants are vulnerable.
- altered hormonal states
  Pregnancy and myxoedema are examples.
- taking of drugs
  This occurs with some hypertensive drugs and with the contraceptive pill.

Clinical features

History

The patient complains of nasal obstruction and

watery rhinorrhoea with sneezing. This is exacerbated by non-specific stimuli such as change of posture and change of ambient temperatures and humidity.

Examination

The nasal mucosa is red and swollen over the turbinates, particularly the inferior ones. The nasal mucosa over the septum is a normal pink colour. This differentiates the condition from infective nasal disease.

Management

Mild cases should not be treated, as they are in fact only the manifestation of a normal autonomic nervous system reflex. Moderate cases will respond to decongestant drops. These should not be given for more than a month at a time (see Section V, p. 65).

In severe cases where nasal obstruction is the principal problem, submucosal diathermy or partial turbinectomy will restore the airway.

In some patients amitriptyline, which has a sedative as well as an anticholinergic effect, is useful.

In a small proportion of patients it is the constant watery rhinorrhoea which is most troublesome. This can be dealt with by sectioning the autonomic nerve supply to the nose – vidian neurectomy.

ACUTE SINUSITIS

Acute sinusitis occurs – in order of frequency – in the maxillary, ethmoidal, frontal and, only very rarely, the sphenoidal sinuses. It is usually part of a general upper respiratory tract infection which is initially due to a virus. A secondary and more prolonged bacterial infection quickly follows.

Causes

Basically all the paranasal sinuses are bony boxes lined by respiratory-type ciliated columnar epithelium and are connected with the nasal cavities by small ostia. The acute rhinitis causes swelling of the nasal mucosa and blockage of the ostia.

The obstruction, along with the swelling of the sinus mucosa and the inflammatory exudate, causes a feeling of tension and even acute pain around the affected sinus.

The primary infection is due to one of the rhinoviruses and the secondary invaders are *Haemophilus influenzae*, *Staphylococcus aureus* and *Streptococcus pyogenes*. Sinusitis can be secondary to dental infection, or to an oroantral fistula.

Acute sinusitis can be either unilateral or bilateral, can affect one sinus only or all the sinuses on one or both sides of the face. Complications arise by spread of infection to neighbouring structures such as the orbit or anterior cranial fossa. This spread can either be by direct extension or by a spreading thrombophlebitis (CP-10, CP-11).

Clinical features

History

The patient complains of partial or complete nasal obstruction with loss of sense of smell. The accompanying nasal discharge will be thin and watery in the earlier stage, but quickly becomes thick and purulent in the secondary bacterial phase. Much of the discharge will run posteriorly into the postnasal space if the maxillary sinus is affected, as its ostium lies in the posterior part of the middle meatus of the nose. There is often a systemic upset.

The pain of sinusitis is due to stretching of the nerve fibres in the walls of dilated blood vessels. It is therefore throbbing in character and made worse by stooping and straining. The amount of pain tends to be in inverse proportion to the amount of pus in the nose. If the ostium is tightly closed by mucosal swelling there will be much pain but little pus escaping into the nose.

The site of the pain depends on the sinus affected. Maxillary sinus pain is felt in the cheek, alveolus, teeth or frontal region. In ethmoidal sinusitis, pain is felt around and behind the eye. Acute frontal sinusitis is characterized by pain in the supraorbital region. It has a diurnal variation – being absent early in the morning, becoming more pronounced in the forenoon and afternoon and easing off in the evening.

Examination

The lining of the nose is red, swollen and obviously inflamed. In particular the colour of the septum is as red as the lining of the turbinates. There may be pus in the middle meatus, spreading to the floor of the nose, and also in the posterior nasal space. The patient usually has a fever.

Although radiology is not a prerequisite for coming to a diagnosis of acute sinusitis, as the symptoms and signs are so specific, X-rays should be taken, as they may show complete opacity, a fluid level or very marked mucosal thickening (X-14–17).

Management

The aim of treatment is to lessen the bacterial infection, and aid the reopening of the sinus ostia. Systemic antibiotics should be given along with decongestant nose drops. A salicylate preparation will reduce the temperature and make the pain bearable.

Complications

The commonest complications are orbital cellulitis and orbital abscess. These are invariably secondary to ethmoidal sinusitis. A spreading thrombophlebitis can give rise to cerebral cortical vein thrombosis and cavernous sinus thrombosis. Osteomyelitis of the maxillary bone may occur in children and, rarely, in adults, where the frontal bone is more often involved.

CHRONIC SINUSITIS

Chronic sinusitis is chronic from the outset, and seldom follows acute sinusitis. This latter condition will occur more frequently, however, in those with underlying chronic sinusitis.

Causes

The nasal mucosa constantly produces mucus to humidify the air and this mucus blanket is moved along in a posterior direction by the cilia. Cilia are paralysed by such things as nicotine and air pollutants and cease to move the mucus as a thin sheet. The mucus therefore lies in the nose, causing a chronic rhinitis. It runs down the nasopharynx as a thick stringy postnasal catarrh. As it lies in the pharynx this infected material causes a reactive hyperplasia in the submucosal lymphoid aggregates of the posterior pharyngeal wall. The results are sore throats and a granular pharyngitis.

The swollen nasal mucosa intermittently blocks the sinus ostia, resulting in a cycle – stasis–infection–oedema–obstruction–stasis. The affected sinus feels full and heavy. Chronic sinusitis is commonly bilateral and may affect more than one group of sinuses.

Clinical features

History

The principal symptoms are thick postnasal catarrh with intermittent nasal blockage and reduced sense of smell. It is important to remember that, while pain is a presenting symptom of acute sinusitis, it is rare in chronic sinusitis. The patient tends to complain of a dull face ache.

As the discharge from the nose is intermittently purulent, in longstanding cases the patient may present with signs of secondary infection – recurrent otitis media, serous otitis media, granular pharyngitis and chronic laryngitis.

Examination

In chronic sinusitis the lining of the nose is red and inflamed. The secretions are thick and stringy and sometimes purulent. There is frequently crusting, especially in the region of the middle turbinate.

The radiological appearances of chronic sinusitis are variable. Opacity of one sinus or group of sinuses is diagnostic, but mucosal thickening is more common. The radiological appearances must be correlated with the finding from the history and the examination, as any condition which causes thickening of the nasal mucosa – such as allergy and vasomotor rhinitis – will also cause mucosal thickening on a sinus X-ray.

Radiological examination is, however, important to exclude abnormalities such as:

- osteomata
  These can block the frontonasal duct causing secondary frontal sinusitis.
- mucocoeles
  These are slowly expanding cysts which can cause erosion. They occur particularly in the ethmoidal and frontal sinuses.

Management

The only effective medical treatment is the use of decongestants – either locally, as drops or sprays, or systemically. Antibiotics have no useful role except during acute exacerbations of chronic sinusitis. If medical treatment fails, surgery has to be considered. Maxillary antral lavage is effective in reopening a blocked ostium and washing out thick mucopurulent exudate. The maxillary sinuses are those most commonly involved and, in pansinusitis, once the maxillary sinus has been treated the ethmoidal and frontal sinuses often improve (Section V, p. 65).

If antral lavage proves ineffective, the maxillary sinus mucosa has probably reached an irreversible state and should be removed in the operation known as radical antrostomy (Section V, p. 65).

NASAL POLYPI

Nasal polypi are pouches of oedematous mucous membrane arising from the sinuses and hanging down inside the nasal cavity.

Causes

Nasal polypi most commonly arise from the ethmoidal sinuses and are frequently bilateral (CP-12). Two contributing factors are allergic rhinitis and chronic sinusitis. The allergy or infection causes thickening of the submucosal layer. In time, the sinus is completely filled by the oedematous lining which then prolapses into the nose. This small polyp is then dragged back and forth by the flow of air within the nose and gradually enlarges. Once polypi appear, although they may alter in size, they never completely disappear. A polyp arising from the maxillary sinus is usually unilateral and hangs down into the nasopharynx. They are called 'antrochoanal polypi' and are commonest in the 10–30 year age group.

There is a great variation in the natural history of nasal polypi. After complete removal, some recur in a matter of months whereas others do not reappear for several decades.

Unilateral swellings in the nose, especially in those over 50 years of age, and in children under the age of 10, should be treated with great suspicion as they are likely to be neoplasms – carcinoma and transitional cell papillomata in the elderly, olfactory neuroblastomata and nasal gliomata in infants.

Clinical features

History

Simple nasal polypi cause nasal obstruction. At first,

this is intermittent and the movement of the polyp can have a valve-like effect. Later there is complete nasal obstruction with anosmia, as air cannot reach the olfactory area.

Examination

Nasal polypi are soft pale bags of extracellular fluid and are relatively insensitive to touch. They can be differentiated from the turbinates as they do not have a bony framework. An X-ray of the sinuses shows opacity of the ethmoids, and mucous membrane thickening is a common finding in the maxillary sinuses.

Tests for allergy should be carried out. This represents a treatable cause once the polypi have been removed.

Management

Polypi should be removed intranasally. If there is radiological evidence of sinusitis the maxillary sinuses should be washed out at the same time, and a course of desensitization injections given if this is applicable. For polypi which recur frequently, an external ethmoidectomy is more effective in reducing the rate of recurrence, and restoring the sense of smell and taste (Section V, p. 65).

BENIGN TUMOURS OF THE NOSE AND SINUSES

The commonest benign tumours are osteomata and transitional cell papillomata.

Nine out of ten osteomata arise in the frontal or ethmoidal sinuses. They are often incidental findings on an X-ray examination, but can give rise to symptoms when they obstruct the sinus drainage.

Transitional cell papillomata arise from the lining of the nose or the maxillary antrum. They have the appearance of a fleshy polyp and cause obstruction. They should be removed completely as they can recur and, in the long term, have the potential of malignant change.

MALIGNANT TUMOURS OF THE NOSE AND SINUSES

Causes

The commonest malignant tumours to occur are:

- squamous cell carcinoma
- adenocarcinoma
  This can be secondary to tumours of the gastrointestinal or genitourinary tracts.
- adenoid cystic carcinoma
  This usually arises from the minor salivary glands

Nine out of ten malignant tumours arise in the maxillary antrum, with or without ethmoid involvement (CP-13). Malignant tumours of the frontal and sphenoidal sinuses are extremely rare.

Clinical features

History

The maxillary antrum is a bony box bordered by the eye, nasal cavity, hard palate, alveolus and cheek. It is rare for symptoms to occur prior to the tumour bursting out of this bony box and affecting one of these structures. The patient may then notice diplopia or proptosis, toothache, ill-fitting dentures, nasal obstruction or epistaxis.

Examination

The eye

Eye signs will include proptosis – displacement of the globe – usually in an upward and outward direction. Diplopia will usually be detected by simple clinical tests, but charting may be necessary. The nasolachrymal duct is frequently blocked, giving rise to epiphora.

The mouth

Swelling can occur in the hard palate or the alveolus may become broader (CP-14). Dental treatment is sometimes sought and extraction of a tooth can lead to a non-healing socket and an oroantral fistula.

The nose

The nose may be obstructed by the tumour itself or by a nasal polyp (CP-15). Both of these bleed readily to the touch.

The cheek

Swelling of the cheek is an uncommon presenting symptom as it tends to occur late in the disease.

Investigations

Over 80% of antral cancers show bone destruction on X-ray when first seen. This means that early diagnosis is uncommon. Tomograms are important in defining the posterior and superior extent of the tumour (X-19).

Immediately carcinoma is suspected, it should be biopsied.

Management

The results of treatment are poor, as the diagnosis tends to be made late. The best results are obtained by a combination of radiotherapy and surgery. Patients selected for treatment receive a full dose of radiation. Six weeks later the maxilla is removed, with the ethmoids and the eye if they are involved (see Section V, p. 65).

Patients with enlarged secondary glands in the neck, or tumours where there has been spread posteriorly to the pterygoid plates, superiorly to the cranial fossa, or laterally to give rise to trismus, should not be treated.

Replacement of the maxilla is achieved by a specially built-up denture (CP-16), but if the eye has to be removed an external prosthesis held on by spectacles is required. The treatment is uncomfortable and can be disfiguring.

CHOANAL ATRESIA

Causes

In early development the nose is closed off from the pharynx by the bucconasal membrane. If this membrane does not disappear, the posterior choana will be occluded by this membrane. It can be unilateral or bilateral, fibrous or bony.

Clinical features

If the atresia is complete and bilateral, severe breathing problems occur at birth. It must be perforated as an emergency, as babies cannot mouth-breathe. Unilateral or incomplete obstruction may go unnoticed for years.

Examination

In an adult, a membrane can occasionally be seen on posterior rhinoscopy. In children, this examination is difficult. A lateral X-ray of skull can show a bony atresia. A membranous atresia can be demonstrated by carefully instilling a radio-opaque dye into the nostril and then taking a lateral X-ray.

Management

This is surgical. The approach to the back of the nose is transpalatal. The obstruction is removed, the choana widened and a tube inserted for 2–3 months.

FOREIGN BODIES

Foreign bodies may be found in the noses of children and mentally impaired adults. They are usually beads, sponge rubber or pieces of paper.

Clinical features

History

The child will sometimes volunteer that he has pushed something up his nose and cannot retrieve it. The foreign body more often makes its presence known by a foul smelling purulent discharge with nasal obstruction. If it remains in the nose for a long time, the discharge will cease and the foreign body and its surrounding debris will calcify to form a stone – a rhinolith.

Examination

This should be carried out gently. There is more chance of identifying the object if the patient can blow the pus out of his nose.

Management

Foreign bodies near the vestibule can be pulled out by the attending doctor. Those further back require skilled attention and perhaps a general anaesthetic.

DEVIATED NASAL SEPTUM

Very few nasal septa are straight. Deviation is most commonly due to uneven growth and trauma. The latter is frequently associated with fracture of the nasal bones.

Clinical features

History

The patient usually complains of the unilateral symptoms of nasal obstruction and stasis and a thick mucoid discharge. In a proportion of cases there are bilateral symptoms where an S-shaped deviation impinges on the airway of both nostrils. A proportion of patients present because of secondary problems such as granular pharyngitis, chronic sinusitis or chronic suppurative ear disease.

Examination

Examination of the nose with a nasal speculum will quickly show the deviation of the septum.

In patients with bilateral symptoms, it is important to ensure that there are no other signs, such as enlarged turbinates, which could contribute to the problem.

Management

Treatment is surgical. The relevant operation is either a submucosal resection or a septoplasty.

SECTION V

Principles of general management and treatment of the nose

PRINCIPLES OF DRUG TREATMENT

Decongestants

There are two ways of administering decongestants, either topically as drops or sprays, or systemically as tablets.

Topical

Drops and sprays are effective and have few side-effects. The nasal lining can, however, become sensitive to them. This leads to a condition called 'rhinitis medicamentosa', where the mucosa is in a state of constant reactive hyperaemia. To avoid this, decongestants should not be given topically for a period of more than 1 month. If they are then found to be ineffective, the condition being treated is probably irreversible. Useful local decongestants are xylometazoline and oxymetazoline.

Ephedrine drops are seldom used nowadays, because of the rebound effect of vasodilatation after the initial vasoconstriction.

Systemic

Systemic decongestants can be used on a long term basis, but should be avoided in patients with hypertension. They are also contraindicated in those taking monoamineoxidase inhibitors. Useful systemic decongestants are pseudoephedrine, phenylephrine and phenylpropanolamine.

Antihistamines

Antihistamines have a specific effect on allergic rhinitis and are given orally. They also have anti-cholinergic side-effects and are therefore decongestant. There is a variable personal response to antihistamines and if the results of the first preparation tried are disappointing, trying another is well worth while. The side-effects of reduction of intellectual function, lengthening of reaction time, and enhancement of the effects of alcohol are well known. Suitable antihistamines are triprolidine, clemastine and chlorpheniramine.

Antibiotics

In upper respiratory tract infections the bacterial organisms responsible occur in the following frequency:

- streptococcus
- staphylococcus
- *Haemophilus influenzae*
- pneumococcus

Penicillin or one of its analogues, to which all streptococci are sensitive, remain the antibiotics of choice. For organisms which are resistant to penicillin, co-trimoxazole (Septrin) is a suitable alternative.

In situations where neither of these antibiotics is suitable, flucloxacillin is effective for Gram-positive organisms.

PRINCIPLES OF NOSE AND SINUS SURGERY

The nose is an efficient organ, with two principal functions relating to the inspired air:

- heating
- humidifying and filtering

It is lined by a sensitive mucosa of ciliated columnar epithelium. This is normally covered with a thin layer of mucus which is slowly moved posteriorly by ciliary movements. In all surgery of the nose and sinuses, the mucosa should be treated with respect and the supporting structure of the tip, principally the nasal septum, must be maintained. It is important that steps are taken to avoid the build-up of adhesions between the septum and lateral walls, and that perforations are not made in the septum.

Cauterization of a nose

The nose should be anaesthetized with less than 2 ml of 10% cocaine on a pledget of cotton wool. This should be held in the nose for 10 minutes.

A small bead is then made by fusing a chromic acid crystal onto a wire probe. The bleeding point is touched with this bead, and excess acid is removed with a dry swab. Trichloracetic acid may also be used, as may silver nitrate sticks.

The patient should instil petroleum jelly into the nose daily for a week thereafter to prevent crusting. This lessens the tendency to pick the nose.

Packing the nose

The nose should be anaesthetized with less than 2 ml of 10% cocaine on a pledget of cotton wool as described before.

As the bleeding point is usually posterior, the pack must extend as far as the posterior choana. Therefore about 1.5 m (5 ft) of 25 mm (1 inch) ribbon gauze should be used for one adult nostril. The pack should be impregnated with an antiseptic or antibiotic to prevent infection, for the natural defence mechanisms of the nose are compromised. It should also contain a lubricant to aid removal. Terracortril and liquid paraffin form a useful mixture for this purpose.

The nose is then packed with double layers of gauze, building up from the floor. The loose ends are inserted last of all into the vestibule of the nose (LD-36).

Nasal packs remain in position for 48 hours. Patients who have lost a lot of blood require admission to hospital. Blood transfusion may be necessary.

As an alternative, proprietary pneumatic nasal epistaxis bags are available – Simpson's epistaxis bag and the Brighton bag. These can be inserted and blown up with air or water. They are easier to handle by the inexperienced but offer no great advantage.

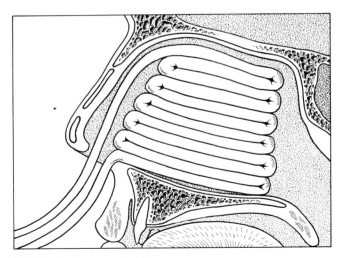

LD-36. *Technique of packing a nose*

Antral washout

The inferior meatus of the nose is anaesthetized with pledgets of cotton wool containing 10% cocaine for 15 minutes. Alternatively, a general anaesthetic is administered. A trochar and cannula are inserted through the thin part of the lateral wall of the nose under the inferior turbinate and about its midpoint. The trochar is removed and the cannula is washed out with sterile saline. This clears the ostium, and removes infected debris (LD-37).

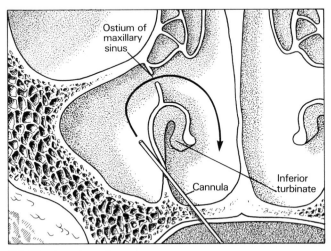

Ostium of maxillary sinus

Cannula

Inferior turbinate

LD-37. *Antral washout*

Antral lavage can be repeated at weekly intervals as an outpatient procedure until the return washout is clear. If pus is still obtained after four visits, further surgery – radical antrostomy – will be required. In the case of an inpatient, if pus is obtained, a small polythene catheter is left in place and can be washed out several times a day by the ward nurse.

Submucosal diathermy

This is done to reduce the bulk of enlarged inferior turbinates which form in response to vasomotor rhinitis or chronic rhinitis.

A Simpson's diathermy 'gun' is passed within the substance of the turbinate to its posterior end. The current is switched on and the diathermy point is slowly drawn forwards, causing a linear loss of vascular space within the turbinate. This should be carried out three times on each inferior turbinate.

As an alternative procedure, the inferior turbinate can be cut off completely – turbinectomy.

Nasal polypectomy

The nasal polypi are gently removed from the nose, using either a snare or blunt forceps. An effort is made to remove some of the lining of the ethmoidal sinuses at the same time. If haemorrhage does not cease quickly, on completion of the operation, an anterior nasal pack should be inserted.

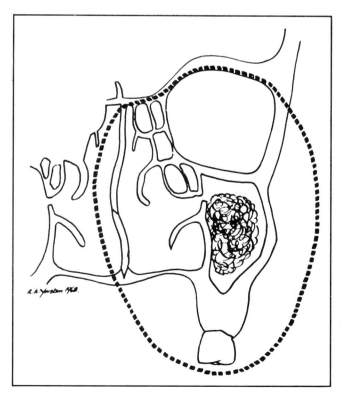

LD-38. *Maxillectomy*

Maxillectomy

The operation for carcinoma of the maxillary antrum is maxillectomy. It is usually carried out 6 weeks after a full course of radiotherapy. It can be partial – leaving the orbital floor, eye, and ethmoids – or radical. The eye and ethmoid sinuses are removed *en bloc* in total maxillectomy.

An incision is made just below the lower lid, down the side of the nose and through the lip. This allows the soft tissue of the face to be retracted laterally. The bony maxilla is removed using chisels and saws. If there is evidence of involvement of the orbit the eye is removed with the ethmoidal sinus cells. The cavity is skin-grafted and the skin flap replaced (LD-38–40).

An upper denture is made which has an obturator attached to its superior surface to close off the cavity (CP-16–19).

Submucosal resection of the nasal septum

This procedure is carried out under general anaesthesia. After incising just beyond the mucocutaneous junction, the subperichondrial layer is entered and lifted off the cartilage and bone on both sides of the septum. The area of deviated cartilage or bone is then removed and the flaps opposed. If the cartilage is repositioned instead of excised, the operation is known as a 'septoplasty'.

LD-39. *Maxillectomy. Tumour filling most of antrum. Removal of palate and orbit*

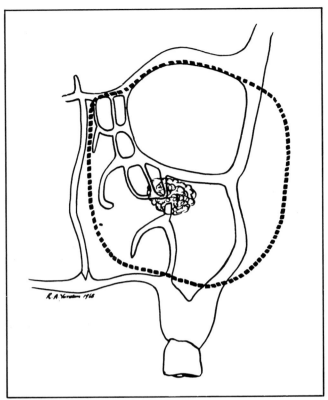

LD-40. *Maxillectomy. Tumour near roof of antrum (± ethmoid). Preservation of palate*

Radical antrostomy

This procedure is carried out under general anaesthesia.

Preoperative packing of the nose with 10% cocaine reduces blood loss.

The anterior wall of the maxillary sinus is opened through the canine fossa. All the diseased mucosa is removed and an intranasal antrostomy for drainage is made from the floor of the sinus into the inferior meatus of the nose at its anterior part.

External ethmoidectomy

This is done for complete removal of nasal polypi if they recur promptly after nasal polypectomy.

The procedure is always carried out unilaterally. A general anaesthetic, preferably with controlled hypotension, is required.

An incision is made in front of the medial canthus of the eye. The ethmoid is entered anteriorly just behind the lachrymal bone, and all the ethmoidal cells are exenterated under direct vision. The sphenoid sinus is entered and polypi removed from the fronto-nasal duct. A radical antrostomy is often combined with this procedure.

TEST-YOURSELF QUESTIONS
Part 2 – The Nose

1. Which of the following bones are involved in the skeleton of the nasal septum?
a) Frontal
b) Nasal
c) Ethmoid
d) Sphenoid
e) Vomer

2. In which of the following diseases is purulent catarrh a feature?
a) Vasomotor rhinitis
b) Influenza
c) Acute sinusitis
d) Allergic rhinitis
e) Choanal atresia

3. Which of the following can cause expansion of the bony walls of a sinus on X-ray?
a) Infection
b) Mucocoele
c) Malignant tumour
d) Benign tumour
e) Allergic rhinitis

4. What is the typical appearance of the nasal mucosa in a patient suffering from hay fever?
a) Red and swollen
b) Red with purulent crusts
c) Pale and swollen
d) Red turbinates and a pink septum

5. Which of the following describes the pathology of a nasal polypus?
a) Malignant tumour
b) Benign tumour
c) Granulation tissue
d) Fatty degeneration
e) Oedematous sinus mucosa

6. Which of the following most readily describes the pain of acute sinusitis?
a) Aching
b) Throbbing
c) Burning
d) Sharp and lancinating

7. What percentage of epistaxis comes from Little's area?
a) 20%
b) 40%
c) 60%
d) 80%
e) 100%

8. What is the safe maximal dosage of cocaine in an adult?
a) 200 mg
b) 2 g of 50% paste
c) 2 ml of a 10% solution
d) 2 ml of a 20% solution
e) 20 mg

9. What is the action of the parasympathetic nervous system on the nasal mucosa?
a) Dilates blood vessels and reduces secretion
b) Dilates blood vessels and increases secretion
c) Constricts blood vessels and reduces secretion
d) Constricts blood vessels and increases secretion

10. Which of the following types of epithelium lines the walls of a healthy maxillary sinus?
a) Cuboidal epithelium
b) Transitional epithelium
c) Ciliated columnar epithelium
d) Squamous epithelium

The answers to these questions will be found on p. 191.

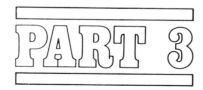

THE PHARYNX

SECTION I

Background to disease of the pharynx

ANATOMY

The pharynx develops from the endodermal lining of the foregut. It is a fibromuscular tube that extends from the base of the skull to the lower border of the cricoid cartilage, where it is then continuous with the oesophagus. At this cricopharyngeal sphincter it is 2.5 cm (1 inch) wide – the narrowest and least dilatable part of the alimentary tract. A foreign body that passes through the cricopharyngeal sphincter is not likely to be arrested further on.

Histology

The pharyngeal wall has four layers.

Areolar layer

This is found on the external surface. It contains the pharyngeal plexus of veins and nerves.

Muscular layer

There are two parts:

- the outer circular layer
  This comprises the superior middle and inferior constrictor muscles.

- the inner longitudinal layer
  This comprises the stylopharyngeous and palatopharyngeous.

Fibrous layer

This is called the pharyngobasilar fascia. It anchors the pharynx superiorly to the medial pterygoid plate, the basi-occiput and the petrous bone.

Mucous membrane

There are two forms:

- pseudostratified columnar ciliated epithelium
  Respiratory epithelium lines the nasopharynx only, as air and not food passes through it.

- stratified non-keratinizing squamous epithelium
  This is adapted for passage of food and saliva.

Functional parts

Opening into the pharynx anteriorly are orifices leading from the nose, mouth and larynx. This functionally divides the pharynx into three parts (LD-41).

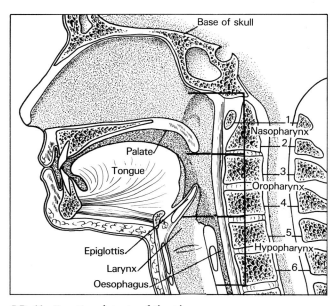

LD-41. Functional parts of the pharynx

Nasopharynx

This lies about the soft palate and posterior to the nasal cavities.

Oropharynx

This lies below the soft palate and behind the mouth and posterior one third of the tongue. It extends downwards to the level of the hyoid bone.

Hypopharynx

This begins where the oropharynx ends at the hyoid bone and terminates at the level of the cricoid cartilage.

Lymphatic drainage

Upper part of pharynx

This drains to the retropharyngeal lymph nodes.

Lower part of pharynx

This drains to the deep cervical lymph nodes.

Nerve supply

This is derived from the pharyngeal plexus. The superior laryngeal nerve supplies part of the hypopharynx.

The pharyngeal branch from the sphenopalatine ganglion supplies the roof of the pharynx.

PHYSIOLOGY OF SWALLOWING

The act of swallowing is divided into two stages — voluntary and involuntary.

Voluntary

The breath is drawn and held. The jaws are closed by the masseter temporal and pterygoid muscles and the food is masticated and made into a bolus. The tongue is raised by the mylohyoids and the styloglossus; and at the same time the hyoid bone and the larynx are also raised.

The tongue is pressed against the roof of the mouth. The bolus of food is driven back into the pharynx and onto the posterior pharyngeal wall, and then descends through the hypopharynx to enter the oesophagus.

Involuntary

This stage is subdivided into two separate phases. The first is in the pharynx and the second is in the oesophagus.

Pharyngeal phase

This is initiated when the bolus contacts the posterior pharyngeal wall which is richly innervated by the glossopharyngeal nerve.

Palatoglossus and palatopharyngeus contract and elevate the soft palate. This prevents food returning to the mouth. The larynx rises with the elevation of the hyoid bone and the epiglottis protects the larynx by contraction of the aryepiglottic and thyroepiglottic muscles. The result is that the bolus glides over the pharyngeal surface of the epiglottis, the aryepiglottic folds and the posterior surface of the arytenoids to enter the oesophagus.

Oesophageal phase

This is entirely a reflex or involuntary phase. Peristaltic waves in the muscle coat propel the food along the oesophagus. Gravity plays very little part.

SECTION II

History and physical examination of the pharynx

HISTORY

Physiological function

Depending on which part of the pharynx is affected, there are four main symptoms:

- nasal obstruction
  This occurs in diseases of the nasopharynx.

- pain
  This mainly takes the form of a sore throat if the nasopharynx is affected, or referred pain to the ear in the case of the hypopharynx.

- deafness
  This occurs if a mass in the nasopharynx (LD-42) blocks the Eustachian tube.

- dysphagia
  This occurs in lesions of the hypopharynx.

Nasal obstruction

Is the obstruction unilateral or bilateral?

Is the obstruction variable?
  Adenoids shrink occasionally and allow an airway, but tumours get progressively worse.

Is there associated bleeding?
  Angiofibromas are the usual source of obstruction plus bleeding.

What is the associated nasal secretion?
  Tumours are not usually associated with discharge, but adenoids are associated with purulent discharge.

Pain

Where is the pain?

Is it referred to the ear?
  This is common in tumours of the hypopharynx.

Is it constant, or intermittent?

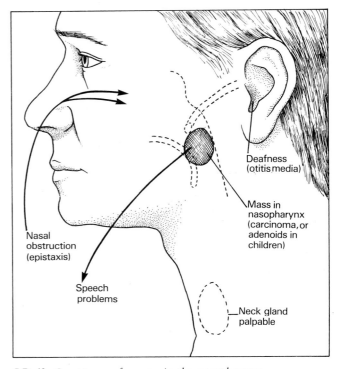

LD-42. *Symptoms of a mass in the nasopharynx*

Is it accompanied by fever?

Is it made worse by swallowing?

Is it progressive?

Deafness

Is it unilateral or bilateral?

When did it start?

Is it accompanied by discharge?
  This would be unusual in tumour obstruction.

Does the patient hear his voice better on the affected side?
  This is known as 'autophonia', and is typical of conductive deafness.

Dysphagia

Where is the obstruction?
    In tonsillitis, the problem is getting food out of the mouth. In hypopharyngeal tumours, the obstruction is felt lower down.

Is it a true dysphagia, or a feeling of a lump in the throat?
    If food sticks then it has a sinister and significant meaning.

Is there weight loss?
    True dysphagia is always accompanied eventually by weight loss.

Is there associated hoarseness?
    Tumours of the hypopharynx often spread to the larynx.

Is there any regurgitation of food?
    This would be typical of a pharyngeal pouch, but also occurs with a severe oesophageal block.

EXAMINATION

Start with a general assessment of the whole patient.
- Does he look anaemic?
- Is there any sign of weight loss?
- Is he in pain?

Once this has been completed a more specific examination can be undertaken.

Inspection

Direct

Oropharyngeal

With a good light source the mouth and oropharynx can easily be seen.
    If the tongue is projected the tip of the epiglottis can often be seen.

A warmed metal spatula is the kindest instrument to aid inspection, but in children a clean finger is less frightening and just as effective.

Nasopharynx

Direct inspection is performed either by drawing aside the soft palate or by the use of a warmed mirror.

Under general anaesthetic, a simple rubber catheter passed through the nose and out through the mouth serves the purpose. A special speculum, called a 'Yankauer's speculum', may be used. This method is particularly useful in eliminating the possibility of neoplasm and for permitting biopsy if necessary.

Hypopharynx

Direct inspection using a simple laryngoscope is easy and allows a biopsy to be taken.

Mirror examination

Specially designed mirrors are used to inspect the nasopharynx and hypopharynx. These should be warmed to prevent steaming. Gagging is not a problem if the patient is approached with consideration. If gagging persists, then spraying the soft palate and pharyngeal wall with cocaine or other local anaesthetic spray is helpful.

Endoscopy

The nasopharyngoscope – a straight instrument – and the fibreoptic laryngoscope – a flexible instrument – can both be passed through the nose under local anaesthesia and give a good view of the nasopharynx and laryngopharynx.

Palpation

This is often forgotten and it can be vital.

Neck

Any patient with pharyngeal disease must have a careful examination of the neck carried out.

Oropharynx

The area of the tonsil fossa and the base of the tongue should always be palpated.
    Tumours in this area are notoriously late in presenting and may only be picked up by careful palpation.

Nasopharynx

Palpation in this area is sometimes feasible but is not advised, as it is extremely unpleasant.

Hypopharynx

Palpation is important, both of the neck and of the hypopharynx under general anaesthetic.

Examination under anaesthesia

This has the obvious advantage of permitting easy access but, nevertheless, should only be carried out after all other routine methods of examination have been performed.

The techniques are known as pharyngoscopy and oesophagoscopy (see Section V, p. 86).

INVESTIGATIONS

Bacteriology

Tonsil swabs

In acute tonsillitis, the haemolytic streptococcus, *Staphylococcus pyogenes* and the pneumococcus are the commonest pathogens.

In young children, *Haemophilus influenzae* organisms are often responsible for infections.

Viral tonsillitis

It is increasingly accepted that viral disorders are associated with many sore throats.

Differential diagnosis

'Sloughing' white areas on tonsils may occur in thrush, infectious mononucleosis, Vincent's angina and diphtheria, as well as in membranous tonsillitis.

Bacteriological studies will usually help in making the diagnosis.

Other blood tests

Full blood count

Anaemia, leukaemia, agranulocytosis or a bleeding diathesis may present with pharyngeal lesions.

Serology

Syphilis and venereal diseases are growing in frequency and should not be forgotten.

Gammaglobulins

Hypogammaglobulinaemia is being increasingly considered to be important in patients with recurrent upper respiratory tract infections.

Biopsy

In the nasopharynx, tumours may be very small and may only be suspected following the excision biopsy of a neck gland in which secondary neoplasm is found.

In the oropharynx, asymmetrical tonsil size must always be looked upon with suspicion.

In the hypopharynx, any abnormal lesion must be biopsied, as the likeliest diagnosis will be carcinoma.

Radiology

Nasopharynx

A lateral view of the nasopharynx will demonstrate the size of an adenoid pad in children (X-20).

Tumours can erode the base of the skull, so special basal views are required (X-21).

Oropharynx

Radiology is rarely helpful but may outline soft tissue shadows at the base of the tongue.

If a lingual thyroid is suspected, a thyroid scan should be done.

Hypopharynx

Radiology is the main investigative tool in hypopharyngeal disease. Plain films may show soft tissue shadows especially on the posterior pharyngeal wall, but the key investigation is the barium swallow. This outlines defects of the piriform fossa and cervical oesophagus.

SECTION III

The presentation of pharyngeal problems and the diagnostic possibilities

DYSPHAGIA

This symptom means 'difficulty in swallowing'. It is derived from Greek '*dys*', meaning 'bad' or 'difficult' and '*phagein*', meaning 'to eat'. Patients with dysphagia are encountered in all branches of medicine.

Swallowing is a vital function – complete dysphagia, when even saliva cannot be swallowed, is a totally disabling condition.

Many patients are referred to otolaryngologists because, with mirrors and endoscopic equipment, they are best equipped to examine the mouth, pharynx and the upper oesophagus.

Childhood dysphagia

The causes here include:
- congenital malformation
- trauma
- ingestion of caustics

Congenital malformations

These may result from:
- malformations of oesophagus
  A blind ending or simply a congenital stricture may be evident.
- tracheo-oesophageal fistula
  The presentation is acute with failure to thrive and development of chest complications.
- dysphagia lusoria
  This is a less acute presentation and is caused by an aberrant right subclavian artery compressing the oesophagus.

Diagnosis of these conditions is made on clinical grounds with the aid of contrast radiography.

Trauma

Foreign bodies may lodge in the pharynx or upper oesophagus. The tonsil, vallecula or piriform fossa are the commonest sites.

The narrowest part of the gastrointestinal tract is the cricopharyngeal sphincter at the upper end of the oesophagus and the larger foreign bodies lodge here.

Foreign bodies vary in nature from sharp objects like fishbones to larger objects such as coins and safety pins (X-22, X-23).

A British twopenny piece (25 mm diameter) will stick in most children whereas a penny piece (20 mm) will pass straight through.

If the foreign body is radio-opaque, then an X-ray will give the answer.

Remember always to take straight and lateral X-rays of the neck and also to X-ray the chest and abdomen as the foreign body may have passed on. Fishbones are rarely seen on X-rays.

Ingestion of caustics

These can present a frightening problem. Children are innately curious and accidents inevitably happen.

Hospital admission is imperative, as the effects may be delayed and skilled treatment is vital. Oedema and a chronic inflammatory reaction may lead to the late development of strictures.

The basis of management is nothing by mouth and careful observation. If there is doubt, cautious oesophagoscopy may be carried out to establish the presence of or the degree of damage sustained. Steroids may be used as they have a part to play in reducing inflammatory oedema.

Adult dysphagia

This is a more difficult problem and requires much clinical judgement.

Clinical approach

Consider:

- Sex

  Middle-aged menopausal ladies may have a hiatus hernia or they may have 'globus hystericus', a condition in which they focus their problems – usually emotional ones – onto their throats.

- Age

- Appearance

  Does the patient look ill?

- Is there any evidence of recent weight loss?

- Is the patient in pain?

- Is there any evidence of any other disease?

  Many neurological conditions present with dysphagia.

History

Can the patient localize the site of the problem?

If there is an acute inflammatory condition of the mouth or oropharynx, this can be easily seen.

If there is an hiatus hernia with stricture, an achalasia of the oesophagus or a malignancy at the lower end of the oesophagus, the patient will usually indicate the site by pointing over the area of the xiphisternum.

If the problem is above the cricopharyngeal sphincter – for example, a foreign body in the piriform fossa, or a neoplasm of the posterior pharyngeal wall – then the patient will localize the site by pressing over one or other side of the thyroid cartilage.

If there is a postcricoid carcinoma, an oesophageal web or a foreign body at the cricopharyngeal level, then the patient will indicate the site by pointing in the midline over the upper trachea.

Clinical classification

By this time the physician will be able in his own mind to fit the problem into broad clinical groups:

- painful inflammatory conditions of the mouth, pharynx or larynx
- a neurological disturbance
- an intrinsic lesion of the oesophagus – benign or malignant
- extrinsic compression of the oesophagus

It is important to note that dysphagia due to a neurological disturbance will usually be as bad for liquids as solids, and that coughing or choking on swallowing is often a problem.

Neurological disturbances are usually associated with signs of involvement of other cranial nerves. Brainstem thrombosis, syringobulbia, motor neuron disease or bulbar poliomyelitis are other possibilities.

The superior laryngeal branch of the vagus supplies sensation above the vocal cords and is therefore often involved in these neurological disorders.

Loss of sensation in the larynx may lead to serious inhalation problems which may be a terminal event in the elderly.

An intrinsic lesion of the oesophagus is usually associated with signs of weight loss.

Extrinsic compression on the oesophagus can follow osteophyte formation in cervical spondylosis, aortic aneurysms, malignant bronchial glands or mediastinal tumours.

Examination

Direct inspection

Any cause of a 'sore throat' will cause dysphagia.

Indirect inspection

With the aid of the laryngeal mirror, a large beefy swollen epiglottis may be seen. This is epiglottitis. It is due to *Haemophilus influenzae*.

Burns, scalds, foreign bodies, trauma, inflammatory conditions and neoplasms of the larynx can all cause oedema and hence dysphagia. Signs of these will be seen on indirect laryngoscopy.

Radiology

Both a plain film of the neck and a barium swallow are necessary in all cases of dysphagia, but a negative examination does not exclude significant pathology.

Examination under anaesthesia

A barium examination should always precede any attempt at oesophagoscopy but, to make a definite diagnosis, oesophagoscopy is usually necessary.

SORE THROATS IN CHILDREN

The commonest cause is tonsillitis. This is often recurrent, lasts 3–5 days and is associated with pyrexia.

Clinical approach

History

A complete history is vital. Parents wishing surgery

for their child may be biased in their account. The time off school is a good yardstick. The number of courses of antibiotics prescribed in 1 year is also helpful.

Remember the possible association with otitis media and sinusitis. The young child is often listless, irritable and off his food.

The course of the condition is important. If there is no improvement with one course of antibiotics then think of a leukaemia, other blood dyscrasias, infectious mononucleosis, thrush or, more rarely, brucellosis.

Examination

The following points should be covered:

- Assess how ill the child is and take the temperature
- Look for a rash or other evidence of exanthemata
- Look for bruising, bleeding or arthropathy
- Feel the neck. Large jugulo-digastric glands are common
- Test for trismus. This is often seen with a quinsy
- Examine nose and ears for adenoid enlargement
- Examine the mouth and pharynx

The size of tonsils is relatively unimportant, except in the young infant where excessive size can lead to a form of cor pulmonale. However, tonsils will be enlarged in exudative tonsillitis, infectious mononucleosis or lymphomas.

Pus in the tonsils is seen in follicular tonsillitis. In leukaemia this is usually associated with necrosis and ulceration.

A white membrane occurs in thrush infection and in diphtheria.

Laboratory investigations

Order a full blood count including differential white count and a monospot or brucella titre if the diagnosis is in doubt. Antistrepsolysin O titres and rheumatoid tests should be requested if there is an associated arthropathy.

The throat swab is of doubtful value – except in thrush – as probably 50% of sore throats are viral in origin.

The significance of IgG and IgA levels is still to be evaluated. Viral studies are too slow to be of value.

SORE THROATS IN ADULTS

Clinical approach

History

The commonest cause is pharyngitis due to postnasal drip or smoking. Chronic tonsillitis is commoner in adults than children, hence an adult is not usually as ill as a child. Always ask about smoking, nasal obstruction and nasal discharge. The frequency, absence or presence of pyrexia is important.

Ignoring a low grade chronic complaint can result in a missed diagnosis of cancer of the oropharynx or hypopharynx. Acute pain may indicate a peritonsillar abscess.

Examination

It is important to:

- palpate neck glands
  These may be enlarged in tonsillitis, infectious mononucleosis, brucellosis, toxoplasmosis, cancer or lymphomas.
- examine the nose
  Exclude allergy, polyps, septal deviations and vasomotor rhinitis. Pus in the nasopharynx is associated with chronic sinusitis and may cause pharyngitis.
- examine the pharynx
  In pharyngitis this will be red and granular with enlarged thickened lateral bands of pharyngeal lymphoid tissue.
- remember that different sizes of tonsils may be due to quinsy or cancer
  The tonsil is pushed medially in quinsy.

It is often difficult to distinguish clinically between tonsillitis, leukaemia, aplastic anaemia, infectious mononucleosis or lymphoma. Examine the hypopharynx. Carcinomas which cause local pain, referred ear pain and enlarged neck glands should be excluded.

Laboratory investigations

A full blood count with differential white count is useful.

If suspicious, order a monospot, brucella titre or toxoplasma titre. X-rays of sinuses and a lateral film of the neck should also be performed.

SECTION IV

Description of specific diseases of the pharynx

ADENOIDITIS

The adenoids are occasionally called the pharyngeal tonsils. They grow rapidly from birth to reach maximum size at age 4–5 years, then regress until shortly after puberty, by which time they are insignificant in size.

Clinical features

These include:

- rhinitis
- a burning sensation at the back of the nose
- nasal obstruction and discharge
- an elevated temperature on occasion
- deafness due to secretory or infective otitis media

Adenoids are frequently involved with virus infections. These include the common cold, mumps and measles. Adenoiditis often occurs with tonsillitis.

Complications

These include:

- cross-infection by droplet spread
- acute infective otitis media
- chronic otitis media
- sinusitis
- bronchitis
- retropharyngeal abscess

Management

Appropriate symptomatic treatment includes bed rest and analgesics, together with antibiotics if relevant. Adenoidectomy should be performed if complications occur or if adenoiditis is recurrent.

TONSILLITIS

This may be acute or chronic.

Acute tonsillitis

Older textbooks distinguished between acute follicular and acute catarrhal tonsillitis. This is an artificial division merely depending on the severity of the condition (CP-20).

Clinical features

These include:

- general malaise
- pyrexia
- fetor and nasal discharge
- pain

If pain is severe and associated with dysphagia it may be referred to the ears.

The tonsils often have white septic spots on their surface and the jugulo-digastric and cervical lymph glands will almost always be enlarged or tender.

Management

Bed rest, adequate fluids by mouth and insisting that a full course of medical treatment be completed are important points in management. Relapses will occur if treatment is incomplete.

Medical management

Analgesics and antibiotics must be given in adequate doses for the age of the patient.

Penicillin for 1 week remains the antibiotic of choice. Fifty per cent of infections are probably viral but it is impossible to tell which. In practice, all are best treated with penicillin.

If thrush is present, nystatin lozenges are useful. If there is a suspicion of infectious mononucleosis, do not use ampicillin as rashes commonly occur.

Surgical management

Adenotonsillectomy in children and tonsillectomy in adults are the common operations. In 1968, 28% of all hospital admissions in the age group of 5–9 years were for adenotonsillectomy (Section V, p. 86).

The indications for surgery are still controversial, but acceptable ones are:

- three or more genuine attacks of tonsillitis in 1 year
- enlarged tonsils or adenoids causing otitis media, secretory otitis media or hyponasality
- a previous attack of quinsy or peritonsillar abscess
- the very few children with cor pulmonale secondary to gross tonsillar hypertrophy

There are no definite rules and only observation and experience associated with common sense and clinical judgement will result in the correct decision becoming apparent.

Contraindications to surgery include:

- a pre-existing pharyngeal infection
- anaemia
- bleeding disorders

PERITONSILLAR ABSCESS OR QUINSY

The original source of infection here is one of the tonsillary crypts. Secondary abscess formation follows between the tonsil capsule and the superior constrictor muscle of the pharynx. It is therefore a peritonsillar, rather than intratonsillar, infection.

Clinical features

This condition is always acute. Generalized toxaemia, pyrexia, pain, dysphagia and, usually, trismus occur.

The affected tonsil is enlarged and pushed medially. The uvula is pushed away from the affected side. The tonsils may be difficult to examine because of trismus, oedema and congestion of the soft palate.

Management

This is usually in hospital. Initially fluids, analgesics and penicillin are given. If this regime fails, then incision and drainage of the abscess under local anaesthesia is performed.

Peritonsillar abscess is an absolute indication for tonsillectomy 6 weeks after recovery, as recurrence is almost inevitable.

PHARYNGITIS

This inflammatory condition occurs to a certain degree in all upper respiratory conditions. It may be acute or chronic.

Acute pharyngitis

It is classically described as being caused by the haemolytic streptococcus – but staphylococci, pneumococci and, perhaps increasingly in children, *Haemophilus influenzae* organisms are also involved. Viruses are other common agents.

Clinical features

This disorder starts with a burning sensation in the throat and back of the nose. There may be a high fever, severe pain and dysphagia.

To reach the diagnosis an adequate history and clinical examination are essential. Culture of a throat swab helps.

Management

This should be vigorous, with fluid replacement, analgesics and broad spectrum antibiotics.

Chronic pharyngitis

This is a common and less clearly defined condition. It

causes a considerable morbidity in the community and is difficult to treat.

Causes

These are usually based outwith the pharynx and include:

- nasal infections – sinusitis or obstructive rhinitis
- oral infections – chronic tonsillitis or dental sepsis
- nasal obstruction
  Polyps, a deviated nasal septum and allergic or vasomotor rhinitis cause chronic mouth breathing, and hence the inhalation of poorly humidified and potentially infected air.
- local irritants
  Alcohol and cigarette smoking are factors. Industrial fumes are a further potential hazard.
- general conditions
  Liver cirrhosis, diabetes mellitus and uraemia are all associated with degrees of pharyngitis.
- emotional and psychological problems

Management

This is directed at the cause. Indiscriminate use of antibiotics is to be avoided. Simple gargles may sooth but rarely cure.

PHARYNGEAL POUCH

This is a posteriorly placed pulsion diverticulum usually presenting on the left side of the oesophagus.

It occurs between thyropharyngeal (upper oblique) and cricopharyngeal (lower horizontal) fibres of inferior constrictor muscle. It is composed of mucous and fibrous tissue only – rarely muscle fibres.

Neoplastic change has been reported but is rare.

Cause

It is thought to be due to neuromuscular incoordination. The male:female ratio is 4:1.

Clinical features

The size is variable but it may present as a swelling in

the neck which can be reduced manually after meals. Usually there is dysphagia and regurgitation of partially digested foul-smelling food.

Sometimes overspill into the larynx occurs with coughing. There are, however, very rarely aspiration problems.

Radiology

Barium swallow radiography demonstrating the classical retort-shaped swelling with a demonstrable septum between oesphagus and pouch is the investigation of choice (X-24).

Management

This includes:

- surgical excision – the commonest method
- endoscopic obliteration

The principle of endoscopic obliteration is to obliterate the oesophageal wall between pouch and oesophagus by diathermy. It is indicated in the elderly and infirm (Section V, p. 86).

FOREIGN BODIES

These lodge commonly in pharynx and hypopharynx. The commonest sites are:

- the tonsil
- the base of tongue
- the valleculae on either side of the epiglottis
- the piriform fossae
- the postcricoid region of the hypopharynx

Clinical features

History

There is usually a definite history of ingestion. Sharp objects lodge in the higher sites. Pain is localized to the affected side in all areas, except the postcricoid area where it will be felt in the midline.

The diagnosis depends on a good history, careful examination with a good light, the correct use of mirrors, and an anaesthetic throat spray if necessary.

In an anteroposterior and lateral X-ray of the neck, small fishbones will not be seen but an X-ray should always be taken (X-22).

Management

This is by removal, either under direct vision with or without an anaesthetic throat spray or under general anaesthesia with an endoscope.

If the foreign body is missed or ignored, local abscesses may form.

PLUMMER–VINSON SYNDROME

This is also known as the Paterson–Brown–Kelly syndrome. It occurs in association with angular stomatitis, glossitis, dysphagia, loss of tongue papillae and koilonychia (CP-21).

Clinical features

Classically, middle-aged women are affected. It is often associated with a microcytic anaemia and a lowered serum iron level. There may be an association with achlorhydria. The barium swallow may be normal or reveal hypopharyngitis, oesophagitis or postcricoid web formation (X-25). Oesophagoscopy and postcricoid biopsy is mandatory.

There is a definite association between this condition and postcricoid carcinoma.

Management

Dilation to relieve dysphagia and correction of the anaemia are important. Careful follow-up is mandatory because of the high incidence of carcinoma.

GLOBUS SYNDROME

Patients who complain of a feeling of a lump in the throat around the level of the cricoid cartilage were often diagnosed as having globus hystericus if, on examination, nothing was found. It is now realized that there are many causes for this other than a psychosomatic one, although this remains the commonest cause.

The other causes include:
- hiatus hernia with reflux
- cervical osteophytes
- the Plummer–Vinson syndrome
- enlarged thyroid gland
- pharyngeal pouch
- postcricoid carcinoma

The diagnosis is based on the history, examination, blood film and barium swallow and meal.

If the lower part of the oesophagus is irritated because of reflux then the cricopharyngeus goes into spasm.

CANCER OF THE NASOPHARYNX

This is the commonest cancer after the age of 40 and occurs more often in males. There is a striking racial distribution. In China and Hong Kong it accounts for 13% of all deaths from carcinoma, whereas in most other countries it is only responsible for 0.5% of deaths. The reason for this is so far unknown.

There is a 30% positive titre to the Epstein–Barr virus in early cases and 100% positive titre in advanced cases.

The tumours are nearly always squamous cell carcinomas, but non-Hodgkin's lymphomas can occur.

Clinical features

Primary tumours are often silent until quite large. They may present, however, with:
- cervical signs
  Enlarged neck glands may be found (CP-22)
- nasal signs
  Obstruction or epistaxis may occur.
- otological signs
  Eustachian tube obstruction with or without secretory otitis media can result.
- neurological signs
  Invasion of the skull base may lead to the jugular foramen syndrome or fifth nerve paresis.

Nasopharyngeal lymph vessels drain to the lateral retropharyngeal lymph nodes which in turn drain to the upper deep cervical nodes. These become palpable and are often the only presenting features.

The diagnosis is based on suspicion supported by radiological investigations. Biopsy under general anaesthesia is always necessary. An unexplained cervical lymph node should direct the surgeon's attention to the nasopharynx.

Lymph node biopsy should not be performed before adequate examination of the nasopharynx has been undertaken.

Management

Radiotherapy is the method of choice, as surgery has nothing to offer owing to the difficult anatomical site. Neck dissection may be required (Section V, p. 86).

Results

Overall about 40% of patients have a 5-year survival.

Result with the lymphoma group are better than with the squamous cell carcinoma group.

CANCER OF THE OROPHARYNX

This includes carcinoma of the anterior pillars of the fauces, the tonsils, the lateral and posterior oropharyngeal walls and the base of the tongue (CP-23).

Squamous cell carcinoma is the commonest. Neoplasms of salivary gland tissue and all varieties of lymphomas are seen less commonly.

The male:female ratio is 5:1, and squamous cell carcinoma is rare before the age of 50. Tobacco chewing, smoking and heavy drinking of alcohol are definitely significant contributing factors.

Clinical features

Fifty per cent present with palpable deep cervical lymph nodes. These are often bilateral if the carcinoma is in the base of the tongue.

Exophytic growths are discovered either by chance or by the patient or dentist or else by interference with swallowing. Deeply ulcerating growths present with pain.

Examination

The lesion is usually seen directly or indirectly with a mirror. Biopsy is often possible without anaesthesia.

Palpation is vital to uncover lesions at the base of the tongue and to assess the overall size of the tumour.

Radiology

X-ray of the chest and mandible are necessary to exclude metastases or direct spread.

Management

Surgery or radiotherapy, or a combination of both, are used. Surgery will usually involve the removal of the affected tissue and the adjacent mandible and a radical neck dissection (Section V, p. 86).

Small tumours less than 1 cm do well with surgery and this is usually preferred as it is quicker and can be conservative. Larger tumours usually involve more mutilative surgery, so radiotherapy is advocated and surgery is reserved for the failures.

Results

The results vary considerably according to tumour size and site. Overall there is an approximate 25% 5-year survival.

CANCER OF THE HYPOPHARYNX

The incidence of postcricoid carcinoma (CP-24) is higher in Great Britain and Scandinavia than in any other part of the world. Almost all these tumours are malignant. The vast majority are squamous cell carcinomas. The hypopharynx extends from the hyoid bone down to the level of the lower border of the cricoid cartilage opposite C6.

It is divided for descriptive purposes into three parts (LD-43):

- the piriform fossa
- the posterior pharyngeal wall
- the postcricoid area

Tumours in these areas tend to behave differently but they often spread to adjacent parts or to the larynx.

Piriform fossa carcinoma is the most common (CP-25). Heavy smoking and drinking are definite aetiological factors.

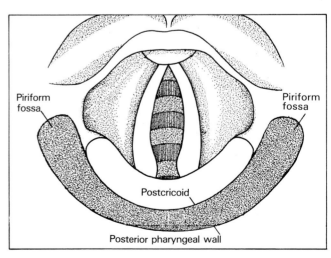

LD-43. *Parts of the hypopharynx*

Clinical features

These tumours present late. There are few symptoms until they are quite large. A total of 60–70% present with palpable deep cervical lymph nodes.

If the tumour is pedunculated or papilliferous, the presentation is usually dysphagia or a feeling of a lump in the throat. If the tumour is ulcerative, pain in the pharynx or in the ear on the affected side may result. This is referred via the glossopharyngeal nerve. Postcricoid carcinoma usually presents with dysphagia and weight loss.

Examination

These tumours are easily seen with a laryngeal mirror. Radiology is vital. Contrast studies – laryngogram or barium swallow – are of value, as well as plain films (X-26).

Direct laryngoscopy or oesophagoscopy under general anaesthetic is always necessary to assess the extent of the tumour.

Management

Surgery or radiotherapy or a combination of both is employed. Neck dissection is often also necessary.

The surgical approaches are numerous. They vary from simple excision through a lateral pharyngotomy approach, to total laryngopharyngo-oesophagectomy (Section V, p. 86).

Results

Radiotherapy alone cannot claim better than 10–15% 5-year survival rates.

The overall 5-year survival rates vary from centre to centre, but are rarely better than 25–30%.

Surgery is associated with a considerable morbidity due to problems associated with reconstruction of a suitable swallowing tube.

SECTION V

Principles of general management and treatment of the pharynx

PRINCIPLES OF PHARYNGEAL SURGERY

Oesophagoscopy

The oesophagus can be inspected under general anaesthesia using a straight rigid oesophagoscope or else under local anaesthesia using a fibreoptic gastroscope.

The latter technique has limitations, as manipulative measures cannot be undertaken, and therefore it is rarely utilized in oesophageal work.

Direct inspection was first reported in 1868 by Kusmarel, who used a rigid tube without anaesthetic. His subjects were professional sword swallowers.

Instruments

Two types of rigid oesophagoscopes are commonly in use:

- Jackson type – this has distal lighting
- Negus type – this has proximal lighting

They vary in size and length.

Indications

These oesophagoscopes are used primarily to identify and inspect oesophageal problems, and secondarily to biopsy a suspicious lesion, remove a foreign body or bouginage a stricture.

Warning

Oesophagoscopy should rarely, if ever, be performed for diagnostic purposes unless a barium swallow X-ray has been carried out and has been seen by the surgeon.

Contraindications

There are no absolute contraindications to oesophagoscopy but to be carefully considered are:

- aortic aneurysms
- severe kyphosis
- gross osteophytes
- a potentially damaged oesophagus that might follow ingestion of caustics

Warning

Oesophagoscopy should not be performed by the inexperienced without supervision. A potential danger of oesophageal perforation always exists and perforation can be fatal.

Technique

General anaesthesia with endotracheal intubation allows adequate relaxation, which is vital to allow easy passage of the oesophagoscope through the cricopharyngeal sphincter.

Complications

Teeth, lips and tongue may be damaged on passing the instrument. Care will avoid this.

Especially in children, the end of the instrument may compress the trachea and produce anoxia. Perforation of the oesophagus is the most dangerous complication. It can occur in the neck or the chest and it can be fatal. It can result in cervical emphysema or acute mediastinitis.

Removal of tonsils and adenoids

This is the most commonly performed pharyngeal

operation. The tonsils are removed by blunt dissection and within their capsule. Haemostasis is obtained by direct ligation of bleeding points. The adenoids do not have a capsule and hence have to be removed by curettage. Haemostasis can only be obtained by pressure.

Complications

Reactionary – or primary – haemorrhage

This occurs within 24 hours of surgery. Deaths are recorded every year in Great Britain as a result of this.

If a trained medical and nursing team can monitor pulse and blood pressure postoperatively, remove blood clot from the tonsil fossa, replace lost blood as required and quickly return the patient to theatre to control bleeding, if required, then these deaths can be avoided.

Secondary haemorrhage

This occurs between the seventh and tenth postoperative days. It is due to infection. It follows the inadequate use of pharyngeal muscles for eating, drinking and talking in the postoperative period. It is rarely serious.

Treatment is with bed rest, antibiotics, analgesics and transfusion if required.

Scarring of the palate

This is rare and usually follows the work of an inexperienced surgeon. It can produce speech problems due to excessive nasal escape.

Removal of pharyngeal pouch

The pouch is filled with gauze from above through an endoscope. This assists in identification. It is approached from the left side of the neck and removed. The resulting hole in the pharynx is closed in layers.

Cricopharyngeal myotomy – division of cricopharyngeal muscle fibres – is carried out to allow relaxation and to avoid recurrence.

The length of time on tube feeding is 6–10 days. The stay in hospital is 14 days. Salivary fistula or oesophageal stenosis can occur as complications.

The jaw/neck or 'commando' operation

This is performed for carcinoma of the dental alveolus, the floor of the mouth or tonsil. It involves removal of the tumour with adequate clearance, with or without part of the mandible. It is performed in combination with a radical neck dissection.

Temporary tracheostomy is required and tube feeding is necessary until the pharynx has healed (CP-26, CP-27).

Complications associated with salivary fistula may lead to a protracted hospital stay.

Pharyngolaryngectomy

This is the most extensive of head and neck surgical procedures. It is reserved for carcinomas of the hypopharynx that have recurred following radiotherapy.

The larynx – due to proximity – is removed *en bloc* with the pharynx and neck dissection is carried out (CP-24).

Problems relate to restoring a functioning swallowing tube. Reconstruction may be attempted with tubed deltopectoral skin flaps or transposition of the stomach or colon into the neck.

Long periods of stay in hospital are often needed. The chance of surviving 5 years is only 20–30%.

TEST-YOURSELF QUESTIONS
Part 3 – The Pharynx

1. Into which part of the pharynx does the orifice open from
a) the nose
b) the mouth
c) the larynx.

2. What questions should be asked of a patient who complains of nasal obstruction?

3. In a patient who complains of dysphagia, for each of the sites on the left localised by the patient, list the likely diagnosis on the right.

a) Over the xiphisternum
b) Over the thyroid cartilage
c) Over the upper trachea

1) Foreign body in the pyriform fossa
2) Hiatus hernia
3) Achalasia of the oesophagus
4) Neoplasm of the posterior pharyngeal wall
5) Postcricoid carcinoma

4. What are the indications for adenotonsillectomy?

5. List five causes of chronic pharyngitis.

6. Which of the following are features of the Plummer–Vinson syndrome?
a) Angular stomatisis
b) Glossitis
c) Dysphagia
d) Onycholysis
e) Koilonychia

7. Which of the following may be found in a cancer of the nasopharynx?
a) Positive titre to the Epstein–Barr virus
b) Epistaxis
c) Eustachian tube obstruction
d) Fifth nerve paresis
e) Enlarged neck glands

8. What anaesthesia is required for endoscopy?

The answers to these questions will be found on p. 191.

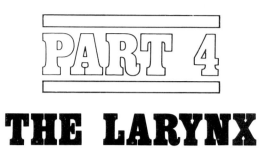

THE LARYNX

SECTION I

Background to disease of the larynx

BACKGROUND

The larynx is situated at the top of the trachea and below the root of the tongue and the hyoid bone. It is the essential sphincter guarding the entrance to the trachea and functions secondarily as the organ of voice. A summary of the relevant background information is found in this section.

ANATOMY

The skeleton

The skeleton of the larynx is made up of:

- the cricoid cartilage attached to the first tracheal ring
- the thyroid cartilage
- the arytenoid cartilage
- the epiglottis
- the hyoid bone attached to the base of the tongue

The inferior horns of the thyroid cartilage articulate with the cricoid cartilage and this allows one to move in relation to the other – a fact that is important in lengthening and shortening the vocal cords. The arytenoids sit on the cricoid arch posteriorly and it is to these and the thyroid prominence that the vocal cords are attached (LD-44). Cords are longer in males than in females and this is why this area (the Adam's apple) is more prominent in males.

The epiglottis

The epiglottis is attached just above the thyroid prominence and is a relic of the time in evolution when it was important to divide totally the respiratory and alimentary tracts so that an animal could both eat

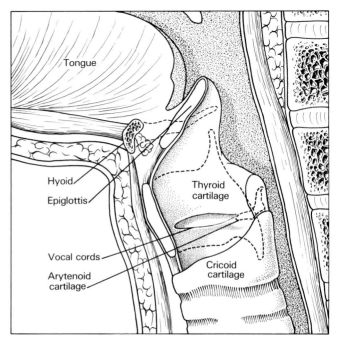

LD-44. *The laryngeal skeleton*

and breathe (smell) simultaneously. Its use in man is debatable and it can be removed in supraglottic laryngectomy with no disability.

The hyoid bone

The hyoid bone completes the skeleton, being attached to the thyroid cartilage by the thyrohyoid membrane and also to the base of the tongue. It is this latter attachment that causes the larynx and thyroid gland to move on swallowing.

The soft tissues

The vocal cords comprise the thyroarytenoid muscle,

which is covered by mucous membrane. It stretches from the arytenoid vocal process to the thyroid prominence at an area called the anterior commissure.

A mucosal fold – the aryepiglottic fold – runs from the side of the epiglottis to the arytenoid cartilage. The lower edge lies above the vocal cord and is named the 'false cord'. The space between the aryepiglottic fold and the medial surface of the thyroid cartilage is the piriform sinus, or lateral food channel. Down this, food passes from the base of the tongue before entering the oesophagus (LD-45).

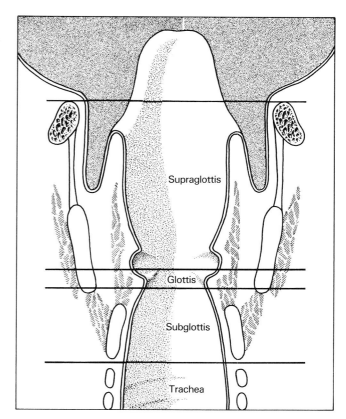

LD-46. *Coronal section of larynx showing the laryngeal compartments*

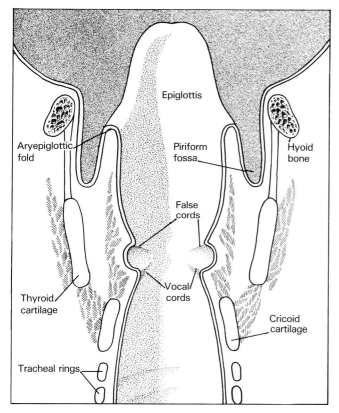

LD-45. *Coronal section of larynx showing the soft tissues*

The compartments (LD-46)

Glottis

The vocal cord area is called the glottis and is important since it has no lymph drainage. It forms a temporary barrier to the spread of supraglottic cancer.

Supraglottis

This compartment includes all the larynx between the hyoid bone and the vocal cords. It has a rich lymphatic drainage and, since it is largely functionless, tumours can grow to a large size before producing symptoms.

Subglottis

The third compartment is the subglottis. It extends from the undersurface of the vocal cords to the lower edge of the cricoid cartilage. The mucosa is lax in children and so laryngeal oedema is commoner in the young. It also has a rich lymphatic drainage.

Movement of vocal cords

The vocal cords are opened (abducted) by the lateral cricoarytenoid muscles and closed (adducted) by the posterior cricoarytenoid and interarytenoid muscles. The thyroarytenoid shortens the cords and the crico-thyroid, which is the only laryngeal muscle attached outwith the larynx, lengthens them. All these muscles are supplied by the recurrent laryngeal nerve, except the cricothyroid which is supplied by the superior laryngeal nerve (CP-28, LD-47).

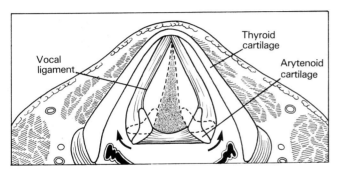

LD-47. *Cord movement. Adducted cords closed by lateral cricoarytenoid and interarytenoid muscles*

The physiology of voice

The larynx produces the sound we know as 'voice'. Speech is produced by changing the sound into words. The teeth, tongue, lips and palate all contribute to the process.

Bernouilli principle

To understand how sound is produced, it is first necessary to understand the Bernouilli principle.

This states that when a fluid or gas passes from a large area to another large area through a constriction, the pressure drops as the flow passes the constriction.

Voice production

To produce a sound, the recurrent laryngeal nerves set the cords together in the midline. The arytenoid bulk, however, normally leaves a tiny gap between the cords and so, when air passes from the lungs (a large area) to the pharynx (a large area), a pressure drop occurs between the cords. This results in the mucous membrane linings of the cords being sucked together in the midline, effectively closing the gap. The subglottic pressure then rises, blows the mucosa apart and allows air to flow. The mucosa is then sucked together again. This opening and closing of the mucosa occurs at speed and the effect on the air column passing through this vibrating area is to produce sound.

If air is blown out of the lungs more forcibly, the sound will be louder. If the cords are shortened, the frequency (pitch) of the sound will be higher. Since their cords are shorter, women and children have higher voices than men. Pop groups who sing falsetto have developed the trick of only vibrating the anterior third of the cords.

Professional singers train and produce a thicker vocal cord than normal, so increasing the vertical depth over which the cords meet. This improves the quality of the voice. Great singers are born rather than trained, because the most important factor is the relationship of the size of the larynx to the resonating chambers (the lungs and pharynx).

SECTION II

History and physical examination of the larynx

HISTORY

When a history is taken from a patient with a laryngeal problem, there is an opportunity of simultaneously examining his or her voice. There are only two vocal symptoms:

- aphonia
  Here there is no voice, a whisper or air wastage.
- dysphonia or hoarseness
  Here the voice is rough.

Specific questions

- How long has the patient had the problem? Find out how the problem started and how it has progressed.
  Vocal cord paralysis causes a sudden loss of voice which gradually improves as the 'good' cord comes across to meet the paralysed one. On the other hand, lesions on the cord such as cancers or polyps cause gradually increasing dysphonia.
- What makes the symptom better or worse?
  It is important to know this, especially in relation to voice usage both at work and at home. Basic voice problems such as voice strain get worse with voice use and get better with rest.
- Does the patient smoke?
- What are his work conditions?
- Is there atmospheric pollution at work?

Pain

Very few laryngeal conditions – apart from cancer,

perichondritis and arthritis – cause pain in the larynx, so this is a symptom to take seriously. It is often referred to the ear and is made worse by swallowing.

Dysphagia

Dysphagia can be due to swollen arytenoids blocking the inlet of the oesophagus or to incoordinate swallowing. This is an inability to close the cords and set up the positive subglottic pressure necessary for swallowing.

In cases of vocal cord paralysis, food goes down the wrong way, causing the patient to cough on eating.

EXAMINATION

Examine the neck to assess the shape, form and mobility of the laryngopharynx. Note any glands that may suggest the presence of an underlying laryngeal cancer. Feel for deviation of the trachea and palpate the thyroid gland.

Examine the ears and nasopharynx for any lesions that could cause paralysis of the vagus nerve such as carcinoma or a glomus jugulare tumour.

Myxoedema often presents as hoarseness, so examine the skin, hair and nails.

Laryngoscopy

Examination of the larynx can be done in the clinic with a mirror (indirect laryngoscopy) or with a general anaesthetic and a laryngoscope (direct laryngoscopy).

Indirect laryngoscopy

Use some form of headlight or reflected light, grasp

the patient's tongue in a swab in the left hand and place a warm laryngeal mirror held in the right hand on the patient's soft palate. Ask the patient to breathe gently in and out and then to try to say 'ee'. The cords should be seen to close on phonation and it should be easy to assess their movement, colour and form. Look at the other laryngeal areas such as the epiglottis, vallecula, aryepiglottic folds, false cords, piriform fossae and the arytenoids (LD-48, LD-49).

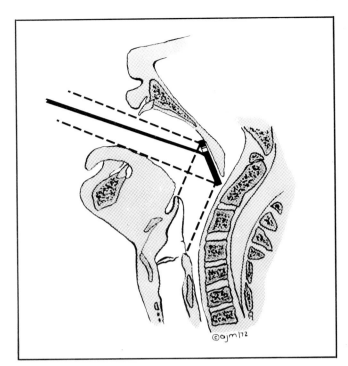

LD-49. Indirect laryngoscopy

Laryngography

This is a method of making a graph of the patient's voice pattern so that his hoarseness can be assessed and the frequency pattern analysed.

Stroboscopic laryngoscopy

This permits examination of the cords in different stages of movement by changing the phase of the stroboscopic light. It is useful in assessing mucosal waves in phonation (CP-29).

Fibre optic laryngoscopy

This is a method of examining the larynx by inserting a fibre optic bundle into the larynx via the nose. It is then possible to watch the cords moving during normal speech.

Respiratory function tests

These may give useful information in certain voice problems, e.g. effectiveness of vocal cord closure.

Thyroid function tests

Suspicion of myxoedema should merit further investigations.

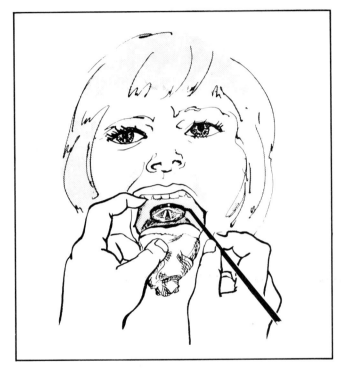

LD-48. Indirect laryngoscopy

Some patients are quite unable to tolerate the procedure and either will require their throat to be locally anaesthetized or will require to come into hospital for a direct laryngoscopy.

Direct laryngoscopy

This allows the larynx to be closely examined and is essential for assessing the extent of tumours for biopsy and for minor laryngeal surgery such as vocal cord stripping or polyp removal.

INVESTIGATIONS

Tape recording

It is necessary to have a recording of a patient's voice problem so as to assess his response to surgery or speech therapy.

RADIOLOGY

Air forms a natural contrast with the soft tissue structures which are moulded on to a radiolucent cartilaginous scaffolding. The vocal apparatus is under voluntary control and therefore lends itself to dynamic studies.

Soft tissue examination

A fairly superficial examination of the larynx can be made by study of the soft tissues. This is especially favourable in the lateral projection where the configuration of the larynx can be seen.

Tomography

In the frontal projection, the larynx overlies the spine and is, therefore, obscured by bone. This problem can be overcome by tomography and a very acceptable appreciation of the coronal anatomy of the larynx becomes available.

Action studies can be made by taking the tomograph in a phonating 'E' position and in the resting position. The outline of the supraglottic and infraglottic spaces can be readily seen (X-27).

Laryngography

A more elaborate and dynamic study of the larynx may be made by introducing non-irritant contrast material into the anaesthetized laryngeal apparatus via a Teimmans catheter.

Under screening control by an image intensifier, the positive contrast is allowed to coat the larynx. The radiologist then has an opportunity to follow the movements of the larynx and to take appropriate spot X-ray pictures to illustrate the most important anatomical recesses.

SECTION III

The presentation of disease of the larynx and the diagnostic possiblities

APHONIA

This literally means 'no sound' and implies that the patient speaks in a whisper or with marked air wastage. The cords have to come together to produce a sound and so if a patient is 'aphonic' his or her cords do not meet.

Causes

These include:

- vocal cord paralysis
- hysterical aphonia
- voice strain
- laryngitis

Clinical approach

Presentation

The onset is nearly always sudden. If the patient has a unilateral abductor cord paralysis, then over a period of a few weeks the normal cord will make some effort to meet the paralysed cord, thus closing the gap and gradually improving the voice. The patient, usually an older man, speaks in a forced whisper as if he is trying hard to produce a voice. His cough will be poor because he cannot close his cords to produce sufficient subglottic pressure. If there is a significant gap, he will also complain of food going down the wrong way. The lack of a positive subglottic pressure causes incoordinate swallowing.

A further presentation of aphonia is the patient who speaks not only in a whisper but also with very little volume so that he is virtually inaudible. He, or

usually she, has no cough or swallowing difficulty and is very often less than middle age. This is the characteristic picture of hysterical aphonia. If suspected, the diagnosis can be made by one simple action – ask the patient to cough. The patient with a vocal cord paralysis will sound 'breathy' and the cough will be ineffective. The hysterical aphonic will give an excellent cough, showing that the cords move and meet normally, and then will lapse back into the barely audible whisper.

Examination

Examination of the first type of larynx with a mirror will show a paralysed cord set well to one side of the midline. On phonation the normal cord will almost close the gap but there will be a chink posteriorly between the arytenoids.

In hysterical aphonia the cords are widely abducted during respiration and also phonation. On coughing however, they meet normally. The diagnosis is easy but the management is difficult.

Speech therapy for a few weeks may help, but if the patient is still aphonic after a month, enlist the help of a psychiatrist.

Investigation

Investigation of a case of laryngeal palsy is aimed at finding the cause. It will be left-sided in nine cases out of ten because the left recurrent laryngeal nerve has a much longer course than the right. The cause is usually found in the chest in association with a bronchial carcinoma, enlarged mediastinal glands or the enlarged left atrium of mitral valve disease. A chest X-ray is therefore the first step.

It is important to check the thyroid for lumps that may have involved the laryngeal nerves. If any are found, a scan and possible biopsy will be necessary.

Oesophageal cancer can paralyse the nerve, but there will usually be marked dysphagia and the tumour will be easily seen on barium swallow. It is important, as well, to look at the ears and naso-pharynx for tumours and also to X-ray the base of the skull.

If all the investigations are negative, then the cause is probably a viral infection or else a small bronchial carcinoma which will declare itself in the ensuing months.

DYSPHONIA

Dysphonia means 'altered sound' and is more commonly known as hoarseness. The mechanism is that the cords come together but the mucosal movement is altered by the presence of a mass on the cord mucosa or else by intrinsic muscle incoordination.

Causes

These include:

- carcinoma of the larynx
- voice strain
- chronic laryngitis
- vocal cord polyp
- vocal cord nodules
- benign laryngeal tumours
- laryngeal trauma
- granulomas of the larynx
- myxoedema
- allergic laryngitis

Clinical approach

Presentation

The onset is usually gradual and, if the mass is increasing in size like a cancer, a nodule or a polyp, then the dysphonia too will increase. If it is due to voice strain or muscle weakness, then the dysphonia will be variable, being better after rest and getting progressively worse on using the voice.

Pain is an unusual feature but its presence suggests a cancer, a perichondritis or an arthritis of the cricoarytenoid joint. Dysphagia is unusual but it is possible that the laryngeal irritation may cause a dry cough.

Examination

Examination is first done with a mirror and the diagnosis should be made at this point. If a mass is seen on the cord, then it must be removed and biopsied. Poor cord movement due to voice strain should be further investigated by special voice tests.

Cords are normally pure white in the larynx. If the larynx is red and inflamed, then the condition is either allergic laryngitis due to an inhalant or acute laryngitis.

If the cords look oedematous, then myxoedema should be excluded.

Warning

If everything else in this book is forgotten, try to remember this! *When a patient has been hoarse for more than 3 weeks he needs his larynx looked at by a laryngologist.* Cancer of the vocal cords has an excellent prognosis if diagnosed early – and hoarseness is its only early sign. The next stage is respiratory obstruction.

STRIDOR

Stridor means 'noisy breathing' and is a symptom to take very seriously. Most patients with stridor need to be in hospital since any further deterioration could cause respiratory obstruction requiring immediate treatment.

Inspiratory stridor is usually laryngeal in origin and expiratory stridor is usually bronchial. This latter type of stridor is not discussed here.

Causes

Table 12 is a useful guide.

TABLE 12 **Causes of stridor**

Congenital	Laryngomalacia	
	Laryngeal web	
	Vocal cord paralysis	
	Vascular anomaly	
	Benign tumour	
Acquired		
Apyrexial	Foreign body	
	Trauma	
	Benign tumour	
Pyrexial	Acute laryngitis	
	Acute epiglottis	
	Acute laryngotracheal bronchitis	

Clinical approach

Stridor in the newborn child

If a newborn child has stridor, then his larynx must be seen so as to diagnose a congenital cause. Prior to doing a laryngoscopy, quite a lot can be learnt by observing him. Listen to the breathing when he is asleep. Stridor is always worse during crying and straining. Infants with unilateral cord paralysis or laryngomalacia will seldom have stridor when sleeping, but both will demonstrate stridor during energetic crying. On the other hand, an infant with a web, a double aorta, a haemangioma or bilateral cord paralysis will have stridor during sleep.

When the infant wakes, he will probably cry and this is the opportunity to assess his voice quality. If the cord has something on it, then the child will have a hoarse cry. Causes for this include:

- a benign tumour
- a cyst
- a web

A normal cry would, however, suggest:

- laryngomalacia
- vascular anomaly
- bilateral vocal cord paralysis

Examination

Direct laryngoscopy, with an examination of the subglottic space, will show many of the above conditions. If the appearances are normal, then the cause is probably laryngomalacia (see p. 103).

Stridor in the child or adult

With no pyrexia

The apyrexial group in childhood presents little problem in diagnosis as the cause is usually evident from the history – an inhaled foreign body, or following trauma. Benign tumours have a history of progressive dysphonia and, in childhood, the commonest type is the papillomata. These are often multiple.

In the adult, acquired stridor is usually due to a narrowing of the airway because of a laryngeal or thyroid carcinoma. More rarely, hypopharyngeal tumours present as stridor. Tracheal tumours are very rare and always present as stridor. Bilateral abductor paralysis of the vocal cords due to surgical trauma, involvement by a thyroid or oesophageal tumour or a brainstem infarct also cause stridor. Diagnosis is usually quite simple after examining the neck and the larynx.

With pyrexia

Stridor with pyrexia is due to:

- acute laryngitis – especially if it involves the subglottis in a child
- acute epiglottis
- acute laryngotracheobronchitis

SECTION IV
Description of specific diseases of the larynx

VOCAL CORD PARALYSIS

The reference line in the larynx is a straight line drawn between the vocal cords in an anteroposterior direction. In normal movements the cords adduct to the line and abduct from it.

A rule which usually applies but is not invariable is that partial lesions of the recurrent laryngeal nerve such as a neuropraxia cause an abductor paralysis and a complete lesion of the nerve causes an adductor paralysis.

Causes

These may be grouped as:
- lesions affecting either vagus nerve
- lesions affecting the left recurrent laryngeal nerve
- lesions affecting the right recurrent laryngeal nerve

Lesions affecting either vagus nerve

These include:
- basal or skull tumours in the nasopharynx or middle ear
- brainstem lesions causing bulbar paralysis
- a viral neuritis
- trauma following surgery or road accident
- metastatic gland enlargement

Lesions affecting left recurrent laryngeal nerve

These include:
- carcinoma of the bronchus
- carcinoma of the oesophagus
- carcinoma of the thyroid gland
- surgical trauma – thyroidectomy, radical neck dissection, pharyngeal pouch removal, or cardiac surgery
- mediastinal gland enlargement
- enlargement of the left side of the heart in mitral valve disease
- aortic aneurysm
- viral neuritis

Lesions affecting right recurrent laryngeal nerve

These include:
- carcinoma of the thyroid
- carcinoma of the oesophagus
- Pancoast's tumour of the apex of the right lung
- surgical trauma – thyroidectomy, pharyngeal pouch removal or radical neck dissection
- viral neuritis

Clinical features

Depending on the lesion four types of clinical picture can emerge.

Unilateral abductor paralysis

In this condition, one vocal cord is fixed in the midline. The patient may not know that anything is wrong with his voice since the normal vocal cord will meet the paralysed cord and leave the voice quite normal. Since the cords are able to close, there is no difficulty in swallowing or coughing. The commonest cause is a carcinoma of the bronchus and, when it affects the nerve, it is usually inoperable.

If no cause is found, then no treatment is indicated since the patient is usually symptomless. If a cause is found, then it is treated if possible.

Bilateral abductor paralysis

In this condition, both cords lie in the midline and, although the patient will have a normal voice, he will also have severe stridor since the airway is severely compromised.

Management

The degree of stridor depends on the patient's occupation. In a sedentary occupation, respiratory embarrassment will not be noted but, if any exertion is taken, then difficulty in breathing will occur as well as stridor. Patients with this condition are at risk if any upper respiratory obstruction supervenes.

Most patients will require a tracheostomy at some stage.

Special tubes can be fitted to the tracheostomy so that the patient will be able to speak normally by directing the airflow through the larynx and yet will be able to breathe normally when air is directed through the tracheostomy. This is made possible by a valve tracheostomy tube.

Alternatively, one of the vocal cords can be operated on and moved to an abducted position. The voice then becomes rather breathy but the airway is restored.

Unilateral adductor paralysis

In this condition the vocal cord will be in the fully abducted or cadaveric position and the patient will present with an aphonia. In a matter of a few weeks the normal cord comes across the midline and almost meets the paralysed cord, but there will always be a gap posteriorly.

No treatment is indicated for about 6 months until the full effects of the increased movement of the normal cord are evaluated. At the end of this time, if the voice is still poor then some teflon can be injected into the paralysed cord to move it nearer the midline.

An alternative method of treatment is surgery to move the paralysed vocal cord into the midline and fix it there.

Bilateral adductor paralysis

This condition is nearly always due to hysterical aphonia. Both cords lie in the fully abducted position and the patient speaks in a very faint whisper. When the patient is asked to cough, however, the cords meet in the midline. The treatment is speech therapy or psychiatry.

Much more serious, however, is when this con-dition is due to a brain stem lesion. If the cords can never be adducted then the patient can neither cough nor swallow properly. Food and drink may be inhaled and very soon a bronchial pneumonia follows.

The patient will require a tracheostomy and may be a candidate for a total laryngectomy if he or she survives the brain stem lesion. The larynx is incompetent and will always act as a sump and a passage for food to go down the wrong way. Fortunately, this condition is very rare.

ACUTE LARYNGITIS

Clinical features

This usually presents as part of a generalized upper respiratory tract infection. In adults it is a harmless condition and is always self-resolving, but in children it can be dangerous because they have a big submucosal space, especially in the subglottic area. Respiratory obstruction due to laryngeal oedema can therefore occur quickly and can be rapidly fatal unless well managed.

On examination the larynx is red and swollen, and pus may be seen in the arytenoid area. The vocal cords, which are usually white, are reddened.

Management

Treatment is voice rest, bed rest if systemic upset is present, and antibiotics if there are signs of secondary infection. Pain is treated with simple analgesics and menthol inhalations may be comforting.

In children, more energetic action is called for and so every patient should receive humidified air. If this is not successful in minimizing laryngeal oedema, then 100 mg of hydrocortisone is given i.v. and repeated in 4 hours if necessary.

Operative interference with the airway is seldom required in simple acute laryngitis (Section V, p. 105).

ACUTE LARYNGOTRACHEOBRONCHITIS

Clinical features

This is altogether a much more severe condition because of the oedema and crusting that affect the entire lower respiratory system. The child has a high temperature, painful cough and respiratory obstruction.

Management

Treatment with antibiotics, inhalations and intravenous hydrocortisone is necessary. If respiratory obstruction occurs inspite of this, then the child should be intubated for 72 hours. If it is not possible to remove the tube without respiration becoming difficult, a tracheotomy should be done (Section V, p. 105).

ACUTE EPIGLOTTITIS

Clinical features

Acute epiglottitis is seen more commonly in children than adults, and presents with a severe deep throat pain, an elevated temperature, dysphagia, muffled speech and submental swelling.

Examination shows a bright-red swollen epiglottis. Since the commonest infecting organism is *H. influenzae*, the antibiotic of choice is ampicillin. The risk of respiratory obstruction is not so high as in acute laryngotracheobronchitis but the same management may on occasion be needed.

All cases of acute epiglottitis require to be in hospital because of the risk of embarrassment to the airway as well as possible septicaemia (Section V, p. 105).

CHRONIC LARYNGITIS

This condition is common and of unknown aetiology. It is usually chronic from the outset and is related to vocal abuse, smoking and atmospheric pollution (CP-30). Many cases are associated with chronic sinusitis and chronic bronchitis.

The whole larynx is lined by respiratory epithelium apart from the vocal cords and tip of the epiglottis. In chronic laryngitis a great deal of squamous metaplasia takes place to convert the larynx into a skin lined tube.

Clinical features

The cardinal symptom is dysphonia, but this is often accompanied by air wastage due to a myositis of the

intrinsic laryngeal muscles. It is commoner in males and never completely clears up.

Examination shows that the interior of the larynx is thickened and hypertrophic. Occasionally patches of leukoplakia are seen. Their appearances are on occasion very alarming and look like carcinoma. The distinguishing feature, however, is that in chronic laryngitis the changes are bilateral and symmetrical. Biopsy is always necessary to rule out cancer since patients with chronic laryngitis have six times the normal incidence of laryngeal cancer.

Management

The treatment is to strip off the hypertrophic mucosa, and for the patient to avoid smoking, vocal abuse and other pollutants and to embark on a course of speech therapy to learn to use the voice properly.

LARYNGEAL TUBERCULOSIS

This used to present as part of pulmonary tuberculosis and involved the posterior part of the larynx and the arytenoids. Nowadays, however, cases present earlier and the laryngeal appearances are similar to those seen in cancer of the larynx, affecting mainly the anterior part of the larynx.

It is always associated with pulmonary tuberculosis and treatment is by chemotherapy.

LARYNGEAL PERICHONDRITIS

Given the large number of cartilages making up the laryngeal framework, it is surprising that perichondritis does not occur more often.

The commonest cause nowadays is radiotherapy for cancer of the larynx. The cartilages start to dissolve and the soft tissues swell owing to oedema. A tracheostomy is often needed. If the condition arises after radiotherapy, it may suggest a residual carcinoma.

If epiglottitis is not well managed then it can also progress to a perichondritis.

LARYNGEAL ARTHRITIS

The cricoarytenoid joints are synovial and so can be

affected by rheumatoid arthritis. The patient presents with pain and hoarseness and the arytenoid cartilages look red and swollen.

Management

Treatment is that of rheumatoid arthritis, but occasionally arytenoidectomy is necessary.

VOICE DISORDERS

Voice strain

This is a common problem and is extremely distressing to those whose voices are essential parts of their professions.

The optimum pitch of the voice is one third of the way up the person's own range.

If cord length, cord tension or breathing pattern are altered, this will alter the function of the thyroarytenoid and interarytenoid muscles. The result is weakness of these muscles which then produce characteristic laryngeal movements. The cords move but fail to meet properly. They have a bowed appearance with a gap posteriorly between the arytenoids.

Clinical features

The symptom is air wastage and a breathy voice which is normal in the morning after rest but which becomes progressively worse on use so that by the evening it has often disappeared.

It usually affects people who pitch the voice too high – baritones who sing tenor parts, contraltos who sing soprano, and nervous schoolteachers.

Management

Treatment is to rest the patient's voice for 2 weeks and then send the patient to speech therapy.

Vocal nodules

These are also called 'singers'' or 'screamers'' nodes and are the result of misuse of the voice, usually by pitching it too high. Thickened areas form at the junction of the anterior third and posterior two thirds of the vocal cord (CP-31).

Management

The nodules are removed by direct laryngoscopy and the patient given speech therapy afterwards.

Vocal cord polyps

A vocal cord polyp is an organized haematoma, usually caused initially by trauma. If traumatic in origin, it only affects one cord, causes dysphonia and should be removed by endoscopy (CP-32).

Bilateral polypi are often myxoedematous in origin and the appropriate investigations should be carried out.

Whatever the cause, the polyps must be removed endoscopically. This is performed in two stages, since bilateral vocal cord stripping is complicated by the cords sticking together at the anterior commissure to form a web.

CANCER OF THE LARYNX

The larynx is divided by the vocal cords (glottis) into the supraglottic area and subglottic area. Cancer in each of these areas behaves differently, presents differently and has a different prognosis. Laryngeal cancer should be diagnosed early, since the prognosis for cases treated then is good. It is a disease of males who smoke cigarettes. Of these tumours, 99% are squamous carcinomas and only 2% metastasize distantly.

Supraglottic cancer

Clinical features

This usually presents as an exophytic wart on the epiglottis and can grow to a large size before symptoms occur. It is often diagnosed during the course of a routine examination or during the administration of an anaesthetic for another condition.

The patient may have a sore throat, slight dysphagia or a muffled voice. Hoarseness is a late symptom since the vocal cords act as a barrier to the spread of the tumour for a long time.

Two out of three patients will have a metastatic neck gland, indicating that surgery should be the primary method of treatment (CP-33).

Management

The surgery should be a supraglottic partial laryngectomy if the tumour is limited in size, or a total laryngectomy if it is large. The neck glands are removed by a radical neck dissection. If metastatic glands are not present the patient should have a full course of radiotherapy (Section V, p. 105).

Glottic cancer

Clinical features

The presenting symptom is hoarseness. The tumours are generally small, for a male vocal cord is only about 2 cm long.

On examination, a white excrescence is seen. It is very important to assess the mobility of the vocal cord for, as the tumour enlarges, the cord becomes more fixed (CP-34).

Management

When the cord is mobile, radiotherapy gives excellent results and leaves the patient with a normal voice.

An alternative treatment is to remove the affected half of the larynx (hemilaryngectomy) and rebuild the cord with the strap muscles. This gives as good results, but the voice is not so good as it is after radiotherapy.

When the cord is fixed or when the tumour has spread into the supra- or subglottis, then the whole larynx should be removed.

When glands are palpable it generally means that spread outside the glottis has occurred, since the glottis itself has no lymph drainage.

Subglottic cancer

Clinical features

This is a 'bad actor'. It declares itself late and usually presents as respiratory obstruction for which a tracheostomy near the tumour is required. By the time it presents it has usually invaded the thyroid gland and the trachea. A little later it involves the oesophagus and the paratracheal nodes in the mediastinum.

Dysphonia is not common, since the vocal cord is not affected until late in the disease. A unilateral abductor paralysis due to involvement of the recurrent laryngeal nerve may occur, but in these cases the voice could well be normal.

One in five cases has metastatic nodes and one in five involves the thyroid gland (CP-35).

Management

The primary treatment is by radiation and, if this fails, a total laryngectomy, thyroidectomy and partial removal of the trachea and paratracheal nodes is required (Section V, p. 105).

To confirm the bad prognosis, these tumours tend to behave like lung cancers and metastasize to bone (a most unusual feature of any head and neck cancer).

Leukoplakia

This presents as dysphonia and shows as white patches on the cords.

Management

All of them must be biopsied to rule out cancer.

If they are hyperkeratotic they are unlikely to be premalignant, but if there is any dysplasia then the whole cord should be stripped endoscopically and the patient followed-up as if he had a cancer. Radiotherapy is reserved for cases that recur with invasive changes.

LARYNGOMALACIA

This causes stridor at birth and can persist throughout the child's first year or two. It is due to laxity in the laryngeal cartilages which causes them to be indrawn during inspiration and allows the larynx to vibrate like an elongated reed. The stridor is worse during crying and exertion.

As the larynx becomes more chondrified it firms up and the stridor is usually gone by the age of 2 years.

It must be distinguished from other conditions causing congenital stridor.

Management

When the diagnosis is established, reassure the parents that nothing dreadful is liable to happen to the child, and that the problem will eventually go away. They should, however, pay a little more attention than usual to upper respiratory tract infections.

LARYNGEAL WEB

This consists of a membrane lying between the vocal cords in the anterior half of the larynx. It represents incomplete laryngeal development. The degree of stridor it causes is in proportion to its size. If it is small, then removal can wait until the child is in its teens, but a large web will require urgent removal.

SECTION V

Principles of general management and treatment of the larynx

PRINCIPLES OF LARYNGEAL SURGERY

Laryngectomy

This is the removal of whole or part of the larynx for carcinoma.

Total laryngectomy

In total laryngectomy, the larynx is removed from the tongue above the pharynx posteriorly and the trachea inferiorly. The open pharynx is converted into a closed tube which is allowed to heal around a nasogastric tube for 10 postoperative days. Thereafter the patient takes a normal diet (LD-50).

The cut end of the trachea is brought onto the surface and left as a permanent tracheostomy in which the patient may or may not wear a tracheostomy tube. A permanent tracheostomy brings no increased risk of infection or lung problems in the long term.

After surgery the patient has speech therapy lessons to learn oesophageal speech.

Partial laryngectomy

This can be done by removing the top half of the larynx – false cords, aryepiglottic folds and epiglottis. This is a supraglottic laryngectomy (LD-51).

The patient has no permanent tracheostomy and has a normal voice. There may be some difficulty in swallowing in the postoperative period, but younger

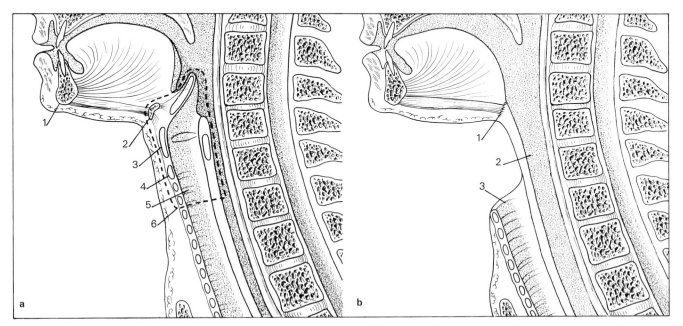

LD-50. *Total laryngectomy.* **a**, *Showing area to be removed.* **1**, *Mandible;* **2**, *hyoid bone;* **3**, *thyroid cartilage;* **4**, *cricoid cartilage;* **5**, *trachea;* **6**, *line of excision.* **b**, *Showing end result after removal.* **1**, *Pharynx sutured to base of tongue;* **2**, *lumen of pharynx;* **3**, *permanent tracheostomy*

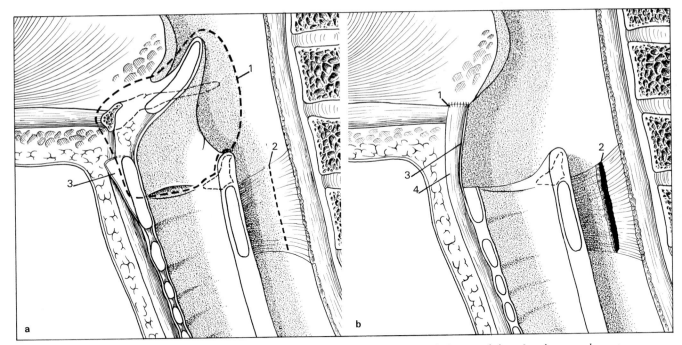

LD-51. *Supraglottic laryngectomy. **a**, **1**, Showing the area of larynx to be removed; **2**, site of the cricopharyngeal myotomy; **3**, perichondrial flap. **b**, After removal of the specimen, the perichondrial flap (**3**) is sutured to the base of the tongue (**1**) and supported by the strap muscle layer (**4**). A cricopharyngeal myotomy is done over a distance of 5 cm (2 inches) (**2**)*

patients rehabilitate well.

If one half of the larynx is removed vertically – false cord, true cord and subglottis – it is called a 'vertical hemilaryngectomy'. The removed side is rebuilt using the small strap muscles. The voice is hoarse but present and usable and the patient does not have a tracheostomy (LD-52).

Endoscopy

By means of direct laryngoscopy under general anaesthesia a large number of minor procedures can be performed. Use is made of the operating microscope so that lesions can be better seen and more carefully removed.

Lesions that are usually dealt with endoscopically are vocal cord polyps, nodules and (removal or biopsy of) leukoplakia.

MANAGEMENT OF RESPIRATORY OBSTRUCTION

Primary treatment should consist of oxygen humidification, antibiotics and steroids. If the stridor persists in spite of this, further steps to improve the airway must be taken.

An old aphorism used to be:

'The time to do a tracheostomy is the time you first think about it.'

Tracheostomy however, is a difficult, dangerous operation if done by someone with no experience. It is especially hazardous in small children since the trachea is narrow and the subclavian vein, the pleura and occasionally the thymus can be in the operating field.

A more apt aphorism for the inexperienced – and if something requires to be done about an airway in a hurry it is usually the inexperienced who are present – is:

'When you think of doing a tracheostomy, intubate and think again.'

Intubation gives several advantages:

- More people can do this more successfully than a tracheostomy
- It is quicker
- If a tracheostomy needs to be done, it is more easily performed on an anaesthetized intubated patient
- With an infective cause, antibiotics and steroids will probably have it under control within 48–72 hours. The patient can then be extubated without having had skin or trachea scarred

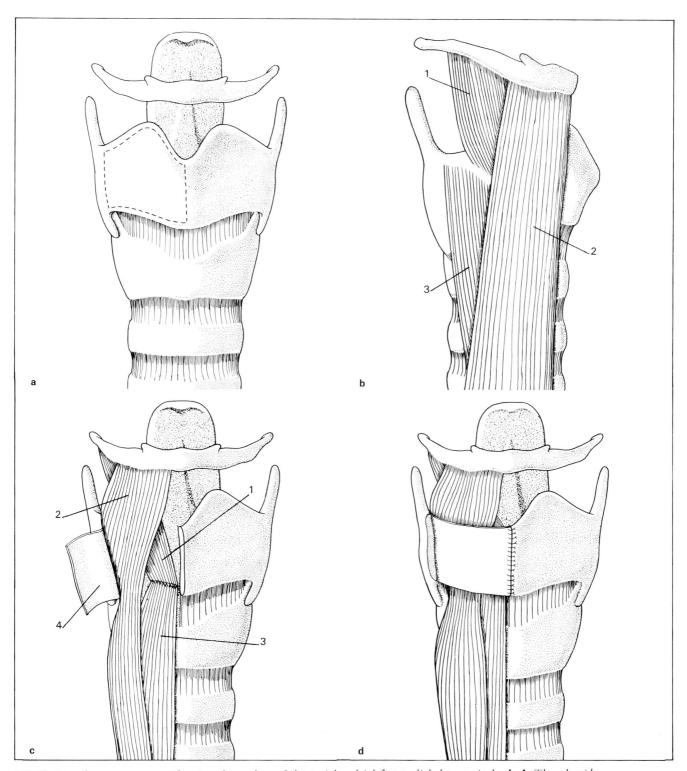

LD-52. *Hemilaryngectomy.* ***a****, Showing the outline of the perichondrial flap pedicled posteriorly.* ***b****, **1**, Thyrohyoid muscle; **2**, sternohyoid muscle; **3**, sternothyroid muscle.* ***c****, After the hemilarynx is removed the muscles are repositioned as shown; **4** is the perichondrial flap.* ***d****, The perichondrial flap is replaced and sutured to the remaining lamina*

• It gives time for someone experienced to be found to do the tracheostomy properly without risking later laryngotracheal stenosis.

If a patient is in severe respiratory distress and breathing is stopped due to a foreign body, then doing a tracheostomy takes too long and intubation may be impossible or impracticable. In such a case a laryngotomy as a temporary measure may be done.

Laryngotomy

This can be achieved by piercing the cricothyroid membrane with a knife or a large bore needle. It is above the thyroid gland and quite safe from haemorrhage. Provided no damage is done to the cricoid or thyroid cartilages then there is little risk of laryngeal stenosis. It should be converted to a tracheotomy within a few hours.

Tracheostomy

Making a hole in the trachea to alleviate respiratory obstruction was originally performed by the ancient Egyptians.

The operation is done via a small horizontal or vertical incision, the strap muscles separated, the thyroid isthmus divided and ligated and an opening made in the 3rd and 4th rings of the trachea (LD-53). In the postoperative period the main complication is crusting due to the unhumidified unwarmed air directly entering the trachea. The most important measure in the first few days is to use an effective humidifier.

*LD-53. Tracheostomy. **a**, Showing structures exposed. **1**, Sternohyoid muscle; **2**, sternomastoid muscle; **3**, cricoid cartilage; **4**, isthmus of thyroid gland; **5**, trachea. **b**, Site of incision in trachea. **1**, Isthmus of thyroid gland divided and ligated; **2**, third ring of trachea; **3**, sternohyoid muscle retracted; **4**, site of incision in trachea*

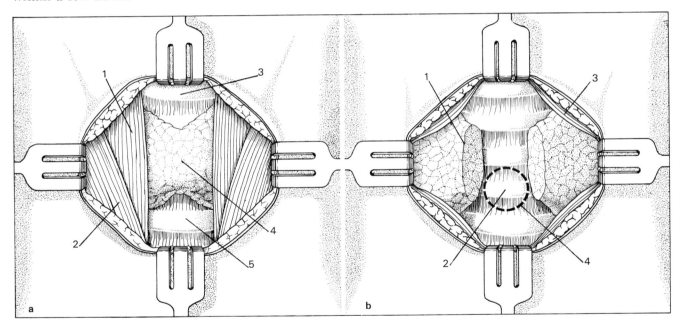

TEST-YOURSELF QUESTIONS
Part 4 – The Larynx

1. Indicate whether the following statements on laryngeal anatomy are true or false:
a) The cricoid is the only complete ring in the respiratory tract.
b) The hyoid is a cartilage.
c) The vocal cord has no lymph drainage.
d) The Adam's apple indicates the level of the vocal cords.

2. The following laryngeal conditions present with pain:
a) Perichondritis
b) Arthritis of the cricoarytenoid joint
c) Laryngocoele
d) Vocal nodules

3. The following conditions may present with aphonia:
a) Bronchogenic carcinoma
b) Subglottic carcinoma
c) Voice strain
d) Myxoedema

4. Stridor may be due to:
a) Subglottic carcinoma
b) Laryngomalacia
c) Abnormal subclavian artery
d) Asthma

5. In unilateral adductor paralysis:
a) The patient may have a good voice but noisy breathing
b) The lesion is at the base of the skull or in the brain stem
c) A tracheostomy is almost always essential
d) Teflon injection of the paralysed cord may restore the voice

6. Supraglottic carcinoma is:
a) Commoner in males
b) A common cause of hoarseness
c) Seldom associated with metastatic neck nodes
d) Best managed by performing a total laryngectomy if no neck nodes are palpable

7. Glottic carcinoma:
a) Is commoner in patients who overuse their voices
b) Always presents as hoarseness
c) Seldom metastasises
d) Is best treated with a partial laryngectomy if the cord is fixed

8. Stridor in the newborn:
a) is most commonly due to laryngomalacia
b) is not due to a lesion on the vocal cord if the child has a normal cry
c) may be due to a web secondary to birth trauma
d) demands that the patient have a laryngoscopy

9. In an emergency presentation of respiratory obstruction, if the cause is laryngeal the following are indicated:
a) A laryngotomy in the thyrohyoid membrane
b) The insertion of a wide bore needle in the cricothyroid membrane
c) Blind intubation
d) A tracheostomy

10. The following conditions may be treated via direct laryngoscopy:
a) Vocal cord polyp
b) Carcinoma in situ of the vocal cords
c) Laryngomalacia
d) Unilateral vocal cord paralysis

The answers to these questions will be found on p. 191.

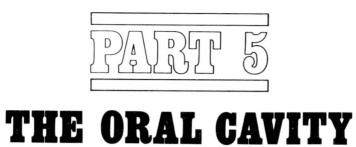

THE ORAL CAVITY

SECTION I

Background to oral disease

INTRODUCTION

The oral cavity is that part of the mouth which is anterior to the soft palate and tonsils. It contains the cheeks, tongue, lower jaw, hard palate and teeth. It is lined with mucous membrane, and the main salivary glands – the parotid, submandibular and sublingual – and the minor salivary glands open into it. The numerous minor salivary glands are situated mainly in the mucosa of the cheek, the floor of the mouth and the hard palate.

ANATOMY

The tongue

The tongue is made up of many interlacing muscles and is attached to the hyoid bone. It is supported anteriorly by the mylohyoid muscle. The anterior two thirds – anterior to the circumvallate papillae – are in the oral cavity, while the posterior third is considered part of the oropharynx.

The tongue is essential for articulated speech and swallowing.

Patients who have had the tongue removed can still swallow but in a different way. They cannot, however, speak intelligibly.

The alveoli

The upper alveolus is part of the maxilla. Therefore some tooth roots are intimately related to the maxillary sinus, leading at times to difficulty in differentiating toothache from the pain of sinusitis.

The lower alveolus is part of the mandible.

With advancing years, and especially after extraction of teeth, the alveoli resorb and can become quite flat.

The hard palate

The hard palate, between the U-shaped curves of the upper alveoli, represents the floor of the nose.

Teeth

Human teeth are composed of three calcified tissues (LD-54):

- enamel
  This covers the coronal portion of the tooth and is the most highly calcified tissue in the body.
- dentine
  This forms the bulk of the tooth. It has a

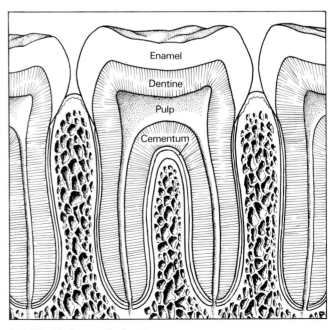

LD-54. *Molar tooth showing structure*

tubular structure through which pass processes from its forming cells – odontoblasts – which lie in the pulp of the tooth.

- cementum
  This covers the root of the tooth and functions as the attachment of the periodontal membrane.

Primary dentition

There are 20 teeth in the primary dentition. These consist of

- two incisors
- one canine
- two molars

in each quadrant of the jaw.

The upper molars are three-rooted and the lower have two roots. Eruption of the incisors occurs at about 3 months and by $2\frac{1}{2}$ years the last molar has erupted.

Secondary dentition

There are normally 32 permanent teeth. These consist of:

- two incisors
- one canine
- two premolars
- three molars

in each quadrant of the jaws.

Eruption commences at about 6 years and is usually complete at about 18 years with the eruption of the third molars. Eruption times for these teeth can, however, be very variable.

Periodontium

The periodontium acts as a supporting structure for the teeth.

It provides a seal or epithelial attachment adhering closely to the enamel surface of the tooth. The periodontal membrane acts as a sling anchoring the tooth in its socket but still allowing slight movement of the root within the socket.

Oral mucous membrane

The oral cavity is lined with mucous membrane which varies in type in different parts of the mouth. The alveolar or attached mucosa is thickly cornified while the gingival or non-attached mucosa is redder and has no stratum corneum. The tongue is highly cornified and is studded with papillae which have a taste function.

The nerve supply

Sensory innervation

The sensory innervation of the oral cavity is by the trigeminal nerve.

Motor innervation

The masticatory muscles are supplied by branches of the motor division of the trigeminal nerve. The tongue is supplied by the hypoglossal nerve.

Secreto-motor innervation

The secreto-motor function of the palatine glands is by fibres from the parasympathetic system which are associated with the facial nerve.

SECTION II

History and physical examination of the oral cavity

HISTORY

In addition to the standard questions on bleeding and past medical history, patients who complain of oral symptoms should be questioned about a number of specific points.

Specific questions

Where is the lesion or condition?

Is the pain localized?

Does the pain radiate?
The distribution of pain gives a good indication of its origin. Temporomandibular joint pain often radiates over the whole of the side of the head. Tongue pain is often referred to the ear.

How long has the symptom or condition been present?

Was there any specific episode which brought the condition on?

What is its relationship to normal movement and function including chewing?

What is the character of the pain?

Is the pain aching, stabbing, dull etc?

Is it constant or intermittent?

Are there aggravating factors?

Are there relieving factors?

Are there associated features?
Clicks or crepitus often occur with temporomandibular joint dysfunction.

Are other joints affected?

Does swelling or pain interfere with sleep?

For denture wearers there are special problems:

- pain
  This can be due to poor support or wrong bite.
- looseness
  This can be caused by the dentures being underextended or because of a wrong bite.
- retching
  The dentures may be too large or may cramp the tongue, or the bite may be wrong.

EXAMINATION

An extraoral examination should be first carried out. Any swelling, erythema or sinus problem should be noted and the cervical lymph nodes palpated. Intraoral examination should consist of examination of the soft tissues, teeth and bone.

In the general assessment, attention should be paid to the state of dental restorations, the presence of carious cavities, plaque and calculus deposits as well as to halitosis.

A more detailed examination should then follow. A number of instruments may be used but the following are particularly useful:

- dental mirror and probe
- tongue depressors

Good illumination is essential and the patient should be seated comfortably to allow inspection of all areas of the oral cavity.

Examination of soft tissues

The soft tissues should be examined systematically.

Lips and buccal mucosa

The lips are examined first. This leads onto examination of the buccal mucosa and the upper and lower sulci. Colour, texture and the presence of lesions should be noted in each instance. Inspection should be followed by bimanual palpation. This reveals mucosal changes as well as lesions in the deeper structures.

Hard and soft palate

The hard and soft palate should now be examined both by inspection and palpation and variations from the normal recorded. The effect of a denture, if worn, should be noted. In the newborn, careful examination should be made to exclude a cleft palate.

Floor of the mouth

The floor of the mouth is examined by raising the tip of the tongue. This reveals the submandibular ducts and papillae. Bimanual palpation, to examine the soft tissues and salivary glands in the floor of the mouth, is necessary. The lingual surface of the mandible should also be palpated to reveal any exostosis or tender areas.

Tongue

Inspection of the dorsum of the tongue may be aided by holding the tip with a piece of gauze. The surface, colour texture and contour should be noted. Special attention should be paid to the lateral surface because this is where 90% of tumours originate. Palpation forms an integral part of this examination.

Examination of teeth

Prior to examination of the teeth, the gingivae and supporting tissues should first be inspected. Look for calculus, plaque and gingival inflammation. Probing of the gingival sulcus for 'pathological deepening' will indicate periodontal disease. Local or generalized hyperplasia of the gingivae is significant. Abnormal pigmentation of the gingivae may be a sign of an underlying systemic problem.

When examining the teeth, deposits should be removed, and the intrinsic colour and staining revealed. The variations in size, form, number and position of the individual teeth should be recorded. Such variations may be related to underlying systemic conditions. Note also abrasions, erosion and fractures of the teeth. Caries usually develops in the pits and fissures of the occlusal surfaces and in the non-self-cleansing areas – the interstitial surfaces.

Percussion testing

Percussion testing with the handle of a dental mirror is a useful method for checking tooth mobility and apical infections.

Testing the reaction of heat and cold

This is useful in determining tooth vitality. It is done by applying hot gutta-percha or ethylchloride on a cotton wool pellet to the tooth.

Examination of dentures

The following points should be checked:
- ulceration
- pressure areas and 'quality' of support
- occlusion
- retention

Palpation of the edentulous ridge is a useful method for determining the suitability of the tissues and underlying structures for denture support. Any uneven contact or denture movement which occurs when the patient bites together should be noted.

Examination of the temporomandibular joint

This requires a specialized and specific examination. The joint and associated muscles should be examined during function. The maximum opening as measured interdentally is an indication of the range of movement.

Joint pain

Palpate the joint for tenderness or crepitus. Similar pain can arise from otitis externa.

Muscle pain

Lateral or forward movement or opening against manual pressure can reveal and localize muscle pain.

Intraoral examination

Points to check here include:
- malocclusion of the teeth
- loss of teeth
- tilting of teeth
- high fillings or 'restorations'

Under normal conditions the opposing teeth meet evenly and simultaneously. If any of the above conditions exist the teeth meet unevenly, putting strain on the muscles or temporomandibular joint.

A stethoscope differentiates between solid, even contacts and slides or deviations. It is also of use in examining for crepitus.

INVESTIGATIONS

Bacteriology

Swabs from the oral cavity are of great value when fungus infection such as candidiasis, or its more severe variation thrush, is suspected. In this instance, however, it is adequate to provide the bacteriologist with a scraping of the white lesion.

Biopsy

Most masses in the oral cavity, all white patches and all ulcers require to be biopsied. The minor discomfort of a biopsy must be weighed against the disastrous consequences of missing an early carcinoma.

Biopsy is usually best performed by infiltrating the area with local anaesthetic and removing a small sample with a scalpel.

RADIOLOGY

Anatomy

Teeth

Radiographically, a tooth shows as an opaque homogenous mass of dentine and cementum (X-28).

Enamel shows as a more opaque cap over the dentine and cementum. The pulp chamber appears as a dark shadow in the centre of the tooth and is larger in the younger than the older patient. The periodontal membrane shows as a dark line separating the tooth from the cortical bone of the tooth socket (lamina dura).

Alveolar process

The alveolar process frequently presents a network of trabeculae joining each other at sharp angles. They are usually finer and closer in the maxilla than in the mandible.

Mental foramen and mandibular canal

In the mandible, the mental foramina appear clearly as radiolucent areas. The mandibular canal can usually be seen as a radiolucent structure, related to the roots of the lower teeth.

Tooth development

At birth, radiographs show the developing teeth lying in crypts below the gums.

By the age of 6 there will be resorption of the roots of the molar and incisor teeth, and the first permanent molars may have erupted.

By 12 years all the teeth, with the exception of the last molars, are usually present in the mouth, but root formation is incomplete.

By 18 years all teeth are present in the mouth although there is considerable variation in the eruption of the third molars. These may be impacted.

Examination

The following points should be looked for when examining dental radiographs:

- continuity and thickness of the lamina dura
- variation in width of the periodontal spaces
- level of the alveolar crest
- periapical radiolucencies
- bony radiolucencies and radio-opacities

Continuity and thickness of lamina dura

Loss of continuity of the lamina dura is a sign of periodontal disease, whereas loss of lamina dura at the apex of a tooth is a sign of reaction of the periapical tissues to infection. In the absence of clinical signs of periodontal disease, the loss of lamina dura may be associated with other X-ray changes suggesting a neoplasm.

Variation in width of periodontal space

Uniformity of width of the periodontal space is evidence of all teeth functioning normally. Widening of this space is evidence of a traumatic occlusion, whereas narrowing may indicate a non-functional tooth.

Level of alveolar crest

The level of the alveolar crest indicates the extent of

periodontal breakdown and is important in determining the prognosis of the teeth in relation to periodontal disease.

Periapical radiolucency

Periapical radiolucency is usually an indication of a non-vital tooth. The usual causes of radiolucency (X-29) are chronic granuloma, periapical abscesses and dental cysts. Rarely, periapical radiolucency may be associated with a neoplasm.

Acute periapical abscesses initially show no radiographic changes. Dental cysts are often surrounded by compact bone and are larger than periapical granulomas.

In any suspected malignancy, assessment of possible bone erosion must be made. In the lower jaw, an orthopantomogram gives the best view while, in the upper jaw, tomograms of the maxillary sinus provide more information.

The temporomandibular joint

Temporomandibular joint pain must be investigated by radiographs, and views of the joint, both in the open and closed position, are often helpful.

SECTION III

The presentation of oral disease and the diagnostic possibilities

PAIN

A patient complaining of pain in the oral cavity may have a lesion in the soft tissues or the teeth and gums and it is essential to locate the cause.

Causes

Since toothache is probably the commonest cause of oral pain it is logical to exclude this first of all.

If the patient has had any direct trauma such as a fractured tooth or has lost a filling then this information is usually easily obtained. Simple examination can confirm the problem.

If there has been a course of dental treatment then a number of possible causes emanate directly from it:

- extraction sockets especially in the lower jaw
  If they remain painful for more than 48 hours, it suggests localized osteitis.
- large unlined metal fillings or fillings composed of acid materials.
  These may cause discomfort or pain. On occasion the latter type of filling can cause a pulpitis.
- dentures
  These can be the source of some of the most common causes of pain on eating.

Galvanism is caused by the difference of electrical potential between two dissimilar but touching metal fillings and gives rise to pain when the affected teeth are in contact.

Dentures

Pain from dentures may result from:

- 'immediate' dentures
  When immediate dentures are made the extraction socket may be painful for a short time afterwards.

- atrophic tissues
  In older patients, the mucous membrane of the alveolar ridges loses its resilience. These patients find dentures very uncomfortable.

- under extended dentures
  Dentures which are too small frequently cause pain, especially in the lower jaw.

- wrong bite
  Pain may also occur if the 'bite' is wrong.

Caries

Every medical practitioner should be able to check for gross caries, since this is the commonest disease to affect man. The pain is often severe and may be aggravated by heat, cold or sweet substances.

Examine the teeth in the area of the pain, looking for fractures or missing fillings, or cavities. The pain from caries occurs when there is pulpitis and this is why temperature change makes it worse (CP-36). Touch the suspected tooth with hot gutta-percha or wool soaked in ethylchloride. This produces a significant temperature change.

When the pulp dies, necrotic material will irritate the apical tissues and at this point moving the tooth or percussing it will aggravate the pain. Chewing can of course make the pain worse.

When the periapical tissues are inflamed the tooth will feel full and will be exquisitely painful. Without treatment, drainage or antibiotics, an abscess will form. At this point pain and swelling may be maximal over the root on the gum margin.

Periodontal disease

Pain as acute as pulpitis can be caused by periodontal disease. Dentine is exposed following wear of occlusal surfaces and with the exposure of roots.

The pain is made worse by cold or sweet substances and also by tooth brushing. As the alveolar margin resorbs, redundant gum tissue forms around the neck of the tooth and food debris can collect in the pockets. This irritates the area and it can progress to abscess formation.

The pain can be differentiated from pulpitis, however, by the fact that movement or percussion of the tooth does not exacerbate the pain.

A similar situation may occur in the gum around an impacted or partially erupted wisdom tooth and there it is termed 'pericoronitis'. There is pain at the back of the jaw, often radiating to the neck, and there is frequently trismus, halitosis and pain on chewing.

Sinusitis

The condition most likely to be confused with toothache is sinusitis, especially if the roots are in close proximity to the sinus lining. Radiographs of both the sinus and the teeth are therefore necessary in almost every case, not only to make the differentiation but also to assess the extent of the dental disease.

ULCERATION

Causes

Carcinoma

Carcinoma is not the commonest cause for an oral ulcer but it is the diagnosis that must be thought of first. On no account should a non-healing ulcer be watched for more than 2 or 3 weeks without carrying out a biopsy.

Presentation

While the traditional picture of a tongue cancer is of an old man with a gland in the neck and a piece of cotton wool in his ear for referred pain, the present-day picture is quite different. There is a rising incidence in young people and also in females. The commonest site is on the lateral border of the tongue. It is extremely rare on the dorsum and tip of the tongue.

The second commonest site for carcinoma is the floor of the mouth where saliva, containing possible carcinogens such as tobacco, continuously bathes the area.

An ulcer on the lip, especially the lower lip in a male over the age of 50, is almost always a cancer. A history of outdoor work, long exposure to sunshine and pipe-smoking is significant. Keratoacanthosis is the main differential diagnosis.

Although rare in the UK, cancer of the buccal mucosa is common in India and the USA. The predisposing factors are chewing tobacco and betel nut.

Trauma

Perhaps the commonest cause of oral ulceration is trauma, and a history of a burn from hot food or accidental ingestion of an acid is important.

Examination may show a broken tooth near a cheek or tongue ulcer. If the patient wears dentures, then a flange of the denture may fit the ulcer (CP-37, CP-38).

Aphthous ulcers

If ulcers are recurrent and in different sites and especially if they are multiple, the diagnosis is likely to be aphthous ulceration. These ulcers have a typical appearance of a grey base surrounded by a fiery red halo (CP-39).

Herpetic ulcers

Acute herpetic ulcers are often accompanied by fever, malaise and lymphadenopathy and in their post-vesicular state may resemble aphthous ulcers.

If vesicles are seen, this confirms the diagnosis. Pemphigoid ulceration should, however, be considered. Virology investigations are not helpful in the diagnosis of herpetic or aphthous ulceration but specific antibodies can be found in pemphigoid.

Vincent's infection

Ulceration around the gums, gingivitis, and a most characteristic and offensive halitosis, are the features of Vincent's infection (acute ulcerative gingivitis). The ulcers are characteristically in the interdental papillae and diagnosis is confirmed by culture.

Lichen planus

Large bullae are characteristic of bullous lichen planus (CP-40) and pemphigoid. The more usual appearance of lichen planus is seen in CP-41. Diagnosis of lichen planus is confirmed by biopsy and of pemphigoid by antibody studies. In its atrophic form, lichen planus can cause the mucosa to appear red and shiny and occasionally small ulcers appear on the surface.

Large areas of red mucosa may also be caused by erythroplakia. This is a definite premalignant condition but fortunately it is extremely rare.

Investigations

As noted previously, any non-healing ulcer must be considered malignant and biopsied after 3 weeks. The commonest site is the lateral edge of the tongue, where eight out of ten tongue cancers start.

LUMPS

Causes

A lump in the oral cavity is diagnosed clinically almost always from its site. Because of the high incidence of cancer in the mouth, the lump must always be biopsied.

Alveolar lump

A lump on an alveolar margin is usually related to a dental cause. If it is firm and painful, then suspect an apical abscess. If it is firm and painless, then suspect a dental cyst, an unerupted tooth or an exostosis.

A soft tissue mass on the gums may arise from denture trauma, in response to phenytoin (Epanutin) therapy or from chronic gingivitis. The gums often hypotrophy in pregnancy – granuloma gravidarum.

Lumps in the floor of the mouth

In the floor of the mouth a stony hard mass is seldom anything other than a submandibular calculus impacted in the duct. This can be verified by radiographs. A ranula is a mass in the floor of the mouth due to either a blocked mucous gland or a cavernous lymphangioma (CP-42).

'Ranula' is a Latin word meaning 'frog's belly' and is very descriptive of this blue domed cyst.

Lumps on the hard palate

These must be taken seriously because they nearly always represent a minor salivary gland tumour. As minor salivary gland tumours are often malignant, all hard palate lumps must be biopsied. These tumours can also occur as lumps on the cheek and the back of the lower lip.

One type of lump on the palate, however, that is common and harmless is the bony hard midline lump called torus palatinus (CP-43). This is merely an exostosis of the palatine bone and requires no treatment.

Lumps in the tongue

While most tongue cancers present as ulcers, it is not unknown for such a lesion to present as a hard non-ulcerative lump. This must always be biopsied, because there is almost nothing else that can cause a non-ulcerative local tongue lump.

A smooth red mass in the middle of the dorsum of the tongue is called 'median rhomboid glossitis' (CP-44) and perhaps represents a fungal infection.

Haemangiomas can occur anywhere in the oral cavity but, due to their characteristic appearance, diagnosis is seldom difficult.

BLEEDING

Causes

Bleeding from the oral cavity, in the absence of a necrotic carcinomatous ulcer, is nearly always dental in origin. Any inflammatory condition of the gums such as Vincent's infection, gingivitis secondary to periodontal disease or pericoronitis can cause either spontaneous bleeding or more usually bleeding on brushing the teeth. In pregnancy the gums may tend to bleed more easily than normal. An haemangioma can be traumatized by tooth brushing and the bleeding will be copious.

The conditions above all others that require to be kept in mind when gums bleed, however, are the bleeding diatheses, and unless a positive clinical diagnosis of one of the dental conditions can be made there should be no delay in proceeding to a full haematological investigation.

PIGMENTATION AND DISCOLORATION

Causes

'Leukoplakia' is a Greek word meaning a 'white patch' (CP-45). It may be premalignant. It can occur anywhere in the oral cavity and is often a response to continued trauma. If it is primarily hyperkeratotic it is not premalignant, but if it shows evidence of dysplasia then it is probably premalignant. The only way that this can be demonstrated is histologically and so every white patch in the mouth should be biopsied.

Lichen planus can also present as a white patch but more often it is represented by white stringlike lines (CP-41).

Raised red patches in the oral cavity may be due to *erythroplakia* which is almost always premalignant but fortunately rare.

Addison's disease may present as a bluish-black or brown-grey pigmentation of the oral mucosa. This should be differentiated from racial pigmentation, that found with heavy metals (bismuth), and tattooing with foreign substances (graphite and amalgam). *Peutz–Jeghers syndrome* also presents with pigmentation of the lips (CP-46).

Tooth discoloration may be the result of tetracycline therapy or from fluorosis during the period of tooth formation.

A black hairy tongue usually results from heavy smoking, excessive use of antiseptic mouthwashes or candidiases (CP-47). There is no specific treatment and perhaps the French have the most pragmatic approach to the problem – they give anxious patients a special comb with which they can keep the hairs clean.

A geographic tongue (CP-48) is characterized by the recurrent appearance and disappearance of red patches. Reassurance is required after the diagnosis has been made.

HALITOSIS

Causes

Offensive breath – halitosis – may arise from either extraoral or intraoral causes. The extraoral causes include diseases of the upper respiratory tract, especially chronic sinusitis with a postnasal drip. Odoriferous substances may be eliminated in expired air:

- food (garlic)
- beverages (alcohol)
- drugs (chloral hydrate)
- tobacco

Abnormal accumulations of waste products can also cause odour:

- urea
- ketones

Hyperacidity and reflux-oesophagitis can cause halitosis, and morning bad breath may be due to lack of salivation during sleeping hours.

Oral causes of bad breath are usually poor oral hygiene and periodontal disease.

Food collects in pockets between the teeth and gums, becoming rancid and resulting in gingivitis. This is diagnosed by finding debris around the tooth roots and in gum pockets. Food can also collect in tonsillar crypts and give the same result. Caries and oral ulcers may also be the cause of halitosis, while oral tumours with ulceration give off a particularly bad smell.

LIMITATION OF JAW OPENING

There are several causes of limitation of jaw opening:

- trauma to the joint or head of condyle
- trismus

  This occasionally occurs after an injection of local anaesthetic in the areas of the pterygomandibular raphe. It may also represent tumour spread into the pterygoid muscles.

- temporomandibular joint dysfunction

  This frequently causes limitation of jaw opening.

- scleroderma
- carcinoma in pterygomaxillary fossa

  In practice this means involvement of posterior maxilla and soft palate from maxillary or oropharyngeal tumours.

- fibrosis following major head surgery

SECTION IV
Description of specific diseases of the oral cavity

ORAL ULCERATION

Aphthous ulceration

Three types of ulcers are recognized:

- minor aphthae
  These are most common (CP-39). They are small painful ulcers occurring anywhere in the oral mucosa, either singly or in small crops.

- major aphthae
  These are much less common. The ulcers are usually single larger and deeper. These ulcers may heal leaving a scar.

- herpetiform ulcers
  A large number of very small ulcers occur in crops. They are very rare and the term used is descriptive rather than an indication of aetiology.

It should be noted that oral ulceration associated with ocular and genital ulceration may be due to Behçet's syndrome.

Causes

The predisposing causes include:

- hereditary factors
- hormonal factors
- emotional factors

Management

Treatment is palliative supported by oral hygiene measures (Section V, p. 127).

Dental traumatic ulcers

If there is a broken tooth or a sharp edge on a filling,

usually in the lower molar region, then the tongue will rub on it and become ulcerated. These ulcers can look very sinister but the cause is usually obvious. Just because an ulcer exists beside a bad tooth does not, however, prove that it is dental in origin. The ulcer must start to heal after the tooth is repaired – if it does not heal a biopsy is required (CP-37).

This pattern of ulceration often occurs with an ill-fitting denture (CP-38).

CANCER

If a mouth ulcer is seen in a patient over the age of 30 – 'think cancer'. Only in this way can the diagnosis be made early enough to get good results from treatment.

There is no excuse for not biopsying an ulcer that is not healing after 2 weeks treatment. There is no differentiating feature between the different types of ulcer and so clinical diagnosis can be erratic.

The lateral edge of the tongue is the most usual site, followed by the floor of the mouth and alveolus, the palate and the cheek.

CANCER OF THE TONGUE

Cancer of the tongue is decreasing in incidence because syphilis and the habit of chewing tobacco are less common. Better dental hygiene has also been a factor (CP-49).

Causes

There are few premalignant conditions; leukoplakia

of the oral cavity is of sinister significance, especially if there is histological evidence of dyskeratosis. Erythroplakia is more frequently premalignant.

A total of 80% of tongue tumours are squamous cell carcinomas. The remainder are lymphomas and salivary gland tumours. The tumour is more common in males than females and the maximum incidence is between the ages of 60 and 70.

Clinical features

The commonest site is the lateral edge of the tongue. The tumour spreads across the floor of the mouth on to the alveolus. More than half of the squamous carcinomas spread to neck glands.

Presentation

The patient presents with a tongue mass which is usually ulcerated, and perhaps with a palpable neck gland.

Pain is a variable feature. The history usually extends back over several months with the patient taking unsuccessful courses of treatment with antibiotics and lozenges. This is unfortunate, for the differential diagnosis of a tongue ulcer is limited. It can only be a cancer, or a dental ulcer for which there should be a very obvious cause. Aphthous ulcers seldom grow very big and occur in crops. Tuberculosis and syphilis are almost never seen now.

Investigations

Diagnosis is by biopsy.

Management

The treatment which gives the best results is removal of part of the tongue along with a radical neck dissection (Section V, p. 127).

If the tumour involves the mandible then part or all of the affected bone will have to be removed. Bone grafting can be carried out to repair the defect.

There is little place for external irradiation but radium needles are often successful.

CANCER OF THE LIP

Causes

This is commonest in East Anglia and north-east Scotland – areas that are mainly agricultural. Outdoor workers tend to get a dyskeratosis of the lower lip which gives the mucosa a whitish appearance – actinic cheilitis. This is now the typical premalignant condition. The contributory role of clay pipe smoking is hardly ever evident now.

Clinical features

The tumour has little variety in its presentation. It is a disease of males over the age of 60, and 99% occur in the lower lip (CP-50).

Almost all are squamous cell carcinomas. Lip cancers grow very slowly and rarely produce glandular metastases. The differential diagnosis is between keratoacanthosis, syphilis and tuberculosis. Before any treatment is undertaken biopsy must be done to establish the diagnosis.

Management

In actinic cheilitis the mucosa of the exposed part of the lip is removed. The remaining mucosa is freed down to the alveolar sulci and advanced forward to be sutured to the skin edge, so forming a new lip. This is called a 'lip shave and vermilion advancement' (see also Section V, p. 127).

In an established cancer, up to one third of the lip can be excised in a V-shape and the lip edges closed together with no loss of function or alteration in appearance.

If more than one third of the lip has to be removed the defect has to be closed by flaps taken from the upper lip.

If glands are present a radical neck dissection is done.

CLEFT LIP AND PALATE

A cleft lip is an ugly deformity. A child with a cleft palate is potentially handicapped by poor speech and hearing. A child born with a cleft lip and palate suffers the disadvantage of both (CP-51).

There is a higher incidence in males when the cleft involves the lip alone. There are also racial variations.

Cleft lip is three times less common in Negroes than it is in whites, and it appears to be most common in Japanese and Malayans. Overall in every 1000 births there is one child born with a cleft lip with or without cleft palate.

The likelihood of this deformity occurring increases to one in 25 if either a sibling or a parent is affected with the deformity.

With cleft palate alone, the incidence is much lower – about one in every 2300 births – and females are affected more often than males in the ratio of 3:2.

Causes

In the normal embryo, the paired nasomedial processes fuse to form the middle or philtrum of the upper lip and the maxillary processes then join the nasomedial process to form the lateral part of the lip. The nasomedial processes also form the alveolus and the palate in front of the incisive foramen.

The normal palate arises from fusion of the two lateral palatal shelves with the nasomedial process. These meet behind the incisive foramen and join from the front backwards. A cleft palate results from failure of fusion of the lateral palatal shelves and, depending on where the fusion ceases, may be of varying degree.

The cleft palate may be accompanied by a cleft lip. It occurs between the fifth and ninth weeks of gestation. The aetiology is not known.

Clinical features

Every child with a unilateral cleft lip has a vermilion-lined notch in the full thickness of the upper lip. This may be wide or narrow, is always to one side of the midline and may extend from the free margin of the lip up into the nasal vestibule. There is always a flattening of the inferior nasal cartilage (alar cartilage) on the affected side. This varies with the width of the cleft. In the bilateral cleft lip, the prolabium and premaxilla may project markedly.

Clefts in the palate may vary from a bifid uvula to a cleft which extends through the hard and soft palate and into the alveolus. The muscles of the soft palate are inserted abnormally into the hard palate and the palate is usually short.

If the lip, alveolus and palate are cleft, the deformity is increased due to the wide separation of the medial and lateral segments in an anteroposterior as well as in a mediolateral direction. The maxilla on the cleft side is often hypoplastic.

Management

Repair of a cleft lip is carried out when the child is about 3 months old. Various flaps have been designed in the area of the cleft to release tissue so that a non-tension closure can be achieved (Section V, p. 127).

Repair of a cleft palate is carried out at about 9 months. Palatal flaps are created and the mucosa is closed over the cleft on both the nasal and palatal surfaces. Thereafter orthodontic and prosthodontic treatment is required to correct the upper jaw appearance.

INFECTIONS OF THE ORAL CAVITY

Infections may affect both the soft and hard tissues. Infection of the oral mucosa may be localized, or it may affect the oral cavity as a whole – when the term 'stomatitis' is applied.

Causes

Bacterial infections

Apart from secondary infections, the following bacterial infections are of importance in the oral cavity.

Acute ulceromembranous gingivitis (Vincent's infection)

This is a mixed bacterial infection of spirochaete vibrios and fusiform bacilli. These organisms are normally commensals, but an altered host–parasite relationship allows tissue invasion.

The presentation is with some bleeding of the gums, a bad taste and halitosis. Necrosis and ulceration of the marginal papillary gingivae are evident. Early in the disease the interdental papillae are destroyed. Their sloughing bases are delineated from the surrounding tissues by a linear erythema. Bacterial investigation reveals the organisms.

Granulomas

Syphilis is an extreme rarity in developed countries but tuberculosis is still occasionally seen. Oral tuberculous lesions are usually secondary to pulmonary tuberculosis. The tongue is the most common site. In syphilis the lesions appear on the lips or tip of tongue as firm ulcers.

Fungal infections

Candida albicans

Local and systemic factors may predispose to candidal infections of the oral cavity. Systemic ingestion of broad spectrum antibiotics suppresses the bacterial flora of the mouth and facilitates candidiasis.

Candidiasis may present as white, removable plaques (pseudomembranous candidiasis or thrush) or as bright-red thinned mucosa confined to the denture-bearing area (atrophic candidiasis – denture sore mouth).

Treatment is by correcting the underlying predisposing factors and by using antifungal agents such as nystatin or amphotericin B lozenges and cream. Ill-fitting dentures should be replaced.

Viral infections

Herpes simplex

The initial infection with herpes simplex – primary herpetic stomatitis – is associated with widespread intraoral vesicles and ulceration. It commonly occurs in infancy and childhood.

For the 10–14 days during which the condition lasts, the patient suffers oral soreness, loss of appetite, fever and difficulty in sleeping. On examination cervical lymph node enlargement may be found.

After the primary infection, herpes simplex presents as a vesicular lesion of the lips – herpes labialis or cold sore. Its appearance is precipitated by sunlight or stress.

Herpes zoster

This condition may affect the oral cavity but is much rarer than herpes simplex infections.

Measles

During the prodromal stage, small white spots with an erythematous margin – Koplik's spots – may appear in the buccal mucosa. These are of no clinical significance other than diagnostic value and no treatment is required.

TEETH AND GUMS

The main diseases affecting the teeth and gums are caries and periodontitis. Both are intimately associated with dental plaque. Plaque consists of large numbers of bacteria embedded in a matrix of protein and carbohydrate derived from saliva, epithelial cells and food debris.

Plaque adheres to the teeth. It forms rapidly on exposed tooth surfaces, especially round the necks of teeth, in tooth fissures and at contact points where there is poor oral hygiene.

Caries

Dental caries is the most common disease affecting man (CP-36).

Causes

There are many causes but three defined conditions must exist before it can develop:

- micro-organisms
  These must be present to form acid and are found in plaque.
- fermentable carbohydrates
  These diffuse into plaque and act as a substrate for the acid-producing organisms.
- tooth substance susceptible to acid
  This is dependent upon the hardness of the teeth, the age of the patient and other factors.

When enamel has been broken down, the caries involves the dentine. The tubules of the dentine allow the transmission of noxious stimuli to the odontoblasts. These respond by laying down a protective layer of secondary dentine. This is an irregular deposition with few, if any tubules present. Within the carious lesion tubular dentine breaks down into irregular masses of debris.

Management

Treatment is removal of the caries and filling the cavity.

In larger cavities the deposition of secondary dentine may be outpaced by the carious advance. The pulpal blood vessels engorge and as the blood vessels of the pulp are contained in rigid walls of dentine, the inflammatory changes produce an increase in pressure. This compresses the blood vessels and may occlude them.

The pain of pulpitis is mainly due to the effect of pressure on the nerve fibres of the pulp.

If pulpal death occurs, necrotic material results. This may irritate the supporting tissues and cause a periodontal or apical abscess. The resulting pain may be acute or chronic (CP-52).

The tooth should be extracted or the root filled (see Section V). Antibiotic therapy is useful before the abscess drains.

Periodontal disease

Causes

Periodontal disease occurs as a result of an interaction of systemic and local factors, the most important of these being dental plaque (CP-53).

If undisturbed, plaque undergoes mineralization to produce calculus. Brushing cannot remove calculus but it can be removed by dental instruments.

Bacteria in the plaque can cause inflammation of the adjacent gingival margins and a loss of the binding power of the collagen fibres between the gingival tissue and the underlying periostium.

Bleeding, swollen gums are a feature of the condition. Bleeding and pain prevents proper oral hygiene and the condition is therefore exacerbated.

Management

A careful scaling and polishing of the teeth should be carried out. Continuing chronic inflammation causes fibrosis of the tissues and the gingival anatomy is permanently damaged. Gum recession occurs with ever-deepening pockets between the gums and the teeth. These become loose and drift out of alignment. (Section V, p. oo). Gingival surgery may be necessary to eliminate the pocket.

A periodontal abscess is a localized exacerbation of infection within the periodontal pocket with pus formation. It is associated with established periodontal disease. Its features are discomfort and a lateral swelling alongside a non-carious or minimally restored tooth. Drainage is indicated.

Oroantral fistula

Causes

An oroantral fistula is an opening between the antrum and oral cavity through which air and fluids may pass (LD-55). It is an uncommon complication following extraction of an upper molar tooth.

Clinical features

Infection is a common and serious complication of an oroantral fistula and, if sinusitis ensues and the fistula remains untreated, the opening becomes permanent.

The symptoms which accompany an oroantral fistula include a salty taste and the passage of fluid from the mouth out through the nose. Pain and swelling in the mouth due to prolapse of the antral lining may occur and blowing the nose may force air into the mouth.

Management

The treatment is by surgery. The edges of the socket are trimmed to make this possible and closure carried out together with a radical antrostomy.

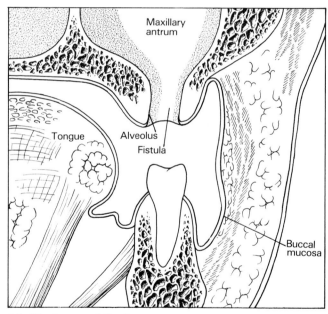

LD-55. *Oroantral fistula*

SECTION V

Principles of general management and treatment of the oral cavity

THE PRINCIPLES OF GENERAL MANAGEMENT AND TREATMENT

Mouth ulcers

The treatment of mouth ulcers is directed at the removal of the underlying cause. Traumatic ulcers heal within 10–14 days after removal of the cause. Any ulcer which persists beyond this time should be regarded with suspicion and biopsy is indicated. A multitude of therapeutic regimes, mostly empirical, are employed in the treatment of recurrent aphthous ulceration.

Topical antiseptics and anaesthetics

These keep the lesions clean and may lessen pain and discomfort. Zinc chloride and zinc sulphate mouth washes have a useful astringent quality and 0.2% aqueous chlorhexidine solution has the added advantage of controlling plaque formation.

The use of surface anaesthetic gels or, in severe cases, xylocaine viscous solution is useful in reducing pain.

Antibiotics

A 2.5% tetracycline mouthwash may be of value for 'herpetiform' aphthous ulcers. However, the very real dangers of upsetting the oral flora and inducing candidiasis must be borne in mind.

Corticosteroids

These suppress inflammatory reactions and may thus limit ulceration.

Corlan

Hydrocortisone sodium succinate as a 2.5 mg lozenge may be placed near an oral lesion and allowed to dissolve slowly. Two or four lozenges per day for 4–12 days is the usual regime.

Betamethasone tablets

These may be dissolved in water and used as a mouthwash 4–6 times a day.

Adcortyl A in Orabase

An 0.1% triamcinolone acetonide in an emollient base (Adcortyl in Orabase) can be applied to lesions 2–3 times a day prior to meals.

PRINCIPLES OF ORAL SURGERY

The lip

Lip shave and vermilion advancement

This is performed to remove all the lip mucosa in actinic cheilitis (see above Section IV, p. 123).

An incision is made along the mucocutaneous border, and the lip mucosa is carefully dissected off the orbicularis oris right down into the labioalveolar sulcus. The flap is then pulled forward, the cheilitic portion cut off and healthy mucosa stitched to the skin edge.

Wedge excision

For a cancer limited to a size that, with 5 mm margins, requires removing less than one third of the total length of the lip, a V-excision is done through the whole thickness of the lip (LD-56). This allows closure to be done in a straight line with minimal scarring.

The tongue

Hemiglossectomy

Up to half of a tongue can be removed without

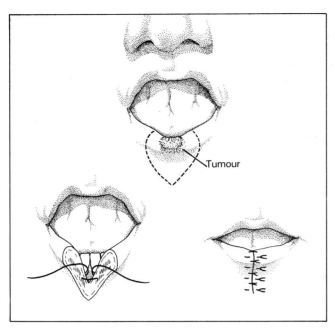

LD-56. V excision of cancer of the lip

crippling the oral cavity. Either the edge of the tongue can be attached to the alveolus, or else a flap of chest or forehead skin can be brought in to give the tongue more mobility (LD-57).

A hemiglossectomy is nearly always combined with a radical neck dissection. The patient should be able to go home eating a soft diet after 2 weeks.

Mandibulectomy

This is often part of oral cancer surgery, if the tumour has spread to the alveolus. It can be partial or complete. Partial mandibulectomy, which leaves a rim of mandible, causes little functional or cosmetic abnormality. Excision of a complete segment of the mandible, however, requires grafting with a piece of rib.

This applies particularly in the anterior arch where loss of tongue support leads to constant drooling and a tragic-comic appearance. This is called the 'Andy Gump' deformity, after a strip cartoon character in the *Boston Globe*.

Cleft lip and palate

Preoperative treatment

If the cleft is complete through lip, alveolus and palate, there tends to be an increasing malalignment of all parts of the cleft. It is then best treated soon after birth by a combination of an intraoral plate and external restraining strapping. This helps to control the projecting premaxilla.

Repair of the cleft lip

The lip is repaired when the child is about 3 months old. In a unilateral cleft lip skin, muscle and mucosa are present on either side of the cleft, although in an abnormal position (LD-58). The lip on both sides of the cleft is freed from abnormal attachments and advanced to cover the gap.

The associated deformity of the nasal cartilage is corrected at the time of lip closure by mobilizing and repositioning the cartilage.

Repair of cleft palate

This is performed soon after the child is 9 months old. As well as closing the lip, the palate is lengthened so that the repaired soft palate can reach the posterior pharynx and occlude the oropharynx from the nasopharynx (LD-59). This prevents nasal escape during speech and acts as a barrier to prevent food from passing into the nasopharynx.

When the child is 4, speech is assessed and can often be corrected by the speech therapist. If there is a

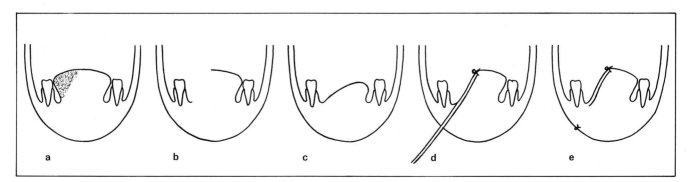

*LD-57. Operation for removal of tongue cancer showing two methods of repair. **a**, Tongue cancer. **b**, After excision of upper alveolus and part of tongue. This may be followed by **c**, primary closure of tongue to buccal mucosa. Alternatively it may be followed by **d**, chest flap sewn to tongue, and **e**, chest flap replaced and cleft closed*

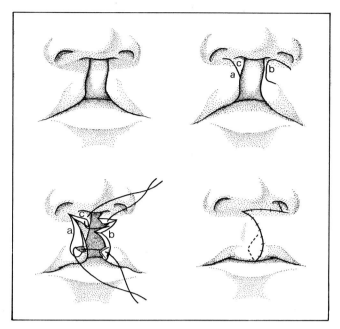

LD-58. Operation for cleft lip. The Millard technique for complete cleft of the lip. Flap a is rotated, flap b advanced and flap c transposed

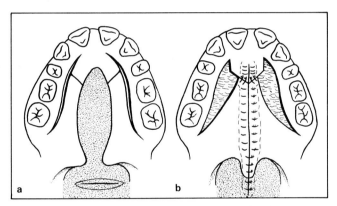

*LD-59. Operation for cleft palate. The Wardill technique. **a**, Outline of the incision and mobilization of the mucoperiosteal flaps. **b**, Complete closure for increased length of palate and greater prominence of Passavant's ridge on the posterior pharyngeal wall*

significant degree of nasal escape due to the soft palate not reaching the pharynx, then an operation which either narrows the pharynx – a pharyngoplasty – or which occludes the junction of oropharynx and nasopharynx – a pharyngeal flap – is performed. This markedly improves speech.

Follow-up

The initial treatment of cleft lip and palate is performed in infancy. The patient should be followed-up into full adulthood by a team consisting of:

- a speech therapist
  Will assess, advise and treat faulty speech.
- an orthodontist
  Will supervise the shape of the growing alveolar arch and correct the commonly occurring malocclusion of teeth.
- an oral surgeon
  Will deal with abnormal teeth and any necessary mandibular or maxillary surgery.
- an otolaryngologist
  Will assess and treat the commonly occurring ear and internal nasal disorders.
- a plastic surgeon
  Will supervise the total care of the patient and perform any necessary secondary surgery.

Prosthetic appliances are constructed not only to seal the oronasal defect, but also to widen the occlusal surface of the upper arch. These restore the bite and the vertical height of the lower part of the face.

In edentulous patients with oronasal defects, retention of the upper denture is obtained from the obturator.

PRINCIPLES OF DENTAL TREATMENT

Conservative dentistry

In the restoration of teeth which have been damaged by caries or accident the aims of treatment are:
- removal of the diseased tooth substance
- preservation of pulp vitality
- restoration of the tooth form and function

If preservation of pulp vitality is impossible, sterilization and sealing to prevent infection should be carried out.

Cavities should be designed to be self-retentive and the margins must be extended into areas which can be readily cleaned.

When dentine has been exposed a lining should normally be placed under the filling. The filling materials commonly used are a silver–tin amalgam in posterior teeth and silicate, or newer composites, in anterior teeth (LD-60). Silicate filling materials are very acid and an adequate lining must be used to protect the pulp from damage.

Techniques
When caries is more extensive, special methods for retention of the filling material have to be used.

In many cases gold inlays can be utilized but, where little tooth substance remains, retention pins can be anchored into the tooth. The filling material is packed round the pins and the tooth contour restored.

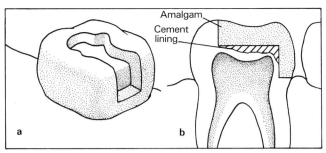

*LD-60. Sectional view of cavity with filling. **a**, Two-surface filling on a molar tooth with the cavity prepared and lined. **b**, Sectional view showing lining and filling and relationship to the pulp*

Crowns

Broken-down teeth may be restored by crowning. The stump of the tooth is prepared to allow the fitting of a crown or cap.

This is fabricated in the laboratory from an impression of the prepared tooth and can be constructed in gold or porcelain. Crowns are frequently used as abutment pieces in bridgework because of their strength.

Endodontics

If the pulp of a tooth dies, the dead space should be eliminated by root filling since the products of tissue degeneration cause apical irritation or infection.

Apicectomy

Chronic periapical infection is frequently difficult to treat by conventional means and surgery may be required.

A full thickness flap of tissue is raised over the buccal alveolus, the alveolar plate pierced, the apex of the tooth removed and the area debrided. Once the residual pulp canal has been carefully root-filled, the wound is closed.

Prosthodontics

Missing teeth can be replaced by fixed or removable prostheses. In addition, the prosthodontist deals with the fabrication of obturators and complex prostheses for cleft palate patients and the orofacial prostheses used after trauma or radical surgery in or around the mouth.

Full dentures

The loss of teeth results in the loss of their specialized supporting structures. Full dentures rest on the mucosa of the gum ridges. This is a tissue poorly adapted to accept the full force of the muscles of mastication.

Dentures must be extended to utilize the maximum available support area and particular care must be taken to ensure that the upper and lower teeth meet evenly. Good dentures should look natural, function well and be comfortable.

Partial dentures

Partial dentures replace single or multiple lost teeth.

Tooth borne partial dentures

In this type of partial denture, the whole weight of mastication is taken by the standing teeth through 'rests' placed on them. Partial dentures are usually firmly clasped in place to the natural teeth.

Tissue borne partial dentures

These dentures are used when insufficient teeth remain to support the masticatory load. They are usually clasped to natural teeth for retention purposes while the stresses of occlusion are taken on the oral mucosa.

As this tissue is compressible, movement of the denture relative to the standing teeth occurs during chewing. If the appliance is closely adapted round the necks of the teeth, the constant rubbing may cause gingival damage.

Periodontal treatment

Dental plaque and calculus are important aetiological factors in periodontal disease. Gingivitis is dealt with by careful oral hygiene, scaling and polishing of the teeth.

Subgingival curettage

This operation is carried out using sharp periodontal hoes to remove the plaque, calculus and necrotic cementum which line the soft tissue margins of the periodontal pocket.

Gingivectomy

This operation is designed to recontour gingival architecture and to eliminate soft tissue pockets (LD-61).

After determining the depth of the pocket, excess tissue is trimmed away using hooked scalpel blades.

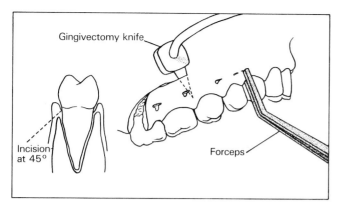

LD-61. *Gingivectomy. A surgical reshaping of the gingival tissues to eliminate pockets*

Flap operation

This is undertaken in cases where the pockets are so deep that gingivectomy is impossible.

A full thickness mucoperiosteal flap is raised from the neck of the teeth into the buccal or labial sulci. The treatment may include bone recontouring. The flaps are replaced and held in place by interrupted interdental sutures.

Dental or minor oral surgery

Minor oral surgery includes extraction of infected or ineffective teeth and roots, the treatment of cysts, and the corrective shaping of the alveolar ridges for dentures. Local anaesthesia is all that is usually required.

Forceps extraction

The blades of the selected forceps are passed well down along the root of the tooth and the crown and root gripped firmly (LD-62). The tooth is moved to expand the surrounding bone and tear the periodontal membrane attaching the tooth to the socket walls. The tooth can then be lifted out. Dead teeth or those with heavy fillings are liable to crumble, while teeth with abnormal roots may resist removal. In such cases, surgical removal is indicated. When root shape and other factors preclude normal extraction, a full thickness mucoperiosteal flap must be reflected. Once the investing bone is exposed, the tooth can be freed by removing bone with chisels or burrs.

Apart from fractured roots and buried teeth, impacted lower third molars are the most frequently encountered oral surgical problem. The cases vary considerably in difficulty depending upon the anatomy and the angle of the tooth.

Cysts are treated by enucleation or marsupialization.

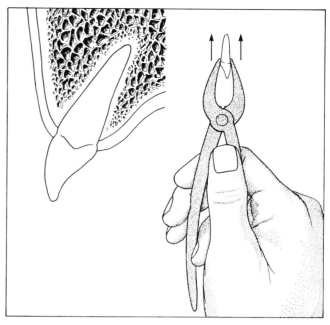

LD-62. *Forceps extraction. The forceps are applied to the neck of a maxillary incisor. Pressure is alternated lingually and labially to enlarge the alveolus. The tooth is then rotated mesially (medially) and lifted from the socket*

Orthodontic treatment

Malocclusion denotes failure of teeth to erupt into the ideal position so that they can meet harmoniously with their opponents in the opposite jaw. The aims of orthodontic treatment are to:

- improve appearance
- improve function

Malocclusions are assessed clinically from the bone relation of the maxilla and the mandible. A more specific approach is Angle's classification. This uses the occlusal relationship of the teeth to classify deviations from normal (LD-63).

Class I

There is normal anteroposterior occlusion of the cheek teeth but there are local abnormalities, e.g. incisor overcrowding.

Class II

The lower teeth meet the upper teeth behind their normal position. The chin is often receded.

Class III

This is the opposite of Class II. The mandibular

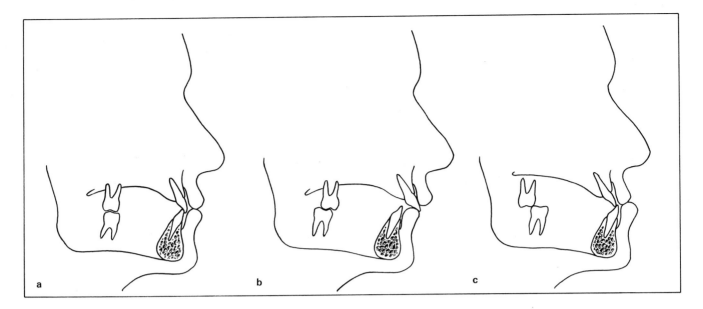

molars meet the maxillary molars in front of their normal position. The chin is often prominent. Both genetic and environmental causes are responsible for malocclusion.

LD-63. *Classification of malocclusions. **a**, Class I skeletal pattern. **b**, Class II skeletal pattern. **c**, Class III skeletal pattern*

Management

Treatment can be divided into preventive and active. Preventive orthodontic treatment avoids malocclusion by careful monitoring of the developing dentition and by serial extraction of deciduous and permanent teeth to prevent any anticipated overcrowding.

Active orthodontic treatment involves the use of various types of appliances which apply light pressure to the tooth or teeth to be moved.

TEST-YOURSELF QUESTIONS
Part 5 – The Oral Cavity

1. Dentine:
a) is the most highly calcified substance in the body
b) is tubular
c) conveys sensory stimuli
d) forms an attachment to the periodontal ligament
e) forms the bulk of the tooth

2. Halitosis can arise from:
a) ingested foodstuffs
b) candidal infection
c) Vincent's infection
d) caries
e) dental apical abcess

3. The symptomatic features of Vincent's infection are:
a) pain
b) white patches on the buccal mucosa
c) halitosis
d) anaemia
e) interdental ulceration

4. Sensory innervation of the anterior $\frac{2}{3}$ of the tongue is from the:
a) glossopharyngeal nerve
b) hypoglossal nerve
c) trigeminal nerve
d) facial nerve
e) lingual nerve

5. The most likely causes of limitation of jaw opening in an 18-year-old female are:
a) trauma
b) scleroderma
c) TMJ syndrome
d) carcinoma of the nasopharynx
e) fibrosis

6. Bleeding gums are frequent occurrence; what are the likely causes in a 25-year-old housewife?
a) gingivitis
b) pregnancy
c) pericoronitis
d) aspirin burn
e) dental caries

7. A loose full upper denture may be the result of:
a) underextension
b) patient is a mouth breather
c) candidal infection
d) hyperkeratosis
e) wrong bite

8. A patient complains of pain when wearing dentures. This may result from:
a) poor fit
b) candidal infection
c) atrophic tissues
d) vitam B_{12} deficiency
e) wrong bite

9. Pain from the teeth with heat or cold is likely to be due to:
a) caries
b) gingivitis
c) exposed dentine
d) sinusitis
e) unlined fillings

10. Intraoral pain from an 18-year-old patient is likely to be due to:
a) caries
b) pericoronitis
c) sinusitis
d) periodontal disease
e) aphthous ulceration

The answers to these questions will be found on p. 191.

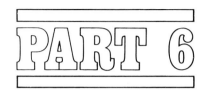

THE SALIVARY GLANDS

SECTION I

Background to salivary gland disease

ANATOMY

There are four main salivary glands – two parotids, which are mainly serous, and two submandibular glands, which are mixed serous and mucus (LD-64).

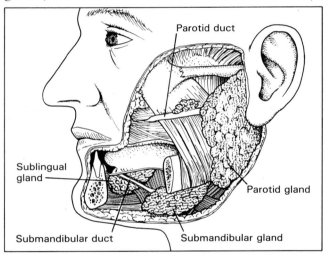

LD-64. *Salivary glands, showing position of the parotid and submandibular glands*

Multiple small collections of salivary tissue, called 'minor salivary glands', occur throughout the oral cavity and laryngopharynx.

The parotid lies on the masseter muscle, extending from the zygoma above to the lower border of the mandible below and running below and behind the lobe of the ear. The parotid duct opens opposite the 2nd upper molar teeth at the anterior border of masseter (LD-65).

The submandibular glands lie under the horizontal ramus of the mandible and the duct opens in the midline on either side of the frenulum of the tongue (LD-66). The gland does not extend further back than the angle of the mandible. This is an important differential diagnostic point between a submandibular and tonsillar gland enlargement.

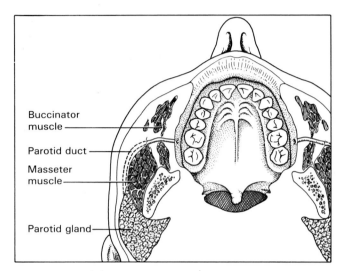

LD-65. *Parotid duct*

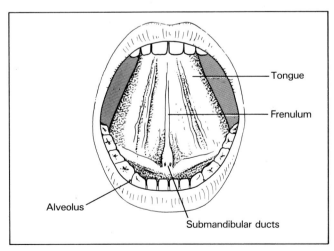

LD-66. *Submandibular duct*

Although in the cadaver (and so in the anatomy books!) the parotid is in two fairly well defined lobes, with the facial nerve between the lobes, it is not like that in the living body. It is better to think of it like a lump of bread dough (parotid) dropped on to an egg whisk (facial nerve) – some runs through, some surrounds the whisk and most lies on top.

Structure

The salivary glands are comprised of acinar cells and a duct system, both intra- and extraglandular, supported by connective tissue. This divides the gland into lobules and supports the neurovascular elements. The control of secretion is complex and is regulated by the autonomic nervous system.

Function

The function of the salivary glands is to produce the saliva which keeps the oral cavity moist, facilitates speech and lubricates food for chewing and swallowing. Saliva is essential for taste acuity and oral hygiene.

The secretion and composition of saliva is variable and many constituents are site dependent. Factors influencing composition include:

- sex
- flow rate
- diet
- hormones
- drugs
- time of day

Saliva has important bacterial functions. By virtue of the local production of immunoglobulin – largely IgA with small amounts of IgG and IgM – the salivary glands may influence the course of oral and dental disease. The factors which alter salivary flow rate include:

- age
- sex
- anxiety states
- drugs

Diurnal variation and environmental factors such as temperature, light and diet are also important.

A consequence of xerostomia (dry mouth) is an increase in oral infection, dental caries and the loss of the important functions previously described.

Sialorrhoea (increased salivation) is rare. Causes of sialorrhoea are acute infections and, especially, neurological disturbance. Here the problems result from difficulty in swallowing rather than excessive production of saliva.

Systemic disease such as fibrocystic disease, thyroid disease, sialosis, hypertension, adrenal disease, diabetes and connective tissue disease may all cause abnormalities in salivary composition. The careful analysis of saliva may thus provide a useful screening and diagnostic test for certain of these conditions.

SECTION II

History and physical examination of the salivary glands

HISTORY

Most patients with disorders of the salivary glands present with a complaint of pain, or swelling, or a mass in a gland.

Specific questions

Pain

If the complaint is of pain, establish the following facts:

- where is the pain?
  Many related structures mimic salivary gland pain – teeth, the temporomandibular joint, the external ear.

- what is its character?
  Sharp pain associated with meals may indicate an obstructive lesion, while deep-seated continuing pain may mean a malignant tumour.

- how bad is it?
  Sialectasis or swelling of the salivary glands can cause such severe pain that eating is impossible.

- how long has it been present?

- is it increasing or decreasing?
  Increasing pain is almost always related to a malignant tumour, usually the adenoid cystic type.

- what makes it worse?
  Eating makes an obstructive lesion worse.

- are there any associated symptoms?
  Some endocrine diseases such as myxoedema, diabetes mellitus and Cushing's disease may be associated with salivary gland disease.

Lump or swelling

If there is a localized lump or a general swelling, then the following questions should be asked:

- how long has the swelling been present?

- is it getting bigger?
  Benign tumours usually grow very slowly but occasionally there may be growth spurts, perhaps due to haemorrhage. This brings the mass to the patient's attention.

- is the swelling single or multiple?
  Sjögren's syndrome usually affects all four main salivary glands. Tumours are almost always unilateral. While a number of glands can be affected by sialectasis, symptoms are only present in one.

- is it painful?

- is there any facial nerve weakness?
  If this has occurred, then the mass is malignant.

- does eating make it worse?

- what drugs has the patient been taking?
  Enquire specifically about Distalgesic (comprising dextropropoxyphene and paracetamol), phenylbutazone, thiouracil and tetracycline, because allergic reactions to these commonly present as salivary gland enlargement often accompanied by pain.

EXAMINATION

Physical examination of the salivary glands should be performed in a systematic fashion. The whole of the cervicofacial region should be inspected and the salivary gland areas palpated, both extra- and intraorally.

The salivary duct orifices should be identified and, when indicated, explored with fine metal probes.

Inspection

For the extraoral inspection, the examiner stands directly in front of and facing the patient about a metre (3–4 ft) away. Signs of asymmetry, discoloration, visible pulsation and the presence of a sinus should be sought. Enlargement, the commonest sign of salivary gland disease, may be unilateral or bilateral and may involve one or all glands. Evidence of minor salivary gland swelling should be sought during the intraoral inspection.

Palpation

Bimanual palpation should be carried out, using the palmar surface of the tips of the fingers. A delicate but firm rotatory motion should be employed. It is often useful for the examiner to stand behind the patient, whose head is inclined forward. The major salivary glands and other neck swellings are thus more easily palpated, since flexion of the neck relaxes the tissues in this region.

The submandibular and parotid glands are palpated bimanually, using both intra- and extraoral approaches. The intraoral minor salivary glands may be palpated by gentle but firm compression.

The patency of the salivary duct orifices may be detected by exerting pressure on the gland and observing the flow of saliva from the orifice. The colour, texture and viscosity of saliva should be noted. A lachrymal probe dilator may be helpful in identifying the duct orifice and in the detection of a duct stricture or calculus.

INVESTIGATIONS

Collection of saliva

This does not form part of the investigation of salivary gland disease except in specialized units.

Samples of mixed or total saliva or separated secretions from the major salivary glands may be collected by a variety of methods. Collecting devices have been developed for the separate major salivary glands.

For parotid or submandibular saliva, a polyethylene catheter suction cup may be employed. A segregator appliance is used to collect submandibular or sublingual saliva. Capillary tubes are used to collect minor gland saliva. Mixed or total saliva is collected using methods such as spitting, drainage, suction or the application of cotton wool rolls.

Laboratory tests

Laboratory tests can be of great value in the diagnosis and treatment of salivary gland disease. Samples of salivary secretions, gland tissue and serum may be submitted for microbiological, histopathological, biochemical and serological examination.

Although its value in clinical practice is limited, measurement of salivary immunoglobulins is possible, using radioimmunodiffusion techniques.

Measurement of serum antibodies such as rheumatoid factor, antinuclear factor and salivary duct antibodies may be of value where salivary gland involvement occurs as part of a connective tissue disorder.

Biochemical analysis of the constituents of saliva in conditions such as Sjögren's syndrome, cystic fibrosis and sarcoidosis may be useful.

A specimen of salivary gland tissue is obtained by incisional, punch or aspiration biopsy techniques.

Radiology

This is the most important investigation in a patient with a salivary gland problem and, next to the history and examination, gives most information.

Plain film radiological examination of the salivary glands is helpful in the diagnosis of calculi in the glands and ducts. Submandibular stones are radio-opaque but most parotid stones are radiolucent (X-30).

Sialography is the radiographic demonstration of the salivary duct system by the introduction of a radio-opaque medium through the duct orifice (X-31).

The salivary glands comprise a main duct and peripheral branching ducts. These, when filled with radio-opaque contrast media, can help locate calcification and space-occupying lesions. In the parotid, the main duct lies lateral to the masseter and at its anterior edge while the submandibular duct descends at the posterior edge of the mylohyoid muscle to enter the submandibular space.

Calcified masses within the gland or duct may be obscured by the teeth and bones of the face. Thus anterior-posterior and lateral oblique films are necessary to throw the glands into relief.

In sialography the medium may be introduced by a hand injection technique, although a hydrostatic method which allows a water soluble medium to flow into the duct system at a constant pressure is favoured. Filling of the gland occurs rapidly and an exposure taken after 5 seconds represents the filling phase film. A secretory phase film is taken a few minutes later after the patient has sucked a lemon. The medium is excreted and normally no retention is observed at this time.

Sialography is a useful technique in the diagnosis of calculi, especially radiolucent stones, duct stricture, chronic inflammatory conditions, fistula and neoplastic disease of the salivary glands. It is contraindicated where there is acute sialadenitis and or where there is a history of allergy to iodine – the main constituent of the contrast medium.

Radioisotopes

Radioisotopes for testing salivary gland function are used in two main ways. Firstly, they may be detected and measured in saliva and, secondly, uptake of the isotopes by the glands themselves may be detected and visualized by scintiscanning and scintography.

Radioisotopes have been used to assess physiological function and to assess function in pathological states, especially neoplastic disease and Sjögren's syndrome. They can also localize ectopic salivary tissue.

The salivary glands concentrate inorganic iodide in saliva to many times the plasma level and this forms the basis of both tests. Salivary radioiodine concentration has been measured in patients with thyroid disease or Sjögren's syndrome and in defects of iodide trapping. Radioisotope visualization, using either the scanner or gamma camera, uses ^{99m}Tc labelled sodium pertechnetate in preference to isotopes of iodine because of its shorter half-life and very low radiation dosage to the tissues.

SECTION III

Presentation of salivary gland disease and the diagnostic possibilities

PAROTID GLAND PAIN

Parotid pain is nearly always accompanied by some degree of swelling and the pain is nearly always made worse by eating.

Causes

These include:

- mumps parotitis
- bacterial parotitis
- calculus
- tumour

Mumps parotitis

The commonest cause is mumps or acute viral parotitis. Although this can be unilateral, nine cases out of ten are bilateral. Complications such as orchitis, pancreatitis or unilateral total deafness occur. Mumps parotitis is very painful to the touch and the gland can become very tense. It seldom goes on to abscess formation.

Bacterial parotitis

Acute bacterial parotitis usually occurs in debilitated patients in the postoperative period but can also occur in fit young adults. It affects the whole gland, is unilateral, and often goes on to abscess formation. Pus can often be seen coming out of the parotid duct.

Calculi

Parotid calculi consist of uncalcified epithelial debris and are therefore radiolucent. They form in associa-

tion with a disease called sialectasis which – second to mumps – is the next commonest disease of the salivary glands. Duct obstruction can occur at any site from the main duct to the periphery. This may or may not be accompanied by swelling, but symptoms are invariably related to and made worse by eating.

Tumour

Discrete lumps that are painful and not related to meals must always suggest tumours. Pain, fixation to skin and facial nerve involvement are the clinical features suggesting malignancy.

Clinical approach

The history and local examination will suggest whether the pain is parotid or extraparotid.

If there is any doubt about the pain arising from the parotid, then the patient should be given some lemon juice to drink. In parotid or submandibular gland disease, the pain will increase markedly. Temporomandibular joint dysfunction or molar tooth problems should be considered. If there is any pus in the duct, then it should be cultured to determine antibiotic sensitivity.

Radiology

Always X-ray to look for stones, to view the temporomandibular joint and any molar teeth that are suspicious. A sialogram should not be done within 3 weeks of a bout of pain as it may cause a resolving parotitis to flare up.

SUBMANDIBULAR GLAND PAIN

Causes

This is almost always due to a stone blocking the main duct with subsequent swelling of the whole gland. It is made worse by eating. The stones may be felt in the mouth or seen on X-ray.

The roots of lower 2nd and 3rd molars lie under the mylohyoid line and are therefore in the submandibular space. Apical abscesses of these can therefore be present as submandibular gland swellings. Mumps very seldom affects the submandibular gland.

If the cause is not within the salivary gland, think of a lymph node lying on the gland and enlarged because of infection within the oral cavity – gingivitis, thrush, aphthous ulcers or a cancer.

Radiology

If it is confirmed that the submandibular gland is involved, then plain films should be taken to look for calculi or apical abscesses. Thereafter, a sialogram should be performed if the plain films are unrevealing.

PAROTID GLAND ENLARGEMENT (PAROTOMEGALY)

The first question to decide is whether the swelling is parotid or extraparotid. Common extraparotid masses are:

- sebaceous cysts
- hypertrophy of the masseter
- lipoma
- high branchial cysts
- winged mandible
- external carotid aneurysm

It is next important to establish if the enlargement is diffuse or localized. Local swellings are almost all tumours. A useful rule to remember about this is the so-called 'Rule of 9'.

- nine out of ten salivary gland tumours are in the parotid gland
- nine out of ten parotid tumours are benign
- nine out of ten benign parotid tumours are pleomorphic adenomas (mixed cell tumours)

Causes

These include:

- pleomorphic and monomorphic adenomas
  These are usually found in the tail of the parotid gland. They are mobile and never involve skin or the facial nerve (CP-54).

- carcinoma
  Pain, skin involvement or facial nerve weakness are the cardinal signs of a carcinoma. This is usually adenoid cystic or mucoepidermoid in type.

- mumps
  The commonest cause of diffuse enlargement is mumps.

- acute parotitis
  This is more usually seen in elderly debilitated patients but is not uncommon in young adults, especially if there is an underlying sialectasis. Pus may be seen coming from the duct (CP-55).

- sialectasis
  This usually presents as an intermittent painful swelling related to eating. It usually clears after a few hours but, if the epithelial debris blocking the duct does not move, then the blocked alveoli will become infected, causing a parotid abscess.

- lympho-epithelial lesion (Sjögren's syndrome)
  Bilateral enlargement is, if not due to mumps, usually due to benign lympho-epithelial lesions. This only gives a mild discomfort and has a typical soggy feeling to palpation.

- sarcoidosis
  Of patients with sarcoidosis, 6% have parotid enlargement. It is often accompanied by uveitis.

- systemic disease
  A number of endocrine diseases can be complicated by parotomegaly:

  myxoedema
  diabetes mellitus
  Cushing's disease.

- drugs
  Drugs such as iodides, Distalgesic (dextropropoxyphene and paracetamol), thiouracil and phenylbutazone can also enlarge the gland.

- gout
  This can occasionally involve the parotid in a diffuse swelling.

Investigations

There are very few laboratory tests which will help in establishing a diagnosis. There may be indications for thyroid and adrenal function tests, blood sugar and mumps antibodies.

Parotid scans

Parotid scans with technetium are of limited value because all the minor salivary glands also take up the isotope.

It is said that all tumours take up the isotope, except monomorphic adenoma which is 'cold' (CP-56).

Biopsy

A diffuse enlargement of the parotid may require to be biopsied. Interpretation of parotid histopathology is, however, not easy.

An incisional biopsy of a local swelling should not be done since there is a risk of skin implantation and therefore recurrence. Any local parotid swelling should be removed by a superficial parotidectomy and then submitted to histology. Frankly malignant lumps require more major surgery – sacrificing, and later grafting, the facial nerve.

Radiology

The most important and useful investigation is contrast radiography. Plain films of the parotid are of limited use since stones are usually radiolucent. Since the parotid produces a serous fluid, this debris does not often calcify, so radio-opaque stones are uncommon.

Sialograms will show filling defects, duct displacement and obstruction by tumours and cysts. In sialectasis, two patterns are commonly seen – multiple small cysts giving a 'snowstorm' appearance (saccular sialectasis) or larger irregular cysts with duct stricture (cystic sialectasis) (X-31).

SUBMANDIBULAR GLAND ENLARGEMENT

Causes

In this area the commonest cause of swelling is a draining apical abscess of a lower molar tooth. It drains into the submandibular space and can closely mimic gland disease. Other painless swellings that occur in the area include dermoids, hamartomas and infected glands due to facial or dental infections.

Localized lumps are rare in the submandibular gland and they have a five out of ten chance of being malignant.

The commonest cause of submandibular gland enlargement, however, is calculus disease. It is usually secondary to sialectasis. Many of these stones block the distal part of the duct and so are visible and palpable in the mouth (CP-57).

They give rise typically to pain and swelling in relation to eating.

Other causes of swelling in this area include:

- metastatic cancer
  The submandibular lymph nodes may have metastases from an ear, oral cavity or neck primary tumour
- benign lympho-epithelial lesion
- primary mandibular tumours
- fatty disposition in the gland due to obesity

Investigations

If a stone is present, it will usually be palpable, but every case requires a plain X-ray. Stones in the submandibular gland are normally radio-opaque.

If no stone is found, a sialogram should be performed to demonstrate duct displacement or sialectasis.

A tumour in a gland should be biopsied at open operation and a frozen section result obtained. If malignant, a wide resection, often including part of the mandible, is carried out.

SECTION IV

Description of specific diseases of the salivary glands

SIALADENITIS

Inflammatory disorders of the major salivary glands which result from bacterial or viral infection are the most common salivary gland diseases. On rare occasions, an allergic reaction may result in sialadenitis.

Mumps, the most common salivary disease, is dealt with later in this section, but it is important to note that parotitis may be caused by other viruses such as Coxsackie virus type A, Echo virus, choriomeningitis virus and parainfluenza 1 and 2 viruses.

Sialectasis, a disease of uncommon aetiology involving destruction of the alveoli of salivary glands, forms a fertile soil for secondary infection.

Acute sialadenitis

Causes

Reduction of salivary flow, which may be a postoperative complication, can lead to infection. It occurs especially with abdominal surgery if the patient is debilitated or dehydrated. Acute sialadenitis may follow the use of drugs such as phenothiazine and its derivatives. They cause xerostomia and thus predispose to ascending infections. The condition may also represent an acute exacerbation of a low grade chronic non-specific sialadenitis.

Clinical features

Acute sialadenitis causes painful swelling of the affected gland, with an alteration in the salivary secretion rate and character. A purulent discharge may be expressed from the duct orifice by digital pressure over the affected gland (CP-55).

The introduction of sulphonamides and antibiotics led to a marked reduction in the incidence of acute parotitis. However, with the emergence of antibiotic resistant *Staphylococcus aureus*, acute parotitis has become more prevalent again.

Chronic sialadenitis

Causes

In practice chronic sialadenitis is not uncommon, especially in the submandibular gland. In general, the aetiological factors are similar to those for acute sialadenitis.

Clinical features

The condition usually is unilateral with pain and swelling in the preauricular, retromandibular or submandibular regions. The affected duct orifice is reddened and a purulent, rather salty tasting discharge may be present.

RECURRENT CHRONIC SIALADENITIS

Clinical features

Recurrent chronic sialadenitis is especially common in children, and is secondary to a congenital sialectasis. The attacks consist of sudden pain and swelling in the region of one or both parotid glands and usually last for a period of 3–7 days. Fortunately, there is a marked tendency for the condition to resolve completely in children once puberty is attained. Those patients whose sialograms show little or no duct dilation, and whose flow rates are within normal limits, are more likely to recover spontaneously.

Management

In the treatment of sialadenitis a culture of saliva or pus from the salivary duct should be carried out so that appropriate antibiotic therapy may be instigated.

Sialography may be performed in chronic cases.

Stimulation of flow by chewing or massage prevents stagnation.

Denervation of the parotid gland by tympanic neurectomy is nearly always successful if conservative measures fail.

INVOLVEMENT OF SALIVARY GLANDS IN SYSTEMIC DISEASE

The salivary glands are seldom involved in specific inflammatory disorders. On rare occasions, however, they may be the site of granulomatous disorders such as tuberculosis, syphilis and sarcoidosis and are affected as part of these systemic disease processes.

'Mikulicz's syndrome' is a term often applied to the condition of bilateral salivary gland and lachrymal gland enlargement due to a known cause, such as the specific granulomata as well as lymphoid neoplasia. 'Mikulicz's disease' is bilateral enlargement of unknown cause. It is synonymous with benign lymphoepithelial lesions and Sjögren's syndrome.

Resolution is usually achieved by appropriate treatment of the systemic disorder.

Salivary gland enlargement as a localized allergic reaction is rare. Among the allergens reported are various foods, drugs such as choramphenicol and oxytetracycline, various pollens and heavy metals.

SIALECTASIS

Causes

Sialectasis is a disease of unknown aetiology, involving degeneration and destruction of the alveolar and duct system of the affected gland. It may be congenital or acquired. The epithelial debris from the alveoli blocks the ducts and may calcify to form stones. These stones cause recurrent bouts of swelling and pain.

Investigations

Pain and swelling associated with eating are the commonest symptoms. Plain films may show stones in the submandibular glands, but parotid stones are radiotranslucent. Sialography is necessary for a firm diagnosis.

Management

Sialectasis in 50% of cases gives so little trouble that it requires no treatment apart from occasional analgesics, gland massage and drinking lemon juice in an attempt to wash out the epithelial debris. In the other 50% of cases, however, more specific treatment is required and the most effective method is to denervate the parotid gland. This is done by dividing a branch of the glossopharyngeal nerve which carries the parasympathetic supply. It runs through the middle ear. Parotidectomy is occasionally necessary and, due to the nature of the disease, it requires to be a total parotidectomy (Section V, p. 149).

CALCULUS DISEASE

Causes

Obstruction to the flow of saliva may follow lesions of the duct papilla, the presence of a salivary calculus (or sialolith), secondary to sialectasis, and pressure from lesions within and outwith the duct wall.

Calcification within duct lumens leading to obstruction can be found in many organs of the human body – most often in the urinary tract, gall bladder and submandibular salivary gland. Calculi also occur in the parotid, submandibular and minor salivary glands. The submandibular gland is much more commonly involved than the parotid (CP-57, X-30).

Clinical features

Adults are more commonly affected, though calculus disease may occur in children. The classical clinical signs and symptoms are those of pain and sudden enlargement of the affected gland, especially at mealtimes. Clinical diagnosis may be confirmed visually by palpation and plain radiographs.

Management

Treatment, depending on the site and clinical features, is by surgical removal of the calculus, although in some cases removal of the gland may be necessary. Minor gland sialolithiasis is rare. With submandibular glands, the calculi are removed via the mouth.

Molars with abscessed apices are also removed. A sialogram is arranged when the swelling and pain have gone to see if there is an underlying sialectasis.

MUMPS

Causes

Epidemic parotitis or mumps is the commonest inflammatory disease affecting the salivary glands. It is an acute, infectious condition. Mumps virus, which has an incubation period of 2–3 weeks, is transmitted by direct contact or in droplets of saliva. Children and young adults are mostly affected.

Glandular tissues are principally involved. The commonest are the parotid glands, but occasionally the submandibular salivary gland, the testes, the pancreas or the ovary may be affected.

Clinical features

The onset of mumps is sudden, with fever and swelling of one or more salivary glands. Classically, one gland is affected first, followed by bilateral involvement which occurs in 70% of cases. The swelling reaches a maximum in 2 days and diminishes over the following week. The diagnosis is made from the history and clinical presentation.

A complement fixation test, which is usually positive 1 week after the onset of symptoms, may assist in making the diagnosis in atypical cases.

Management

Treatment is symptomatic, and mouthwashes should be prescribed as dryness of the mouth is invariably present. Patients should be isolated until glands are symptom-free and enlargement has subsided.

A durable immunity results from mumps and may be detected in adults by the presence of complement fixing antibodies in serum and by a positive reaction to a skin test antigen.

SALIVARY GLAND TUMOURS

Salivary gland tumours are relatively uncommon,

comprising fractionally more than 3% of all tumours. Tumours of the parotid gland are approximately ten times more common than the other salivary gland tumours. The sublingual glands are rarely affected by tumours but, in the mouth, the palate is the commonest site for tumours.

Salivary gland tumours are classified as:

- adenomas
  The pleomorphic adenoma
  The monomorphic adenoma
    adenolymphoma
    oxyphil cell adenoma (oncocytoma)
- muco-epidermoid tumour
- acinic cell tumour
- carcinomas
  adenoid cystic carcinoma
  other malignant tumours

Adenomas

Pleomorphic adenoma

Clinical features

The pleomorphic adenoma is the commonest type of salivary gland tumour. It is usually solitary and begins as a small, painless swelling which grows slowly in size. There is no fixation to skin, mucous membrane or deeper structures.

The tumour has a characteristic histological pattern with cuboidal duct-like tumour cells proliferating in clumps, sheets and cords. A pseudocapsule is formed by condensation of the connective tissue. Small clumps of tumour cells, however, may be present within the pseudocapsule.

Management

Enucleation of such lesions is condemned since recurrence is almost inevitable. The tumour is relatively radio-resistant, and thus careful local excision with a margin of normal tissue is the treatment of choice.

Monomorphic adenomas

The monomorphic adenomas are characterized by the regularity of their cell structures and pattern.

Adenolymphoma

The adenolymphoma arises almost exclusively in relation to the parotid gland, usually in a superficial location towards the lower pole. The tumour is often multifocal, and occasionally bilateral gland involvement is present.

Histologically the tumour has a papillary cystic pattern, lined by columnar eosinophilic cells. Varying amounts of lymphoid tissue with follicle formation characterize the stroma. Rather than being a true neoplasm, this lesion may represent a metaplastic process leading to a tissue reaction of the delayed hypersensitivity type.

Oxyphilic adenoma

The oxyphilic adenoma is a rare tumour composed of granular eosinophilic cells.

The basal cell adenoma and the clear cell adenoma are rare monomorphic adenomas.

Muco-epidermoid tumour

The muco-epidermoid tumour is a non-capsulated and generally slow-growing tumour. The behaviour of the tumour is difficult to predict. They account for 3–9% of all salivary tumours. Seventy per cent occur in the parotid.

Histologically, the tumour is characterized by the presence of squamous cells, mucus-secreting cells and cells of an intermediate type. Depending upon the relative proportion of these cell types, the tumour may range from a solid variant to one in which cystic spaces lined by mucus-secreting cells predominate.

Management

Muco-epidermoid tumours invade locally and, on rare occasions, may metastasize. The prognosis is based on distinguishing between well and poorly differentiated types, but is uncertain. Complete excision of the parotid gland is, however, associated with a good prognosis.

Acinic cell tumour

The acinic cell tumour arises from cells similar to the serous acinar cells of salivary tumours and the majority arise in the parotid gland. Rarely the tumour invades locally or metastasizes. They should be completely excised.

The tumour cells have either an acinar arrangement or occur in sheets having a solid pattern.

Carcinomas

Malignant disease of the salivary glands is relatively rare. The clinical signs associated with a malignant neoplasm at this site are rapid growth, pain, fixation to adjacent tissues and nerve paralysis (CP-58, CP-59).

Adenoid cystic carcinoma

The adenoid cystic carcinoma accounts for 6% of all salivary tumours. It is rare in the parotid but occurs relatively commonly in the submandibular and minor glands, comprising up to 25% of all tumours at these sites.

Histologically the tumour has a characteristic cribriform pattern. The tumour cells are small, polygonal and basophilic and are arranged in such a fashion as to enclose cyst-like spaces of varying size. Rarely, a more solid pattern may be present.

Management

The adenoid cystic carcinoma grows slowly, has a tendency towards perineural lymphatic spread and metastasizes late. It should be excised widely.

Other malignant tumours

Adenocarcinoma, epidermoid carcinoma and undifferentiated carcinoma are rare neoplasms. They are highly malignant and may metastasize widely. On occasion, a neoplasm is encountered in which there is definite evidence of malignancy, such as invasive growth and cellular atypia together with histological areas consistent with pleomorphic adenoma. This lesion is called 'carcinoma in pleomorphic adenoma' – malignant mixed cell tumour (CP-60, CP-61).

Non-epithelial tumours such as haemangioma, neurofibroma and lymphangioma may occur in the salivary glands. Rarely, metastatic malignancy may affect the salivary gland.

SALIVARY DUCT FISTULA

A salivary duct fistula allows secretion of saliva externally onto the skin surface, where it presents as a troublesome and distressing condition for the patient. Alternatively, a fistulous tract may open into the oral cavity but, in this situation, it is asymptomatic and of little consequence.

Causes

A salivary duct fistula usually occurs as a complication of trauma – for example, a deep laceration of cheek or following major gland surgery.

Inflammatory, obstructive or neoplastic disease of the salivary glands may lead to ulceration of the overlying skin and so give rise to a fistula.

Management

Sialography can determine where the duct has been involved. Treatment is primarily by surgical repair which involves freeing the proximal portion of the duct and transferring it to the buccal mucosa. The external scar is removed by a plastic procedure.

In some instances, it may be necessary to ligate the proximal portion of the duct as it leaves the gland, thus producing atrophy of the gland, proximal to this point. Extraoral fistulas of the submandibular and sublingual glands usually require excision of the affected gland.

SJÖGREN'S SYNDROME

Sjögren's syndrome consists of the triad of xerostomia, keratoconjunctivitis sicca and a connective tissue disorder, usually rheumatoid arthritis. The diagnosis is made when two of these three features are present. The term 'sicca syndrome' is applied when the connective tissue disorder is absent – only xerostomia and keratoconjunctivitis are present. Enlargement of the salivary and the lachrymal glands may be present. Middle-aged females are primarily affected (CP-62).

The cause of Sjögren's syndrome remains unknown but it seems likely that a combination of genetic, immunological, viral and/or environmental factors play a role in pathogenesis.

The remarkable prevalence of circulating autoantibodies, both organ and non-organ specific, is a striking feature of the syndrome. Viral-like particles have been noted at a fine structural level in endothelial cells of kidney, parotid and labial glands.

Clinical features

The symptoms, signs, laboratory findings, and radiographic changes of patients with rheumatoid arthritis complicated by Sjögren's symdrome closely resemble those of classical rheumatoid arthritis.

Multisystem abnormalities are noted in patients with Sjögren's syndrome. Nasal, pharyngeal, vaginal and skin dryness may be present in addition to dryness of the mouth and eyes. Various gastrointestinal, pulmonary, renal, neurological, muscle, cardiac and endocrine abnormalities may occur.

Malignant lymphoma may complicate Sjögren's syndrome in 6–7% of cases and is more common in those with the sicca components only.

Investigations

Salivary gland dysfunction is demonstrated by markedly reduced salivary flow rates. Scintiscanning and scintography can reveal reduced isotope uptake. Protein abnormalities in saliva may be present and, in the serum, an autoantibody to salivary duct cell cytoplasm may be detected in 50% of cases. Biopsy of major or minor salivary glands reveals focal lymphocytic adenitis and duct hyperplasia.

Keratoconjunctivitis sicca is diagnosed by demonstrating diminished lachrymation, using the Schirmer tear test, and by finding filamentary or punctuate keratitis on slit lamp examination of the cornea.

Management

The treatment, both local and general, requires a broad approach. The symptom of xerostomia may be alleviated by glycerine and lemon mouthwashes, and fluid intake should be increased. Local oral infections, especially candidiasis, should be detected and treated with appropriate antifungal agents.

SECTION V

Principles of general management and treatment of the salivary glands

PRINCIPLES OF SALIVARY GLAND SURGERY

Parotidectomy

Two forms are employed. Superficial parotidectomy involves removing the parotid tissue superficial to the facial nerve. Total parotidectomy involves dissecting the facial nerve and its branches off the deep lobe and removing the deep lobe. Any parotid surgery is therefore a dissection of the facial nerve and its branches. To remove the deep lobe, the whole facial nerve from the main trunk to the divisions of the upper and lower main branches has to be carefully dissected on its deep surface so that it can be lifted upwards to allow the deep lobe to be removed by blunt dissection from the pharyngeal space.

The main trunk of the facial nerve is found just below the external meatus about 2.5–3.5 cm (1–1½ inches) below the skin surface. As it is followed forward, and the parotid tissue removed from its lateral aspect, the terminal branches will be reached and the whole superficial lobe removed.

Facial nerve paralysis

If a facial nerve paralysis is noted immediately after surgery, then the nerve and its branches should be re-explored to uncover the site of any injury. Haematomas of the sheath can be evacuated. Sutures involving parts of the nerve can be removed and, if the nerve has been cut, the ends can be sutured together.

Submandibular gland removal

A horizontal incision is made at the level of the hyoid bone. The fascia is dissected off the gland and retracted away from the operative field. This protects the mandibular branch of the facial nerve which lies in the fascia. If this is damaged the mouth is pulled to the opposite side giving an unattractive appearance.

The gland is dissected off the digastric and mylohyoid muscles and is removed, identifying and preserving the lingual and hypoglossal nerves. The facial artery runs through the gland posteriorly and has to be divided.

Tympanic neurectomy

By dividing the tympanic branch of the glossopharyngeal nerve that runs across the promontory of the middle ear the parasympathetic supply, which is secreto-motor, to the parotid gland is interrupted.

It is a simple procedure done by turning the ear drum forwards, identifying and dividing the nerve and replacing the drum.

MANAGEMENT OF FACIAL NERVE PARALYSIS

This is a most disfiguring condition and requires rehabilitation or else the patient may withdraw from social contact. There are a number of approaches.

Facial nerve grafting

If a small area of facial nerve is damaged then it can be excised and a graft sewn in place. If this is successful then some movement and tone may return in about 6 months.

Facial nerve bypass

If the main trunk of the nerve is damaged close to the mastoid bone, making grafting difficult, the ipsilateral hypoglossal or accessory nerve can be divided, rerouted and anastomosed to the distal segment of the facial nerve. If this is successful, the face is liable to move when the patient moves his tongue (if the hypoglossal nerve has been used) or his shoulder (if the accessory nerve has been used).

Cross-face nerve anastomosis

If only the terminal branches of the nerve remain (e.g. after a major cancer excision), a nerve graft (LD-67) can be joined from terminal branches on the sound side so that axons grow up it. It is then joined to the terminal branches on the paralysed side in the hope that the newly grown axons will reinervate these. The nerve usually taken for this graft is the sural nerve from the leg. The branches to which it is joined on the unparalysed side lose function but sufficient are left not to paralyse the good side.

Free muscle grafts

The plantaris and palmaris muscles may be taken from the foot or hand and implanted around the paralysed eye or mouth. There is evidence that this can reinnervate and create some movement.

Tarsorrhaphy

The main complication after a facial paralysis (apart from cosmetic disfigurement) is that the patient cannot close his or her eye and so is at risk of a corneal ulcer. This is prevented by sewing the lateral sides of the eyelids together thus narrowing the palpebral fissure.

Face lift

A unilateral face lift goes some way to pulling up the lax tissue on the paralysed side and gives a temporary improvement.

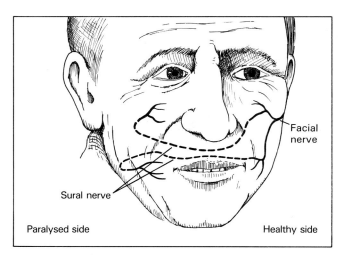

LD-67. *Cross-face nerve anastomosis*

TEST-YOURSELF QUESTIONS

Part 6 – The Salivary Glands

1. The following diseases of salivary glands are exacerbated by eating:
a) Sialectasis
b) Pleomorphic adenoma
c) Sjögren's disease
d) Calculi

2. The submandibular gland:
a) has a duct that opens opposite the lower canine tooth
b) extends below the hyoid bone
c) is mainly a serous gland
d) does not extend behind the angle of the mandible

3. The following conditions may mimic enlargement of the salivary glands:
a) Hypertrophy of the masseter muscle
b) Hypertrophy of the temporalis muscle
c) Tonsillar lymph node enlargement
d) Branchial cyst

4. Pain in the salivary glands is usual with:
a) Viral parotitis
b) Adenoid cystic carcinoma
c) Warthin's tumour
d) Sarcoidosis

5. The following endocrine conditions may cause parotomegaly:
a) Thyrotoxicosis
b) Myxoedema
c) Addison's disease
d) Diabetes insipidus

6. Stones in the salivary glands:
a) are more common in the submandibular than the parotid
b) are always radio opaque
c) reflect an underlying sialectasis
d) only cause pain when in the main duct

7. Pleomorphic adenoma of the parotid gland:
a) has a high potential for recurrence
b) usually presents in the preauricular region
c) is made more painful by eating
d) may cause facial nerve paralysis

8. Sjögren's syndrome:
a) is commoner in females than in males
b) needs a positive sublabial biopsy for definitive diagnosis
c) may be accompanied by keratoconjunctivitis sicca
d) is often associated with osteoarthritis

9. The following viruses may cause parotitis:
a) Echo virus
b) Choriomeningitis virus
c) Rhinovirus
d) Coxsackie type A virus

10. Facial nerve paralysis:
a) Occurs with all types of malignant tumours of the parotid gland
b) If total, presents greatest risk to the eye because of corneal ulceration
c) If total, the mouth is pulled to the paralysed side
d) If rehabilitated with a nerve graft will show no movement for up to 6 months

The answers to these questions will be found on p. 191.

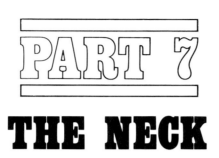

THE NECK

SECTION I

Background to disease of the neck

ANATOMY

The anatomical structures of the neck can be conveniently divided into midline and lateral components.

Midline structures

These consist of the supporting cervical vertebrae posteriorly and the laryngopharyngeal apparatus and thyroid gland anteriorly.

The laryngeal skeleton consists of the hyoid bone, the thyroid cartilage and the cricoid cartilage together with their soft tissue attachments. The trachea is the inferior continuation of the larynx (LD-45, LD-46).

The hyoid bone is attached to the base of the tongue by the hyoglossus muscle and to the thyroid cartilage by the thyrohyoid membrane. The strap muscles are attached to the anterior surfaces of these structures and consist of the thyrohyoid, sternothyroid and sternohyoid muscles.

The pharynx

The constrictor muscles of the pharynx are attached to the larynx and form an incomplete circle. The lower segment of the inferior constrictor muscle, the cricopharyngeus, acts as a sphincter.

The cricopharyngeus forms the lower limit of the hypopharynx and is continuous with the cervical oesophagus.

Recurrent laryngeal nerves

The recurrent laryngeal nerves run between the trachea and oesophagus and enter the larynx at the level of the cricopharyngeus. They supply motor fibres to all the muscles of the larynx except the cricothyroid which receives its supply from the superior laryngeal nerve. In the lower neck the nerves are at risk of damage from surgery or by tumour spread from the larynx, trachea, or thyroid.

The thyroid gland

The thyroid gland, which envelops the upper trachea and oesophagus, consists of two lobes which are joined by the isthmus which lies across the 2nd–4th tracheal rings.

The thyroid gland, although low in the neck, develops as a downgrowth from the foramen caecum in the tongue.

Lateral structures

Carotid sheaths

These lie immediately lateral to the laryngopharyngeal apparatus. Contained in them are the common carotid arteries, the vagus nerves and the internal jugular veins.

The carotid arteries lie medial to the internal jugular veins and the vagus nerve lies between the two and slightly posterior. The sympathetic trunk lies posterior to and outside the sheath (LD-68).

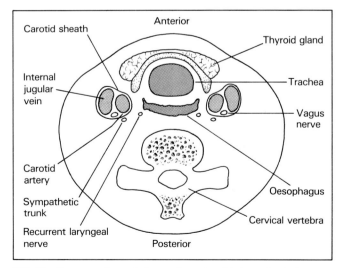

LD-68. *Cross-section of the neck at the third tracheal ring to show the relationship of the thyroid gland, carotid sheaths, nerves and trachea*

Sternomastoid muscle

This covers the carotid sheaths. Posterior to this muscle lies the posterior triangle of the neck.

Anterior triangle

This is bounded inferiorly by the clavicle, posteriorly by the sternomastoid muscle and anteriorly by the midline of the neck (LD-69). It contains the submandibular gland, fat and lymph nodes. These lie under the mandible, and the tail of the parotid gland lies between the angle of the mandible and the mastoid bone.

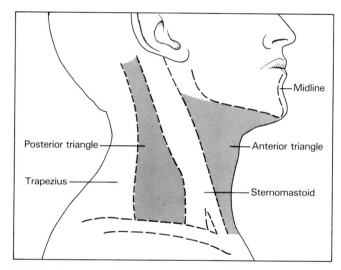

LD-69. *Anterior and posterior triangles of the neck*

Posterior triangle

This is bounded by the clavicle, sternomastoid and trapezius. It contains fat and lymph nodes and is crossed by the accessory nerve.

Lymph nodes

There are 80–100 lymph nodes on each side of the neck. These are named in groups according to their position (LD-70).

Submental and submandibular nodes

The submental nodes lie under the mandible anteriorly while the submandibular group lie on the submandibular salivary gland.

Deep jugular nodes

The deep jugular chain of nodes lies along the carotid

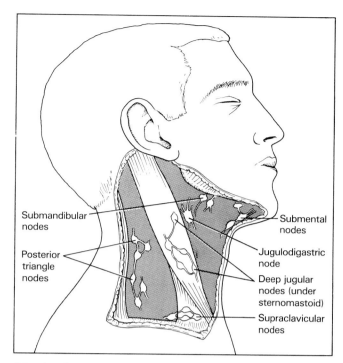

LD-70. *The main groups of lymph nodes in the neck*

sheath. These nodes are often involved in head and neck cancer, tuberculosis and lymphomas. The upper node in this group is the jugulodigastric node which is frequently enlarged as a result of tonsillar infection.

Carcinomas of the nasopharynx and piriform fossa may present as an enlarged node in the deep cervical chain with no other symptoms.

Posterior triangle nodes

The posterior triangle group, lying between the sternomastoid and trapezius, may similarly be involved in carcinoma, lymphoma or tuberculosis. Metastatic carcinoma in this area is a bad prognostic sign as it indicates distant tumour spread and a poor immune response. Infectious mononucleosis, and rarely, brucellosis, may also cause lymphadenopathy in this area.

Supraclavicular nodes

The supraclavicular nodes are often enlarged in carcinoma, metastasizing from the chest or abdomen.

The nodes in the right supraclavicular fossa drain the whole of the right lung and the left upper lobe and are often enlarged in lung cancer. Those on the left drain the gastro-oesophageal area and may be the first sign of carcinoma in these organs.

SECTION II
History and physical examination of the neck

HISTORY

Lumps or swellings

In general practice the commonest neck lump is an enlarged tonsillar lymph node which is inflamed secondary to an upper respiratory tract infection. In hospital practice the commonest cause of neck lumps is disease of the thyroid gland. The following factors can give some help in discovering the causative disease:

- age
- general health
- pain
- duration of symptoms
- precipitating factors
- associated symptoms

Age

The age of the patient will give you a first guide to the diagnosis.

Age below 20 years

Under the age of 20, inflammatory nodes or congenital masses are most common:

- the tonsillar nodes
  These may be enlarged and tender secondary to tonsillitis or a dental abscess.
- congenital masses which occur in the midline
  These are usually thyroglossal cysts or dermoids.

Branchial cysts, which are also congenital, are usually placed more laterally under the anterior border of the sternomastoid muscle.

Age 20–40 years

In this age group, salivary gland disease or thyroid disease is more common. Lymphoma and chronic infections must also be considered.

Salivary gland enlargement may be due to a tumour or there may be enlargement secondary to an obstructing calculus in the duct. A localized thyroid swelling is likely to be a tumour whereas a more diffuse swelling may be due to thyroiditis.

Chronic infections, such as toxoplasmosis, tuberculosis or brucellosis occur rarely. Other rare infections, such as tularaemia or actinomycosis, may have to be considered outside the UK.

Age above 40 years

Above the age of 40, a neck mass appearing for the first time should be regarded as being malignant until proved otherwise.

General health

Ask about the patient's general health. If the cause is inflammatory, the patient may often have a fever.

Vague malaise may be the only symptom of toxoplasmosis or infectious mononucleosis.

Pain

Pain with a red lump is usually associated with acute infection or salivary gland obstruction. The commonest cause is a lymphadenitis secondary to tonsillitis.

An infected thyroglossal cyst will present as a tender, swollen midline mass. Similarly, a branchial cyst can present for the first time as a lateral neck abscess. A stone impacted in the submandibular duct will give rise to pain and swelling of that gland (CP-57).

Duration of symptoms

Ask how long the lump has been present and if it is getting bigger or smaller.

A constant size suggests a congenital mass unless infection supervenes. A reduction in size might suggest removal of an obstruction such as a calculus; an enlarging mass or masses suggest malignancy.

Precipitating factors

Ask if anything makes the mass bigger.

A blocked salivary gland enlarges while the patient is eating, while a laryngocoele may only be present when the patient is blowing.

Associated symptoms

If metastatic disease is suspected, ask about dysphagia, hoarseness or deafness. Weight loss may be associated with metastatic disease or thyroid dysfunction. If the thyroid is enlarged the patient's thyroid function should be carefully assessed.

Carcinoma of the nasopharynx commonly gives rise to deafness by obstructing the Eustachian tube.

EXAMINATION

Inspection

Ask the patient to strip to the waist or at least to the shoulders. Inspect the neck from the front and sides in a good light.

Palpation

Stand behind the patient, who should be seated, and follow this scheme of examination. Start by palpating the tip of the mastoid bone and follow the line of the trapezius down to where it joins the clavicle. Now come upwards again, palpating any glands in the posterior triangle under the flats of the finger until the mastoid process is reached again.

Next come down the line of the sternomastoid muscle to the clavicle palpating deep under the muscle. Glands in this area are about an inch (25 mm) from the surface of the skin and may be difficult to palpate. At this point you are in the midline and so should now examine superiorly, palpating the trachea and thyroid gland.

Continue superiorly and palpate the laryngopharynx and hyoid bone. In the submental region go more laterally and palpate the submandibular glands and finally the parotid glands (LD-71).

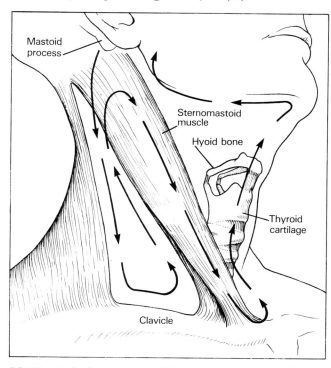

LD-71. *Method recommended for palpation of the neck*

Enlarged lymph nodes should be assessed with regard to mobility, texture and tenderness.

Fixed lymph nodes are suggestive of advanced malignant disease. Tender or inflamed nodes are more indicative of an inflammatory cause. Carcinomatous lymph nodes are usually hard, while nodes involved in lymphomas are more rubbery in consistency.

The thyroid gland is normally not palpable in health as it is soft and is partially covered by the strap muscles and the platysma.

INVESTIGATIONS

Laboratory tests

All patients should have a full blood count and film. The film will be useful in infectious mononucleosis, leukaemias and perhaps in the lymphomas. Immunoglobulin estimations may be also useful in the lymphomas.

In thyroid masses a full thyroid investigation should be done. This includes a thyroid scan, serum T_4 and T_3 levels and a free thyroxine index.

If tuberculosis or sarcoid is suspected, a Mantoux or a Kveim test should be performed. If there are multiple glands in the posterior triangle, then blood should be sent for cytomegalovirus, toxoplasma and brucella titres and a Monospot test.

Scanning techniques

Thyroid scan

This is carried out whenever a nodule is found in the thyroid gland. The material used is ^{131}I, which is a radioactive isotope of iodine.

'Cold' areas arouse the suspicion of malignancy but 'hot' areas are less often malignant.

Other causes of 'cold' areas are haemorrhage or degeneration in a cystic goitre.

RADIOLOGY

Plain radiography

Neck

Anteroposterior and lateral views of the neck are useful in demonstrating calcified tuberculous nodes, cervical ribs, tracheal compression or deviation, and thyroid enlargement.

Postcricoid carcinomas may be suspected from the lateral film if the soft tissue shadow is greater than the depth of a vertebral body. If a laryngocoele is suspected, the patient is asked to do a Valsalva manoeuvre, then a large air shadow is seen as the air sac fills.

Chest

Chest X-rays are taken to rule out pulmonary tuberculosis, mediastinal lymphoma or bronchial carcinoma.

Skull

Base of skull and lateral skull films are taken to see if there is any bone erosion due to nasopharyngeal carcinoma.

Carcinoma of the nasopharynx is one of the commonest causes of a metastatic lymph node where there are no other symptoms.

Tomograms

Tomography of the base of skull or larynx may be necessary to define the extent of tumours in these areas.

Tomography of the larynx is particularly useful in showing the extent of subglottic spread in a laryngeal tumour (X-27).

Contrast radiography

Barium studies

A barium swallow and meal will show filling defects in the oesophagus, stomach or oesophageal displacement by intrathoracic tumours.

Carcinomas of the hypopharynx, piriform fossa and oesophagus may be seen on the barium swallow.

Angiography

Carotid angiography is essential in pulsating neck masses and also to see if involvement of the carotid tree by metastatic tumour has compromised further surgical treatment.

Laryngograms

Laryngograms may be done in cases of laryngopharyngeal tumours to outline their extent.

Propyliodone (Dionosil) is trickled into an anaesthetized larynx. The procedure is especially useful in determining the lower extent of supraglottic tumours.

Lymphangiography

In cases of proven lymphomas, lymphangiography is required to assess the spread and stage of the disease. It is seldom of use in assessing spread in metastatic lymph nodes.

Biopsy

Diagnosis of a neck lump still depends primarily on clinical skill and diagnostic acumen, rather than being dependent on laboratory or radiological tests. Biopsy of a mass is not a basic clinical skill and a biopsy at an early stage is not recommended for the following reasons.

If metastatic disease is suspected, there is an 85% chance of the primary being found in the head and neck. If the gland is biopsied and the primary missed, the survival potential of the patient is reduced.

Biopsy of the gland may also lead to tumour implantation in the skin.

The correct treatment policy is to find the primary and to treat the whole area as one, with definitive surgery or radiotherapy.

If a gland from a primary piriform tumour is biopsied without finding the primary, then the survival potential of the patient is reduced by 66%.

If a metastatic gland from a symptomless tonsillar tumour is biopsied and tumour implanted in the skin, the 5-year survival rate is reduced from about 40% to 14%.

SECTION III

The presentation of lumps in the neck and the diagnostic possibilities

LUMPS IN THE NECK

A patient with a lump in the neck presents a diagnostic challenge in which clinical skill far outweighs any help obtainable from ancillary investigations.

Clinical approach

Presentation

The first step is to take a history and examine the neck. The following points should be answered:
- relation to skin
- position of mass

Relationship to skin

It is important to decide whether the lump is in or attached to the skin or deep to it, before embarking on further investigations. A sebaceous cyst below the ear may closely resemble a small parotid mixed cell tumour, for example.

Midline masses

Midline masses are usually single and can only be thyroid adenoma or carcinoma, a chondroma, a thyroglossal cyst or a dermoid (LD-72).

Thyroid masses move on swallowing but not on sticking out the tongue, while thyroglossal cysts move during both manoeuvres. Thyroglossal cysts are always below the hyoid bone but dermoid tumours are usually above it.

Chondromas are bony hard and associated closely with the thyroid or cricoid cartilage.

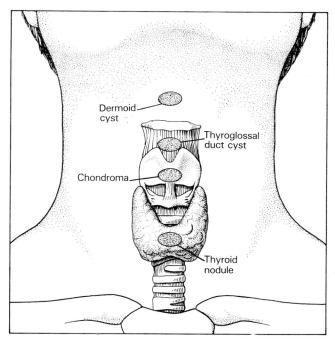

LD-72. Position of commonly encountered midline neck swellings

Posterior triangle masses

In the posterior triangle, cervical ribs are sometimes palpable but, apart from this, most masses in this area are due to lymphadenopathy. Large rubbery firm matted nodes can be due to tuberculosis or lymphoma (LD-73). Small mobile multiple nodes may be caused by infectious mononucleosis.

Other causes may be toxoplasmosis, brucellosis and cytomegalovirus.

Supraclavicular fossa masses

Enlarged glands in the right supraclavicular fossa are usually secondaries from a bronchial carcinoma, whereas glands in the left supraclavicular fossa are often from gastro-oesophageal neoplasms.

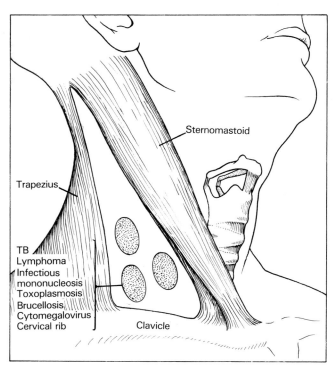

LD-73. *Differential diagnosis of a mass in the posterior triangle*

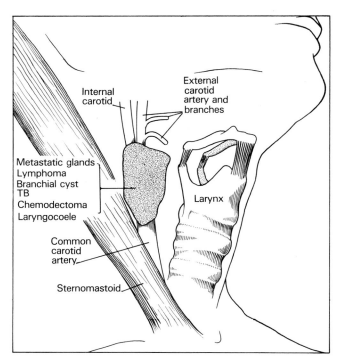

LD-74. *Differential diagnosis of a lateral neck mass*

Metastases from head and neck cancer are usually squamous carcinomas. Gastro-oesophageal neoplasms are usually adenocarcinomas.

Submandibular masses

Submandibular gland enlargements may be discrete if due to tumour or metastatic glands, or diffuse if due to calculus disease or sialectasis.

Parotid region swellings

Swelling of the tail of the parotid gland is usually due to a benign tumour and may present behind, below or in front of the lobes of the ear. Swelling in front of the ear may sometimes be confused with an enlarged jugulodigastric node but these are usually near the angle of the mandible.

The commonest benign parotid tumour is a benign mixed cell tumour.

Lateral neck masses

Lateral neck swellings nearly always occur near the carotid bulb and present a difficult diagnostic problem, especially if they pulsate. The differential diagnosis is branchial cyst, tuberculous nodes, lymphoma, metastatic glands, carotid body tumour, or a laryngocoele (LD-74).

Branchial cysts are generally fluctuant (LD-74). They are nearly always situated at the junction of the upper third and lower two thirds of the sternomastoid at its anterior border.

Tuberculosis and lymphoma nodes are rubbery and often multiple, whereas metastatic nodes are very hard.

Laryngocoeles arise from the ventricle of the larynx. They are made worse by blowing but usually empty easily.

Carotid body tumours can be moved from side to side but not up and down. They are very rare but, if suspected, angiography must be carried out before proceeding to biopsy. Angiography must be performed in every case of a painless pulsating lump. It is the only certain way of diagnosing a carotid body tumour.

Investigations

By this stage it should have been possible to diagnose the following:

- sebaceous cysts
- dermoid cysts
- branchial cysts
- thyroid masses
- parotid masses
- submandibular masses
- acute infections causing lymphadenitis

- chronic infections
- chemodectomas

Difficulty arises with non-pulsating neck masses arising from the deep-jugular group of nodes and the supraclavicular nodes. The diagnosis is likely to be one of the following:

- a metastatic lymph node from a head and neck primary or a bronchial or alimentary source
- a lymphoma
- tuberculosis

Radiology

The following X-rays may help in the diagnosis:

- chest X-rays
  These may show evidence of pulmonary tuberculosis, mediastinal lymphoma or bronchial carcinoma.
- soft tissues of the neck
  This X-ray can show evidence of postcricoid carcinoma, hypopharyngeal carcinoma and, occasionally, laryngeal carcinoma.
- X-ray of the nasopharynx, base of skull and sinuses
  Masses in the nasopharynx, or bone erosion of the base of the skull or walls of the sinus are very suggestive of local malignancy.

- barium swallow and meal
  This can show lesions of the hypopharynx, oesophagus, stomach and perhaps evidence of mediastinal masses.

Panendoscopy

If all approaches are negative, the patient is submitted to panendoscopy under a general anaesthetic. This procedure involves an oesophagoscopy, a pharyngoscopy, a laryngoscopy, a bronchoscopy and a nasopharyngoscopy. If no obvious lesion is found, biopsies are taken from the base of tongue, tonsil, piriform fossae and nasopharynx. Carcinomas in these areas can be small, but present as metastatic lymph nodes.

Biopsy

If carcinoma is demonstrated in one of the areas biopsied, a definitive policy of surgery or radiotherapy is adopted. If the biopsies reveal normal tissue the patient is returned to theatre, the gland excised and a frozen section taken. If the frozen section report is tuberculosis or lymphoma, the wound is closed and the appropriate treatment is instituted. If the gland contains squamous carcinoma, the incision is extended and a radical neck dissection performed.

SECTION IV

Description of specific diseases of the neck

THYROID MASSES

Clinical features

The commonest cause of thyroid enlargement is a simple goitre with or without hypothyroidism.

Solitary nodules of the thyroid should always be fully investigated. They may be benign or malignant. The benign nodules are usually adenomas. Malignant nodules may be due to papillary carcinoma, follicular carcinomas or medullary carcinoma.

Uniform enlargement of the thyroid gland with tracheal compression and recurrent laryngeal nerve paralysis is commonly due to a lymphoma of the gland. Undifferentiated thyroid tumours and squamous cell carcinomas may also present in this way.

A swollen painful thyroid is suggestive of thyroiditis.

Management

Single thyroid nodules should generally be excised. If carcinoma is suspected a frozen section is advisable and, if confirmed, a total thyroidectomy is performed. Thyroiditis is treated symptomatically – unless acute, when antibiotics may be required.

INFECTIONS (EXCLUDING TUBERCULOSIS)

Causes

The second commonest cause of lumps in the neck after thyroid enlargements is lymphadenopathy secondary to an infection.

Enlarged jugulodigastric nodes are frequently found and are secondary to an upper respiratory tract infection, usually tonsillitis (CP-63). Oral problems such as dental caries and mouth ulcers can also cause enlarged lymph nodes, as can infected skin lesions. Otitis externa may cause pre- or postauricular lymphadenopathy.

Multiple glands in the posterior triangle can be caused by infectious mononucleosis or rubella but a more common cause, especially among children in large cities, is scalp infestation.

Other causes are brucellosis, toxoplasmosis and cytomegalovirus. These also cause lymphadenopathy in the deep jugular chain of nodes.

Fungal infections may affect the skin and subcutaneous tissue of the neck. These are less common and include actinomycosis and blastomycosis.

Management

Treatment is by appropriate chemotherapy. Brucellosis usually responds to tetracyclines, and toxoplasmosis to sulphonamides, but cytomegalovirus does not respond to any drugs at present available.

CONGENITAL LUMPS

Cystic hygroma

A cystic hygroma is due to maldevelopment of the lymph spaces and lymph trunks on one side of the face and neck.

Clinical features

This is always obvious at birth and presents as a large lump on the side of the neck and face (CP-64).

It is brilliantly transilluminable and although rare is easily diagnosed.

Management

The only effective treatment is removal. This is tedious and difficult since the lymph spaces may permeate important structures such as the carotid sheath, skull base and facial nerve.

Dermoid cysts

Clinical features

These cysts are found in the midline, usually above the hyoid bone (CP-65). They occur along the lines of fusion and, if suprahyoid, usually move on swallowing and on sticking out the tongue.

Management

Treatment is by local removal, which is usually simple and effective.

Thyroglossal duct cyst

Cause

This is the commonest midline neck lump. It occurs when there is failure of obliteration of the thyroglossal duct in the fetus during descent of the thyroid from the tongue to its position in the neck (CP-66).

The thyroid develops at the base of the tongue and as neck growth proceeds it descends in the neck but remains attached to the tongue by the thyroglossal duct. If this duct fails to obliterate normally and cystic spaces develop in it, a thyroglossal duct cyst occurs.

Clinical features

Thyroglossal duct cysts are usually below the hyoid bone and in the midline and move on swallowing and on sticking the tongue out. This is because the duct always joins the tongue behind the hyoid bone and it is, therefore, attached both to the tongue and the thyroid cartilage.

Management

Treatment is by excision.

Branchial cyst

Cause

A branchial cyst represents failure of disappearance of part of the branchial cleft apparatus. It may, therefore, have an internal opening just behind the posterior pillar of the tonsil or between the bony and cartilaginous external auditory meatus.

Clinical features

This is the commonest lateral neck mass. It occurs anywhere along the anterior border of the sternomastoid but most usually at the junction of the upper third and the lower two thirds (CP-67). It often presents as a fluctuant, mobile neck lump but, if infected, will present as an abscess. If fluid is aspirated from an uninfected cyst, it is found to contain cholesterol crystals.

Management

Treatment is by local removal, making sure the tract is followed to its internal opening.

On very rare occasions, malignant change can occur, giving rise to a branchogenic carcinoma.

Laryngocoeles

Causes

They arise from the ventricle of the larynx which is a remnant of the primitive air sacs; they expand through the thyrohyoid membrane.

A person may have a large ventricle at birth and, if he takes up a 'blowing' hobby or occupation, the latent laryngocoele will come to light.

Clinical features

These present as painless neck lumps, usually made worse by blowing. They empty easily. They are said to occur in trumpet players and glass blowers but this impression is not substantiated. They have a characteristic X-ray appearance when full of air (X-32). If the mouth of the sac gets blocked and infection supervenes, it may present as a pyocoele.

Management

Treatment is by excision.

CERVICAL RIBS

These, if large, can simulate a bony hard lymph node in the lower part of the posterior triangle. No treatment is required.

PRIMARY TUMOURS

Chemodectoma

Clinical features

This is a very rare benign tumour of the receptor cells in the carotid bulb. They nearly always pulsate and because of their attachment to the artery move from side to side, but not up and down.

They can be diagnosed clinically but definitive diagnosis is always by angiography.

They grow slowly and generally cause no symptoms.

Management

In old people they are best left alone but in young people they should be resected.

Surgical removal is difficult and dangerous and should be done with full precautions for doing a carotid artery replacement.

Neurogenous tumours

Causes

These usually arise from the vagus and – being deep to the sternomastoid muscle, parotid tissue and occasionally the great vessels – they are difficult to palpate.

They are usually neurofibromas or neurolemmomas and are nearly all benign.

Neurofibromas can also occur in association, in the skin of the neck as flat raised areas, sometimes associated with café-au-lait spots.

Clinical features

Presentation is often as a mass in the lateral pharynx pushing the tonsil medially and forwards.

Management

Treatment is to explore the neck and to peel the tumours off the vagus nerve.

The nerve is sometimes sacrificed with the benign tumours and is invariably sacrificed with the very occasional malignant tumour. Postoperatively the patient will then have a vocal cord paralysis and often a Horner's syndrome due to involvement of the nearby sympathetic fibres.

Horner's syndrome is paralysis of the cervical sympathetic causing sinking in of the eyeball, ptosis of the upper eyelid, slight elevation of the lower lid, constriction of the pupil, narrowing of the palpebral fissure and anhidrosis.

Cartilaginous tumours

Clinical features

These occur on the cricoid or less commonly on the thyroid cartilages. Chondromas are benign and present as hard midline swellings which move on swallowing.

Management

Treatment is by local excision.

The malignant variety, *chondrosarcoma*, should be suspected where there is rapid growth and invasion of the larynx.

Treatment is by laryngectomy.

Lipomas

These benign tumours of fat occur usually in the supraclavicular area and seldom require treatment.

Sebaceous cysts

Although not true tumours, these cysts can be mistaken for them unless the punctum of the cyst is looked for and identified (CP-68).

Skin tumours

These include squamous cell carcinoma, basal cell carcinoma and melanoma and can occur with or without enlarged metastatic lymph nodes.

METASTATIC GLAND ENLARGEMENT

Clinical features

Primary squamous carcinoma of the head and neck will metastasize to neck glands long before distant spread. In most cases, the primary tumour gives rise to symptoms (CP-69).

Carcinoma of the glottis usually presents early, as hoarseness, and pharyngeal carcinomas cause pain or dysphagia. Some areas, however, are notoriously silent – such as the piriform fossa, the posterior surface of the epiglottis and the nasopharynx.

The site of the mass gives little help as to the probable site of the primary. This is especially true of the deep jugular chain nodes. The exceptions to this rule are the supraclavicular nodes. Right-sided node enlargement suggests a bronchogenic primary while left-sided enlargement suggests a gastro-oesophageal primary.

GRANULOMATOUS LESIONS

Tuberculosis

Clinical features

This is not as common in Britain as it was but still occurs, usually affecting glands in the deep jugular chain and occasionally the posterior triangle (CP-70). Only a few have coexisting pulmonary tuberculosis, but a full examination must be done to rule it out. The route of entry is thought to be via the tonsil.

Management

The treatment is to excise the gland for biopsy and thereafter to start appropriate chemotherapy.

Sarcoidosis

This can present in a manner similar to tuberculosis. Diagnosis is confirmed by histology, by the Kveim test or gland biopsy.

LYMPHOMAS

Clinical features

These very commonly present in the head and neck region and can affect lymphoid tissue in the nasopharynx, tonsils, salivary glands or posterior triangle. Occasionally the glands reach a massive size very quickly and become matted together (CP-71). A massive neck node enlargement should be regarded as lymphoma until proved otherwise.

On cut section the glands have a typical smooth white appearance.

Management

This entails establishing a diagnosis by excisional gland biopsy. It is best, if possible, to excise a whole gland as this enables the histopathologist to study the entire gland architecture.

The extent of spread of the disease is next determined and, depending on the degree of spread, treatment by radiotherapy or cytotoxic drugs is instituted.

Every patient should have a lymphangiogram and many also undergo laparotomy to enable the disease to be staged.

SALIVARY GLAND ENLARGEMENTS

These are included with the neck swellings, since the submandibular gland lies wholly within the neck as does the tail of the parotid. Lumps that are associated with eating are probably due to calculi, but painless discrete lumps are usually benign tumours.

The 'Rule of 9' applies to salivary gland tumours:

- nine out of ten salivary tumours are in the parotid gland
- nine out of ten parotid tumours are benign
- nine out of ten benign parotid tumours are pleomorphic adenomas

If these glands are diffusely enlarged, then Sjögren's syndrome is a possibility (p. 148).

Painful lumps involving skin and/or facial nerve are probably malignant tumours.

The commonest histological types are squamous carcinoma, adenoid cystic carcinoma and muco-epidermoid carcinoma.

Other causes of diffuse enlargement are thiouracil or iodide overdosage and diabetes.

SECTION V

Principles of general management and treatment of the neck

PRINCIPLES OF SURGERY

Incisions

These, where possible, should be made in the lines of the skin creases. Incisions placed in these lines heal better and will be cosmetically less noticeable. Neck incisions should therefore be made horizontally wherever possible and not vertically.

Thyroidectomy

This is carried out through a horizontal incision made 2.5 cm (1 inch) above the clavicles. The strap muscles are retracted laterally and the thyroid gland revealed (LD-75). The vessels are ligated, the recurrent laryngeal nerve identified and the gland removed.

The vessels which have to be accounted for are the superior thyroid arteries and veins, the middle thyroid veins and the inferior thyroid vessels.

Thyroglossal duct cyst removal

A horizontal incision is made over the cyst and the tract excised.

The cyst, duct and the body of the hyoid bone must all be removed to ensure excision of the attachment to the base of the tongue, thus preventing recurrence.

Radical neck dissection

This is sometimes called 'block dissection'. It involves removal of all the lymph nodes from the neck. This is accomplished by removing all the structures anterior

to the prevertebral fascia except the carotid artery and the vagus nerve. Various incisions have been described (LD-76) and in spite of the extent of the excision there is very little morbidity.

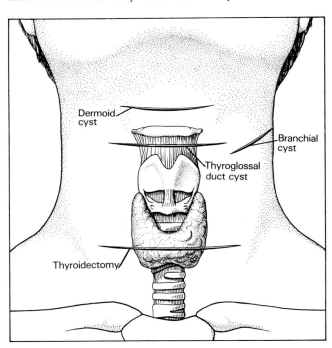

LD-75. *Incisions used in common procedures*

The following structures are removed: the sternomastoid muscle, the internal jugular vein, the fat of the posterior triangle, the accessory nerve, the digastric muscle, the tail of the parotid and the submandibular gland.

Removal of a branchial cyst

A horizontal incision is made over the cyst, which is dissected off the jugular vein and carotid artery. The tract of the cyst is then carefully dissected out and transected.

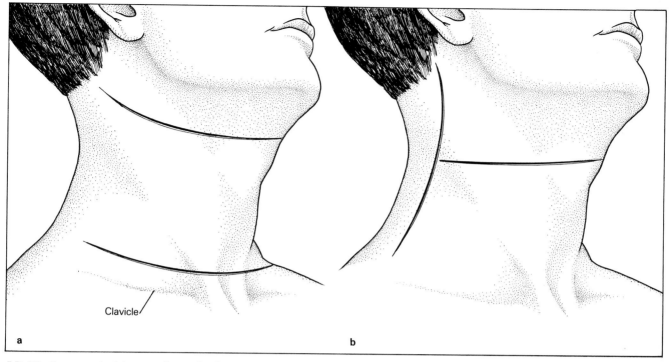

LD-76. *Common incisions used in radical neck dissection.* **a**, *McFee incision.* **b**, *Schechter incision.*

The sternomastoid has to be retracted laterally and the tract has usually to be followed superomedially between the external and internal carotid arteries and above the hypoglossal nerve. It is followed as far as possible before being transected.

Removal of a laryngocoele

A horizontal incision over the thyroid cartilage is required and the sac is completely removed.

The upper half of the thyroid lamina on the affected side is removed, the neck of the sac identified, the sac removed and its neck ligatured in the ventricle.

Gland biopsy

The following points should be kept in mind:

- never biopsy a malignant gland and close the skin
  There is a risk that implantation will follow and the cure rate will fall dramatically.

- give the pathologist a whole gland
  This is particularly important with lymphoma.

- care is needed with tuberculous nodes
  They are often stuck in the wall of the internal jugular vein.

- beware of a chemodectoma
  Never biopsy any lump intimately associated with the carotid bulb without a preoperative angiogram.

- biopsy first in the posterior triangle
  If there are multiple glands this is the best site, for there is little to damage there.

- obtain the best specimen
  Glands from the periphery of an area or necrotic material from the main mass of glands are unlikely to be helpful to the pathologist.

- the finding of a malignant gland on frozen section means a full radical neck dissection

TEST-YOURSELF QUESTIONS

Part 7 – The Neck

1. Which of the following muscles are attached to the laryngopharyngeal apparatus?
a) Sternomastoid
b) Hyoglossus
c) Thyrohyoid
d) Trapezius
e) Frontalis

2. The posterior triangle of the neck contains the following structures:
a) Carotid sheath
b) Accessory nerve
c) Vagus nerve
d) Lymph nodes
e) Thyroid gland

3. A 50-year-old man presents with a painless swelling in the area of the right jugulodigastric node. This is likely to be:
a) Secondary metastases from a nasopharyngeal carcinoma
b) Hypertrophy due to recurrent tonsillitis
c) Secondary metastases from a gastrointestinal neoplasm
d) A thyroglossal duct cyst
e) A laryngocoele

4. Which of the following investigations are appropriate in investigation of a thyroid mass?
a) Chest X-ray
b) Laryngogram
c) Lymphangiography
d) Thyroid scan
e) Kveim test

5. Movement on swallowing is a feature of:
a) Thyroid masses
b) Thyroglossal duct cyst
c) Chondroma of the thyroid cartilage
d) Branchial cyst
e) Dermoid cyst

6. A 30-year-old-man presents with a painless lump situated in the posterior triangle of the neck. There is no skin fixation and no other symptoms. Which of the following should be considered in the differential diagnosis?
a) Cervical rib
b) Chemodectoma
c) Benign parotid tumour
d) Tuberculous lymph node
e) Laryngocoele

7. Squamous carcinoma metastases in a deep jugular lymph node can originate from:
a) Stomach
b) Nasopharynx
c) Maxillary sinus
d) Pyriform fossa
e) Tongue

8. Antibiotic treatment is indicated in:
a) Cytomegalovirus infection
b) Infectious mononucleosis
c) Toxoplasmosis
d) Dermoid cyst
e) Chronic thyroiditis

9. The features of a branchial cyst are:
a) It is situated at the junction of the lower $\frac{1}{3}$ and upper $\frac{2}{3}$ of the sternomastoid muscle
b) It can present as an abscess
c) It never becomes malignant
d) It arises from the primitive air sacs of the laryngeal ventricle
e) It is fluctuant and mobile

10. Removal of a neurolemmoma from the vagus nerve in the neck can result in:
a) Ptosis of the eye on the ipsilateral side
b) Abducent palsy on the ipsilateral side
c) Hoarseness
d) Dilatation of the pupil on the ipsilateral side
e) Hyperhidrosis of the face

11. A swelling of one parotid gland with intact facial nerve function is most likely to be due to:
a) Sjögren's syndrome
b) Adenoid cystic carcinoma
c) Lymphoma
d) Pleomorphic adenoma
e) Tuberculosis

12. Which of the following statements are true?
a) During a thyroidectomy the recurrent laryngeal nerve is at risk
b) A branchial cyst is removed via a vertical incision
c) Chemodectomas can be biopsied safely
d) The first step in investigation of a suspected metastatic lymph node is biopsy of the node
e) A radical neck dissection is indicated if a frozen section of a node shows lymphoma

The answers to these questions will be found on p. 191.

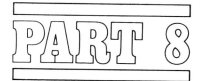

TRAUMA

SECTION I

Background to trauma of the face and neck

INTRODUCTION

This chapter is about trauma of the face and neck. It specifically excludes injury to the eye, the brain and cervical spinal column, the bones enclosing the brain and the cervical vertebrae. It is not concerned with the trauma which results from operations on the head and neck.

The face

Facial trauma is now one of the most common reasons for surgery. The injury may be minor, such as a small skin cut, or may involve a massive disruption of the facial bones with damage to the eyes, nose and mouth. However, no matter how great or small the injury is, it is important that the repair is performed carefully so that the best functional and cosmetic result is obtained, for after surgery the injured person has to go out and 'face' the world.

In 1901, at the age of 31, a French surgeon called Le Fort published three papers in which he described the midface fracture lines produced when the head of a corpse was struck by a wooden club with blows from different directions and of varying severity. From this work developed the present classification of facial bone fractures named after him.

Rather curiously the pattern of bone fracture that occurs when a face is struck is very constant, therefore only the major types of middle third fractures are described (see Section IV, p. 177).

A minor blow will damage the most prominent part of the central middle third of the face – the nose. A lateral blow will cause two main types of fracture and again the pattern is fairly constant.

The mandible is the lower third of the face and can be fractured by both central and lateral blows but the pattern of fracture is less constant than in the maxilla.

Since both the maxilla and mandible are tooth bearing structures, an important sign of a facial fracture is altered dental occlusion, and repair is largely controlled by placing the teeth in correct alignment.

The neck

The anatomy of the neck is considered in Part VII, p. 154). The two significant areas of injury are the carotid sheath and the larynx. Injury to the first kills by blood loss and to the second kills by airway obstruction.

The carotid sheath is well protected by the sternomastoid muscle and it has to be a very determined and painful suicide attempt actually to sever it.

The larynx is not so well protected and it can either be perforated, giving rise to internal oedema and respiratory embarrassment, or it can be pushed back and compressed against the cervical spine causing it to fracture. During sports such as basketball and karate it is liable to injury when it is unprotected. The commonest cause of a laryngeal fracture is hitting the neck on the steering wheel or dashboard in an automobile accident.

The ear

The external ear may be injured in many different ways – from indiscriminate ear piercing to having it bitten off in a rugby scrum. Fortunately the excellent blood supply allows quick healing.

More serious is an injury to the skull that fractures the petrous temporal bone in which the middle and inner ear are found. Damage to the ear ossicles and drum produces conductive deafness either because of disruption of the ossicular chain or the development of a haemotympanum. Sensorineural deafness, usually total, is produced when the cochlea is damaged. The facial nerve runs through the petrous temporal bone and may be bruised or divided, causing a facial nerve paralysis.

Perhaps the most serious consequence of this fracture is a cerebrospinal fluid (CSF) leak. This follows a dural tear in the middle fossa at the fracture site.

THE TYPE OF TRAUMA

Trauma of the head and neck may be caused by sharp injury, blunt injury or combination of both, or by a burn.

There may be loss of tissue in all of these types of trauma. In a sharp injury this can follow a tangential laceration or removal of part of the face by a dog or human bite. After a blunt injury, tissue may be lost by severe contusion and damage to blood vessels. Very severe violence such as gunshot wounds may cause loss of bone and soft tissues.

Sharp injury

In a sharp injury, typically seen when the head and neck go through a windscreen or after a knifing, the edges of the lacerations are cleancut and bony damage is rare.

Blunt injury

Bursting, ragged lacerations, fractures of the facial bones and fractures of the cartilages of the trachea and larynx may occur after a blunt injury such as a punch, kick, or when the rapidly moving face is stopped by an immovable object.

This commonly occurs when the head or neck hits the dashboard or steering wheel in a road traffic accident.

Burn injury

Burns of the head and neck may cause much loss of tissue.

Partial thickness burns involve the epidermis and heal rapidly. Deeper burns involve the full thickness of the skin while more severe burns may cause destruction of the aural and nasal cartilages and charring of the orbits and facial bones.

PREVENTION OF TRAUMA

The incidence of head and neck trauma in peacetime would be greatly reduced if it were made compulsory for car users to wear front and back seatbelts. Serious head and neck injuries have been reduced in the UK since the introduction of seat-belt legislation in 1983.

Provoking and teasing of dogs is a common cause of injury to children that could be avoided.

Burns of the head and neck in children are often due to scalds and can be prevented if the container of hot fluid is kept well out of reach of small but inquisitive fingers.

Epileptics, drug addicts and alcoholics are at risk of losing consciousness, when they may sustain severe burns. Some degree of prevention can be attained by ensuring that there are protective guards around fires. These patients, however, are always at risk. Burns of the head and neck in healthy adults are usually due to lack of care in the handling or use of inflammable materials. Wearing non-inflammable garments does reduce the risk of serious burning if clothes should catch fire.

SECTION II

History and physical examination of trauma of the face and neck

HISTORY

It may not be possible to obtain a history if the patient is unconscious and it may only be brief and limited if he is semiconscious. The examination and treatment of bleeding and airway obstruction take precedence over the history but some facts must be obtained quickly, if not from the patient then from relatives, friends or witnesses.

The accident

The details of the accident are important and although some assessment can be made of the severity of the trauma it must be remembered that very severe injuries can be due to apparently minor causes.

The patient

It is important to enquire about any past illnesses or surgery that the patient has had. A drug history should be obtained and a search made, if necessary, of his or her personal effects for cards or other evidence that may indicate epilepsy, diabetes mellitus, steroid or anticoagulant therapy etc.

Questioning about each area in the head and neck is postponed until any life-threatening injuries to the brain, chest or abdomen have been excluded or treated.

EXAMINATION

General assessment

Facial injuries

Points to elicit include:

- Do the teeth meet properly?
  If the maxilla or mandible have been fractured, then the teeth will feel out of alignment. Many patients' teeth look squint and it is only the patient who can tell if they feel different from normal.

- Is the bite normal?
  Mandibular and zygomatic fractures can cause abnormalities.

- Can the patient breath through the nose?
  This is unusual after a nasal fracture.

- Was the nose squint before?

- Is there evidence of diplopia?
  Several fractures involve the bony orbital walls and so alter the position of eye muscles and ligaments.

- Is there any abnormal nasal discharge?
  This may appear anteriorly or trickle down the throat. Remember CSF rhinorrhoea.

- Can the patient see normally?
  It may be difficult to assess this with black eyes but some fractures may involve the optic nerve.

Neck injuries

Points to elicit are:

- What is the voice like?
  A fractured or injured larynx will cause hoarseness.

- Is breathing difficult?

- Is it sore to swallow?

Ear injuries

Points to elicit are:

- Can the patient hear properly?

- Can the patient move his face on both sides equally?
- Is there any discharge from the ear?

Local assessment

It cannot be stressed too strongly that local examination should never take precedence over general assessment of the patient and getting priorities correct. This is described further in Section III, p. 175.

Facial injuries

The points to elicit include:

- Is the dental occlusion normal?
  Is there overbite or underbite?
  Are there any teeth fractured or missing?
  Did the patient wear a partial or complete denture?
- Are there lacerations in the mouth?
- Is there a mobile segment of the upper alveolus?
  This should signify a Le Fort fracture.
- Is there a mobile segment in the mandible?
- Can the patient completely close or open the mouth?
- Is the nose squint?
- Is there any clear nasal discharge?
- Is the nasal airway clear?
- Is the orbital rim fractured?
  This would occur with both lateral fractures and a Le Fort type II fracture (see p. 180). Bony irregularities can be detected on palpation.
- Is there diplopia?
  If there is diplopia on upward gaze this is diagnostic of a blowout fracture of the orbit with trapping of the inferior rectus muscle.
- Does the patient have a black eye?
  Haematoma of the orbit can be due to simple contusion or to nasal factors – Le Fort II and III and lateral and middle third fractures.
- Is there any facial flattening?
  Le Fort fractures produce a 'dish-face' deformity with depression of the middle third. Fractures of the zygoma produce flattening of the cheek.
- Is there severe bleeding?
  Assess the size, depth and position of facial lacerations. Decide if the bleeding is arterial or venous.
- Is there any respiratory obstruction?
- Is there any flattening of the larynx?
  A loss of the Adam's apple prominence could indicate a fracture.
- Is there any surgical emphysema?
  This could follow a fractured sinus but it could also be due to a fractured larynx.
- Is there any injury to the cervical spine?

Ear injuries

The points to elicit:

- What is the external ear like?
  Are there pieces missing and can they be found?
- Is the eardrum intact?
- Is there blood in the middle ear?
- Is there any clear discharge from the ear?
- Is there deafness as judged by voice tests?
- Is there a partial or complete facial paralysis?
  This is a most important assessment to make, because a bruised nerve may later fail to conduct, causing paralysis. This lesion will always respond to steroids but they can only be given safely if it is known that some facial movement existed initially. If this is not the case, a facial paralysis means open surgical exploration.
- Is it conductive or sensorineural?
- Is the patient dizzy and is there nystagmus?

INVESTIGATIONS

Laryngoscopy

In a fractured larynx a direct laryngoscopy will have to be carried out to assess the damage and the safety of the airway.

Tests for cerebrospinal fluid

Any clear discharge from the nose or the ear should be regarded as a possible CSF leak. Although sophisticated radioisotope tests are available, a simple Clinistix test usually suffices. CSF contains enough sugar to give a positive result if a Clinistix is dipped into the discharge.

Facial nerve tests

These should be undertaken, as soon as practical, whenever any facial nerve weakness is observed. Electroneuronography will usually indicate whether the lesion is a neuropraxia, an axonotmesis or an neuronotmesis. It is essential to have a baseline, for the treatment is different in each case.

Audiometry

This is not very important until the acute stage is over. It will show the severity of deafness and whether it is conductive or sensorineural.

Vestibular function tests

These are not done in the acute phase, but will be necessary to assess the extent of damage from any petrous bone fracture.

RADIOLOGY

Apart from simple nasal fractures, if there is a clinical suspicion of a facial bone fracture, X-rays of the face should be taken.

The standard views include:

- posteroanterior (X-33)
- lateral (X-34)
- 30° occipitomental (X-35)
- submentovertical (X-36)

Additional views for the mandible include:

- lateral oblique (X-37)
- orthopantomogram (X-38)

An erect chest X-ray (X-39) should be taken at the same time as the facial bone X-rays. This X-ray may show concurrent pulmonary disease or teeth or bone chips if they have been aspirated.

X-rays of the face are often difficult to interpret. Fractures can be seen if the bony outlines of one side of the face are compared with the other (X-40–42). An opaque maxillary antrum usually means that the maxilla or malar bone has been fractured. The extent of bony and soft tissue damage in some cases of severe facial trauma can only be discovered at operation.

When a laryngeal fracture is suspected, plain films should be taken to see if there is any surgical emphysema that was not discovered on clinical examination. A laryngogram will outline any internal derangement of the soft tissues.

With any injury to the ear, plain films of the petrous bone are necessary but a fracture line is very seldom seen unless tomography is performed.

SECTION III

Presentation of trauma of the face and neck and the diagnostic possibilities

CLINICAL APPROACH

After ensuring that the patient is not in respiratory difficulty and that any severe bleeding has stopped, a brief history of the accident should be obtained from either the patient or witnesses. Thereafter a general and specific examination should be carried out.

Airway obstruction and haemorrhage

Airway obstruction and haemorrhage takes precedence over a careful history and examination.

Airway obstruction

Airway obstruction may be due to:
- blood clots or debris in the oropharynx
- laryngeal trauma or oedema
- tracheal trauma or oedema
- swelling of the tongue and floor of the mouth
- an unstable tongue falling back and occluding the oropharynx

Facial burns predispose to oedema and lingual instability occurs after bilateral anterior mandibular fractures.

It is important, therefore, to inspect the mouth, removing loose teeth, dentures, blood clots and debris.

Turn the patient on his side so that the tongue falls away from the oropharynx.

If there is still difficulty in breathing, the patient should be intubated or a tracheostomy performed.

Haemorrhage

Serious haemorrhage is not common in facial trauma

and can usually be controlled by firm pressure. Occasionally a large vessel, usually the facial artery, requires ligation. Bleeding from a neck wound may be massive and fatal if it is not quickly controlled. Massive bleeding is usually from the internal jugular vein, the carotid arteries or the great vessels in the root of the neck.

As a first aid measure, firm direct pressure must be applied. The neck should be explored and the bleeding vessel identified. Lacerations of the great vessels in the root of the neck should be repaired with vascular sutures. The common and internal carotid artery must be repaired if possible to prevent cerebral ischaemia. However, the external carotid artery and its branches and the veins in the neck, including the internal jugular vein, can be safely ligated, for there is a rich vascular anastomosis in the head and neck.

History

Establish when, where, how and why the injury did occur. If the patient is conscious a full history should be taken.

Note if there has been pre- and posttraumatic amnesia, or pain and discomfort of the head and neck. The previous health, current medications and allergies of the injured person should be recorded.

Examination

General examination

The head and neck are examined after a quick, but thorough, examination of the rest of the body. The points that should be answered by this examination include:

- Are the limbs marked?
  Is there normal sensation and movement in them?
- Is the trunk marked?
  The seat belt or steering wheel may leave marks.
- Is there perineal bruising?
  Can the pelvic girdle be painlessly compressed?
- Is there abdominal pain?
  Are there signs of tenderness or rigidity and are the bowel sounds present?
- Is breathing easy?
  Do both sides of the chest expand equally or is the apex beat displaced?

Examine the spine and pay special attention to the cervical vertebrae. These are often fractured after a road traffic accident. If these fractures are not diagnosed early, there may be serious or even fatal consequences.

Specific examination

After the patient has been generally assessed and the various life support systems set up, more specific attention can be given to the head and neck. Apply the examination techniques described in Section II.

Face lacerations

All debris must be removed and a minimal debridement done. Assess and document the facial lacerations and note any that will require specialist help for repair. They include those involving:

- eyelids
- lips
- nasal ala

- facial nerves
- salivary ducts

Face fractures

Establish whether or not there is a facial bone fracture. Try to identify the type.

Central middle third fractures will require an oral surgeon to establish proper dental occlusion and to make temporary dentures. Radiographs are required to confirm the clinical findings. A facial fracture should be treated as soon as possible before swelling makes assessment and treatment more difficult.

Laryngeal fractures

If a laryngeal fracture is suspected, then appropriate radiographs should be undertaken. A laryngologist should carry out immediate exploration and repair.

Acute laryngeal fractures are relatively easy to treat. If, however, they are allowed to scar, then treatment may be impossible – thus condemning the patient to a life with a tracheostomy tube.

Ear trauma

If the ear is injured, then the petrous bone should be X-rayed. The facial nerve function should be accurately recorded, using the other side for comparison. The otologist may well consult a neurosurgeon if there is a CSF leak. The only indication for immediate surgery is if the facial nerve is totally paralysed. This indicates complete division.

Other measures

When the airway is secure, bleeding controlled and the examination of the patient complete, the appropriate form of tetanus prophylaxis is given.

If more than 4 hours have elapsed since the injury or if there is obvious wound contamination, a course of antibiotics should be started. Blood transfusion may be necessary.

SECTION IV

Description of specific trauma of the face and neck

FACIAL SOFT TISSUES INJURY

Causes

The face may be lacerated in an infinite number of ways. Typical lacerations from sharp trauma are cleancut and those of blunt trauma have ragged skin edges (CP-72).

Clinical features

Examination

All facial lacerations, bruising and swelling are carefully examined and their relationship to deeper structures such as the facial bones, facial nerve, sensory nerves, parotid gland and duct established. Particular note is made of injury to the lips, eyelids and ear and of any skin loss.

Facial skin retracts when incised and skin loss, especially in the young, is more apparent than real.

The facial muscles are tested to exclude damage to the facial nerve or its branches. The eyes are inspected and any loss or alteration in vision noted.

Lacerations, fractures and burns around the orbit may result in such gross eyelid swelling that the eye is closed. The eyelids must be prised apart and the eye inspected.

Throughout the examination, the injured side of the face is constantly compared with the uninjured side.

Management

Most facial wounds are small and confined to skin and are easily sutured using a local anaesthetic. They must, however, be scrupulously cleaned and explored to exclude injury to deep structures (CP-73, CP-74).

Deep tissues are united with 3/o or 4/o catgut.

Mucosal wounds are sutured with 3/o and 4/o catgut. These stitches are not removed.

The skin is carefully closed with interrupted sutures of 5/o silk or 6/o nylon. Landmarks like the skin–vermilion border of the lip, eyebrow hair and the rim of the nose are noted and accurately aligned. Skin sutures are removed 4–7 days after insertion to ensure a fine scar.

Tissue loss

Occasionally a bit of the face is completely detached. If available, it should be sewn back on (CP-75–78).

Pieces of ear and nose are commonly bitten off. If found, they should be brought to the hospital, washed in sterile saline and kept in a sterile saline solution on ice. As soon as possible, they are sutured back into place. Because of the excellent blood supply of the face, they often survive. Similarly, any flap of skin, no matter how long and thin, should be stitched back on to the face.

Anaesthetic

In patients, especially children, with extensive wounds and when there is also intraoral and bony damage, repair is usually best performed under a general anaesthetic.

· *This anaesthetic should be given by an experienced anaesthetist capable of passing an endotracheal tube under difficult circumstances.*

After appropriate anaesthesia, the wounds are scrubbed with a nailbrush to remove dirt and blood clots.

The injury can then be thoroughly assessed and carefully repaired.

FACIAL BURNS

Burns of the face can involve the full or partial thickness of the skin.

Partial thickness burns heal well and quickly if left exposed. After 3 weeks there is usually only an erythema over the burned areas.

Full thickness burns require removal of dead skin and replacement with skin grafts or skin flaps (CP-79).

Management

The mucosa of the oral cavity and the upper respiratory tract may be involved in burns of the head and neck. The resultant swelling and damage can cause respiratory obstruction.

Patients sustaining burns of the head and neck should be carefully observed for signs of airway obstruction or respiratory difficulty. The inhalation of smoke may cause severe damage to the lungs. Intubation or tracheostomy may be needed and, if there is pulmonary damage, the patient may have to go onto a respirator. The advice of an anaesthetist should be sought early, as inhalation of smoke with respiratory failure is one of the common causes of death in the burned patient.

Small discrete full thickness skin burns may be excised and grafted immediately. Larger burns are treated as soon as the facial swelling has subsided and the general condition of the patient is satisfactory. To protect the cornea after full thickness burns of the eyelids, an early temporary tarsorraphy or eyelid skin grafting may be done.

*LD-77. Common mandibular fractures. **a**, Fracture: **1**, at neck of condyle; **2**, at mandibular angle; **3**, through body of mandible. **b**, Fracture: **1**, through neck of condyle; **2**, at mandibular angle; **3**, through body of mandible; **4**, at symphysis*

FACIAL BONE FRACTURES

The face has three main bony complexes. They are the mandible, which is the lowest part of the face, and the malar, maxillary and nasal bones which make up the midface. The upper face is mainly formed by the frontal bones.

Undisplaced facial fractures often need no surgical treatment provided there is no impairment of function.

Fractures of the mandible

Mandibular fractures commonly occur at the symphysis, through the body, at the mandibular angle and at the neck of the condyle (LD-77). The bone fractures at the impact site or else the force is transmitted to a weaker part of the mandible – usually the condyle – which then fractures.

Posterior to the first lower molar tooth, the muscles of elevation of the mandible – the masseter, medial pterygoid and temporalis – are inserted. Anterior to this tooth the depressor muscles – the digastric, mylohyoid and geniohyoid – are inserted. Thus vertical fractures of the body of the mandible result in elevation of the posterior fragment and depression of the anterior fragment. This is exaggerated when the fracture line runs obliquely posteroinferiorly to anterosuperiorly. If the fracture is in the opposite direction, it may be stable (LD-78, LD-79).

Blows on the chin often produce an indirect bilateral condylar fracture. The lateral pterygoid muscles pull the mandible forwards; the upper and lower molars then become the first teeth to meet, causing the patient to gag. An open bite results.

Fractures of the mandibular body usually end in a tooth socket. This is a potential route for infection to spread to the fracture site.

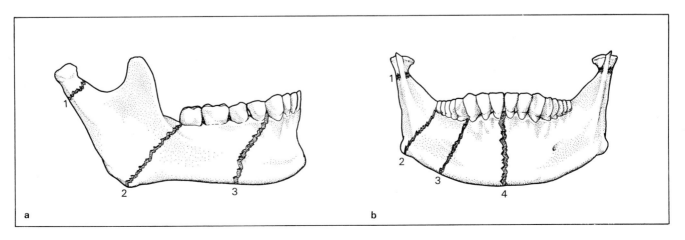

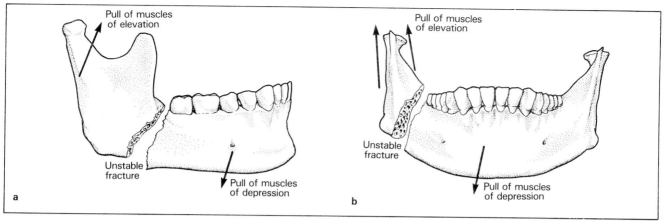

LD-78. *Unstable mandibular fracture*

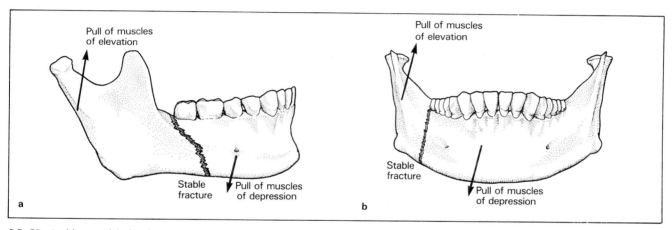

LD-79. *Stable mandibular fracture*

Clinical features

Diagnosis is usually obvious since the patient has great difficulty in opening the mouth and speaking. The fracture may be compound into the mouth. This will produce a great deal of bleeding and dental disruption. Crepitus and pain may be elicited on moving the bony fragments. The mandible should be palpated bimanually, with one finger inside the mouth and the other outside. If a fracture of the jaw is suspected and the patient feels and the examiner observes that the dental occlusion is not normal, a fracture is present.

An X-ray will confirm the fracture.

Management

If the injury is compound into the mouth it is liable to infection and so a suitable antibiotic should be given.

Mandibular fractures are reduced and kept immobilized in the correct position for at least 4 weeks.

Accurate reduction can be achieved, for when the teeth are in normal occlusion, the mandibular fracture is correctly aligned. The fractured fragments are kept in that position by wiring the teeth together. Usually 'cap' splints are made, fitted on to the upper and lower teeth and wired together (CP-80). In the edentulous, splints or dentures have to be secured to the alveoli. Occasionally the fracture is directly wired or plated (X-43).

Fractures of the maxilla

The midface bones include the maxilla, malar and nasal bones. Fractures of the maxilla may be through any part of the bone, but commonly are at three levels and are often continuous with the other bones of the midface. The maxilla acts as a buffer and absorbs most of the force of severe facial trauma, saving the cranial bones from fracturing and thus lessening cranial damage. The maxillary fracture lines, described by Le Fort, are called Le Fort I, II and III fractures (LD-80–82).

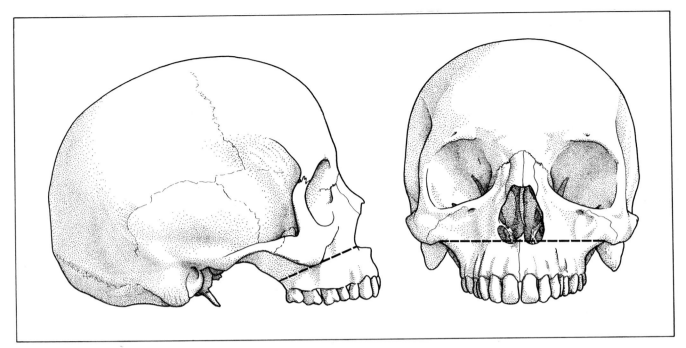

LD-80. *Le Fort I fracture*

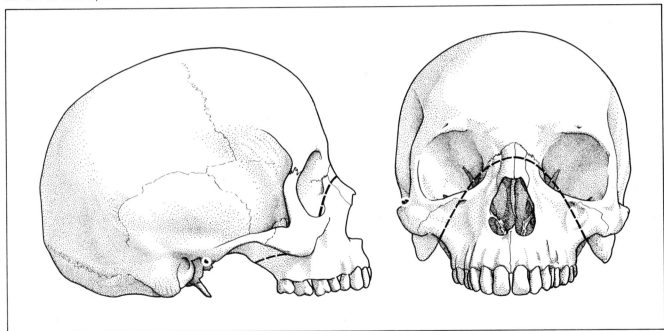

LD-81. *Le Fort II fracture*

Le Fort fractures

Le Fort I

In the Le Fort I fracture (LD-80) the palate is separated from the rest of the maxilla. The fracture line passes through the base of the antrum, divides the septum from its attachment on the nasal floor and stops at the inferior end of the pterygoid plates.

Le Fort II

The Le Fort II fracture (LD-81) separates the maxilla from the orbit. The fracture line goes through the upper half of the pterygoid plates, passes between the maxilla and the malar bone, through the infraorbital margin and across the weak lachrymal bone to the bridge of the nose (CP-81, CP-82).

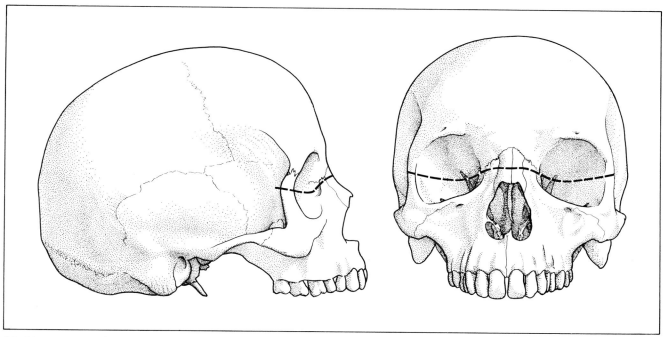

LD-82. *Le Fort III fracture*

Le Fort III

The most severe midface fracture is the Le Fort III fracture (LD-82). This results in a separation of the facial bones from the cranium. The fracture line is through the zygomatic arch, the lateral orbital margin and the posterior part of the orbital cavity and into the ethmoid sinus. The cribriform plate is usually fractured. This leads to a temporary cerebrospinal fluid leak and anosmia which may be permanent.

Usually the Le Fort fractures are symmetrical, but any combination of fractures such as a left Le Fort III and a right Le Fort I and II may occur. An associated midline fracture of the palate is often present (CP-81, CP-82). The type and severity of the maxillary fracture depends on the direction and force of the injury and the strength of the bones.

Clinical features

The facial bones are palpated for irregularity, deformity and tenderness. If one of these features is present, it is assumed there is a fracture.

Fractures of the maxillomalar complex produce an elongation of the face and are accompanied by much facial swelling. Conversely, a bony deformity may be masked by a nearby soft tissue injury.

The maxilla is tested by stabilizing the forehead with one hand while the fingers of the other hand grip the hard palate and upper alveolus, rocking them gently anteroposteriorly. Any movement is abnormal and is due to a maxillary fracture (CP-83).

Radiographs of the sinuses will demonstrate the fracture lines.

Management

Maxillary fractures are reduced and immobilized for at least 4 weeks. Reduction is achieved when the teeth are in occlusion. Immobilization is obtained by wiring the maxillary alveolus to the mandible and then securing the fractured segments by rigidly splinting them to an area above the fracture. These splints may be internal or external.

The external splint or rod is attached inferiorly to cap splints and superiorly to a frame of either the 'box' or 'halo' type. These frames are screwed into the skull – the 'halo' frame – or into the skull and mandible – the 'box' frame (CP-84–86, X-44). Internal fixation is used widely in the USA. In this technique wires are passed from an upper cap splint directly to the skull, instead of indirectly via a frame. These wires are usually attached to the zygomatic arch or the upper part of the lateral orbital margin.

Occasionally fragments of the maxilla are directly wired together.

Fractures of the malar complex

The malar complex is made up of the zygomatic arch, the malar bone and part of the lateral and inferior orbital walls. It is usually fractured by direct violence. Occasionally the orbital floor is fractured indirectly by an object compressing the soft tissues of the orbit – a blowout fracture.

The sudden increase of pressure in the orbital cavity results in the orbital walls fracturing at their weakest point – the orbital floor behind the infraorbital margin. The floor is 'blown out' into the maxillary antrum (LD-83).

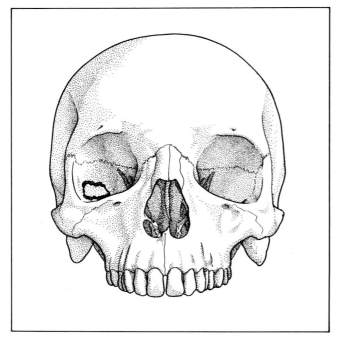

LD-83. Fracture of orbital floor behind infraorbital margin. The fragment drops into the antrum

More commonly the malar complex is fractured through its margins. There may be a discrete fracture of the zygomatic arch (LD-84). The malar buttress may be broken off intact, with fracture lines through the infraorbital rim and zygomatic arch and through the maxillomalar suture (LD-85).

Direct trauma to an orbital margin may produce comminution of that margin (LD-86).

Clinical features

These fractures usually cause local swelling, diplopia and infraorbital anaesthesia.

Diplopia is due to the ocular muscles being trapped by fractured bone. This is more noticeable on upward gaze.

Infraorbital anaesthesia results from pressure on the infraorbital nerve by the displaced fractured bone.

In severe orbital floor fractures there may be

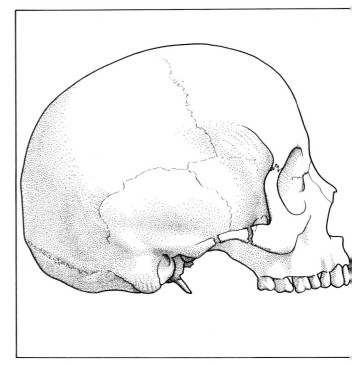

LD-84. Discrete fracture of zygomatic arch. The medially driven fracture may cause trismus

enopthalmos and the eye may be displaced inferiorly. This is due to the orbital contents dropping into the maxillary antrum through an orbital floor defect.

Certain fractures of the zygomatic arch may cause trismus due to pressure on the coronoid process of the mandible.

Management

Malar fractures are reduced by:

- direct exposure of the fracture
- levering the bone into position
  This is achieved by an indirect approach.
- pushing the bone into position
  This is achieved by packing the maxillary antrum (LD-87).

Some malar fractures are stable when reduced. Some require wiring or support of the fractured bone with an antral pack for 2 or 3 weeks (X-41).

Orbital floor fractures often result in part of the orbital contents dropping into the antrum. The contents may be returned by opening the antrum through a Caldwell–Luc approach, replacing the contents into the orbit and supporting the reduction of the orbital floor fracture by packing the antrum. The orbital floor fracture can also be exposed directly by an infraorbital incision. Bone loss of the orbital floor can be corrected by an autogenous bone graft or a sheet of silastic.

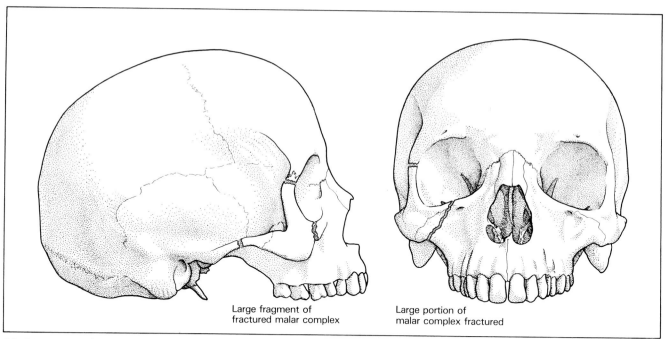

Large fragment of
fractured malar complex

Large portion of
malar complex fractured

LD-85. Fractured malar complex

LD-86. Fracture of the orbital margin

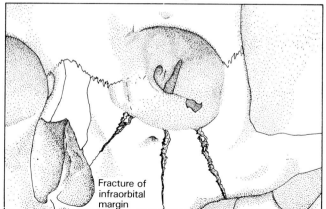

Fracture of
infraorbital
margin

LD-87. Methods of approach to a malar fracture

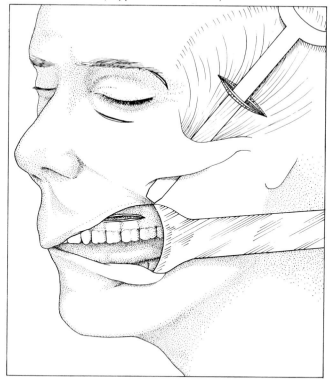

Fractures of the nasal complex

The nasal complex consists of an upper bony part, a cartilaginous lower part and in the middle a bony-cartilaginous septum. The nose may be injured by a lateral or frontal force.

When the nose is broken by a lateral force, the nasal bones and septum become impacted and there is an additional lateral displacement of the whole of the nose (CP-87).

A frontal blow forces the nasal bones backwards beneath the frontal bone. A flattening of the midface results. This may be accompanied by a widening between the medial canthi if the force fractures the ethmoid and lachrymal bones, and disrupts the insertion of the medial canthal ligaments.

Clinical features

The nose is carefully palpated for tenderness or undue mobility in the bones or cartilage. Alteration in shape of the nose is recorded.

The nasal mucosa is inspected for tears, displacement and swelling of the nasal septum. A swelling in the septum indicates a haematoma. A watery colourless or bloodstained nasal discharge may indicate probable cerebrospinal fluid leak down the nose from a dural tear in the cribriform plate area.

Management

The fractured, displaced nasal bones and septum are manipulated under anaesthetic into a correct position and the fracture immobilized.

A septal swelling due to haematoma, if not drained, often gets infected. The septum may then necrose and cause collapse of the nose.

During manipulation, the septum is inspected for swelling.

Immobilization is by a combination of nasal packing for at least 5 days and an external plaster of Paris splint for at least 1 week.

The ethmoidal and lachrymal bones may be fractured as well as the nasal bones. This produces disruption of the insertion of the medial canthal ligaments and an apparent widening between the orbits. In these injuries the bony fragments and the canthal ligaments have to be wired back into position.

If cerebrospinal rhinorrhoea occurs after a fracture of the midface an antibiotic which penetrates the blood–brain barrier must be given, to prevent ascending infection of the meninges and brain.

Timing of surgery in facial trauma

When the injury is confined to bone, reduction and fixation should be carried out in the first few hours before the face swells or between the third and seventh day when such swelling has subsided. If treatment is delayed for more than 10 days, accurate reduction may be difficult because the fragments will have started to unite in a faulty position.

Soft tissue injuries should be repaired promptly to prevent wound infection.

Under exceptional circumstances such as a history of prolonged loss of consciousness, the soft tissue repair can be postponed for up to 24 hours, provided a broad spectrum antibiotic is given.

Postoperative care in facial trauma

A fluid or soft diet is given and excessive talking is discouraged. Rest for the healing face is vital if the jaws are fixed together. Facial trauma is not very painful, but some analgesia may be needed. Frequent oral toilet is carried out. This is especially important when the jaws have been fractured.

After the repair of severe facial trauma, appropriate intravenous hydration may be required.

Facial fractures in the young

Facial fractures seldom occur in the young, as they are less exposed to the violence of adult life and their bones are more pliable. The patterns of fracture and the management are similar to those of adults.

Prompt recognition and early treatment is important as facial growth may be affected by inaccurate reduction. But even with precise reduction, future growth may be altered by damage to the developing bone and cartilage.

INJURIES OF THE MOUTH

Causes

A blow around or on the mouth may cause direct damage to teeth and to the alveoli and indirectly may result in extensive oral mucosal lacerations. The damage is due to the teeth being forced against the mucosa.

Lacerations of the lower and upper labial sulci result from shearing forces stripping the soft tissues of the mandible and maxilla at the weak point of the mucosal reflection of the alveolus.

Clinical features

Careful local examination of the teeth, alveoli and intraoral mucosa is essential. The sulcal lacerations are often deceptively extensive and may communicate with the nasal vestibule.

X-rays of the jaws and chest should be taken if there is injury to the bone or teeth.

Management

The wounds are carefully examined, cleaned and sutured. Bleeding tooth sockets may require suture. Tooth replantation may be considered.

INJURIES OF THE EAR

Causes

Common causes of ear injury are foreign bodies in the ear and blows to the side of the head.

Blows may cause bleeding of the cartilage of the external ear and result in a haematoma. They may also cause pressure waves to build up inside the external meatus and rupture the ear drum. An explosive blast ruptures the drum in the same way.

Lacerations of the ear and bites – canine and human – can cause tissue loss.

Road traffic accidents and falls may fracture the temporal bone.

If the head is compressed in an anteroposterior direction, then the petrous bone fractures longitudinally. Side-to-side compression of the head causes transverse fractures of the petrous bone.

Clinical features

There may be a bloody or a clear discharge from the ear. The latter is typical of a leakage of cerebrospinal fluid.

The ear drum should be inspected for a perforation or a bulging blue drum which suggests a haematoma of the middle ear.

There may be nystagmus and vertigo.

The facial nerve may be damaged, causing either a partial or complete facial paralysis.

Tuning fork tests should be performed to try to establish whether any deafness is conductive or sensorineural. Audiometry is done early to establish the degree and confirm the nature of the deafness.

Conductive deafness follows damage to the drum or ossicular chain or it may be due to a middle ear haematoma. Sensorineural deafness is due either to concussion or to fracture of the cochlea.

Damage to the vestibule or semicircular canals results in dizziness or vertigo. Caloric tests and an electronystagmogram are required to assess the severity of damage.

Management

With trauma to the external ear, the lacerations are sutured. The ear has such a good blood supply that even narrow based flaps should be sewn back and any detached bits should be replaced.

A watery discharge from the ear following trauma is due to loss of cerebrospinal fluid. Antibiotics which cross the blood–brain barrier should be given, and the patient kept in bed for a few days with a sterile absorbent dressing over his ear.

A CSF leak usually settles spontaneously and the patient should be covered by antibiotics until it does. If it persists, then the dural tear will have to be repaired.

If the drum is perforated it may heal on its own, but if healing does not occur within 2 months then a myringoplasty will be required.

A haemotympanum usually resolves and drains via the Eustachian tube but if it does not then a myringotomy is required.

Ossicular discontinuity is treated by a tympanotomy and reconstruction of the damaged chain.

There is very little to be done about the vertigo that results from inner ear damage. It will eventually settle but it may take up to 6 months to do so.

Rehabilitation can be speeded by Cooksie and Cawthorne exercises. These exercises are designed to help to re-establish equilibrium by enhancing the part played by the eyes and limb proprioceptors.

Facial nerve paralysis

If facial paralysis is partial, the patient should receive steroids until recovery commences. The steroids reduce swelling of the nerve and so stop it being compressed in its bony canal. If paralysis is complete, it probably means that the nerve is divided and, in this case, the mastoid bone must be explored and the divided nerve ends resutured or grafted.

INJURIES OF THE NECK

Causes

Injuries of the neck are caused by blunt or sharp injury or by a combination of both.

Blunt trauma

The main causes of blunt trauma are direct blows on the neck and failure to wear adequate seat belts.

If a person involved in a car smash is wearing a lap-type seat belt or no seat belt at all, then when the car stops, the upper part of the body will continue with the same momentum to hit the dashboard or steering wheel.

If the neck hits the steering wheel, the larynx is pushed back against the cervical spine and splayed apart. If the larynx is uncalcified then the thyroid prominence breaks, to produce a palpable fracture. Since the vocal cords and the epiglottis are attached in this area, their detachment compromises the airway to a greater or lesser extent.

If the thyroid cartilage is calcified, then when it hits the cervical spine it will shatter, causing a flattening of the neck and a similar detachment of the vocal cords and epiglottis. More severe injury may produce a shearing-off of the cricoid and thyroid cartilages from the first tracheal ring. This is likely to produce total airway obstruction.

Sharp trauma

Lacerations of the neck rarely occur accidentally. Knifings and suicide attempts are the commonest causes.

In the latter, the neck is often extended before the incision is made and thus the large sternomastoid muscles protect the main neck vessels – the internal jugular vein and the common, internal and external carotid arteries. Conversely, if the neck is flexed these vessels are liable to be injured.

Penetrating stab wounds of the neck may injure distant vital structures in the neck and chest.

It is important to examine the chest, as neck wounds may involve the thorax causing pneumothorax or haemothorax as well as damage to the great vessels.

Clinical features

Examination may show:

- swelling
- difficulty in swallowing
- difficulty in breathing or stridor

Swelling may be due to a haematoma from a cut vessel or it may be due to surgical emphysema. This important sign occurs when the larynx is fractured and the airway is opened into the tissues of the neck. The first cough that the patient gives expels air into the neck tissues and causes surgical emphysema. With blunt trauma, the signs may be minimal.

Dysphagia may be due to swollen bruised arytenoids or pressure of blood on the oesophagus.

Difficulty in breathing may be due to direct damage to the larynx and trachea or due to pressure from blood collecting around these structures.

Management

If the condition of the patient permits, an X-ray of the neck and an erect chest X-ray should be taken. Blood should be sent for cross-matching. If the airway is at all affected, it must be made secure by either intubation or tracheostomy.

If the neck wound is deeper than the platysma and there is swelling, dyspnoea or bruising of the neck, then the wound should be explored under endotracheal general anaesthesia.

The wound should be exposed to allow good access and enlarged if necessary. All the veins in the neck except the subclavian and innominate veins in the root of the neck may be safely ligated. The external carotid artery and its branches may also be safely ligated. But damage to or ligation of the internal or common carotid artery and the great veins in the root of the neck may have serious functional consequences, and vascular reconstruction with the help of a vascular surgeon should be considered.

The larynx

If the larynx is injured, it is repaired as soon as the general condition of the patient permits. An open reduction of the fracture within the larynx and reattachment of the vocal cords and the epiglottis is performed. These fracture reductions are carried out around a laryngeal mould or keel to prevent later laryngeal stenosis.

Injuries of the oesophagus should be repaired and if necessary a thoracotomy may have to be performed if there is an injury to the lungs, heart or great vessels.

SECTION V

Principles of general management and treatment of trauma of the face and neck

TECHNIQUE OF SUTURING FACIAL WOUNDS

Equipment

A small needleholder, a pair of toothed forceps, some artery forceps and a pair of scissors are essential. An assistant is useful.

The deep layers of the wound are closed using 3/0 or 4/0 chromic catgut with the knots inverted. The skin is sutured using 5/0 silk or 6/0 nylon. An atraumatic, curved, fine cutting needle should be used.

Procedure

The needle pierces the skin 2–3 mm from the wound edge. It passes through the epidermis and dermis to emerge slightly more distant from the wound than the skin entry point. The needle is then inserted in the dermis of the opposite side of the wound and brought up through the skin in the mirror image of the other side. The wound edges are thus slightly everted. The knot is tied with at least two throws for silk and three for nylon. When the knot is bedded down on the skin, a fine adjustment of the wound edges can be made with pressure from the tips of the needleholder.

It is usually easier to stitch from a mobile piece of skin to a less mobile piece of skin.

Removal of stitches is performed with fine sharp-pointed scissors or a Number 11 blade. The stitch is pulled towards the suture line to avoid wound disruption. After suture removal, the wound may be supported by adhesive paper tape for a few days.

TARSORRAPHY

This is a procedure in which the upper and lower eyelids are joined together – usually to prevent the cornea being injured by exposure. In its simplest form, it involves passing a stitch through the free margins of the eyelids immediately behind the eyelashes. Care is taken to prevent the lashes turning in against the globe.

INTERMAXILLARY FIXATION

It is important to keep the jaws together in proper occlusion when there has been a fracture of one or both jaws. This is called 'intermaxillary fixation'. The precise nature depends on the presence or absence of teeth.

If teeth are present, loops of stainless steel 0.4 mm in diameter are passed between the necks of adjacent teeth, from within out. The ends of the wire are passed through the spaces between the teeth on each side of the loop and the long ends are brought through to the front of the teeth and twisted to the loop and themselves. This is repeated on several teeth of the upper and lower jaws. From the loops and protrusions made by the wire, the upper and lower teeth can be held together by wire or elastic bands (LD-88–90).

A more exact technique of intermaxillary fixation is to make accurately fitting splints which cap the teeth. These cap splints are carefully made from impressions of the upper and lower dentition. They are cemented onto the teeth and can be fixed together by wire or elastic bands passing from hooks incorporated into the labial surface of the splint.

In the edentulous patient, dentures without teeth are made after impressions have been taken. These are called Gunning splints and are held in place by being wired to the alveolus. The upper and lower Gunning splints are fixed together in the same way as cap splints.

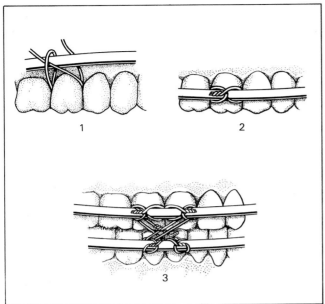

LD-88. *The steps in arch wiring*

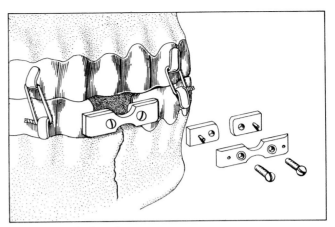

LD-89. *The locking bar*

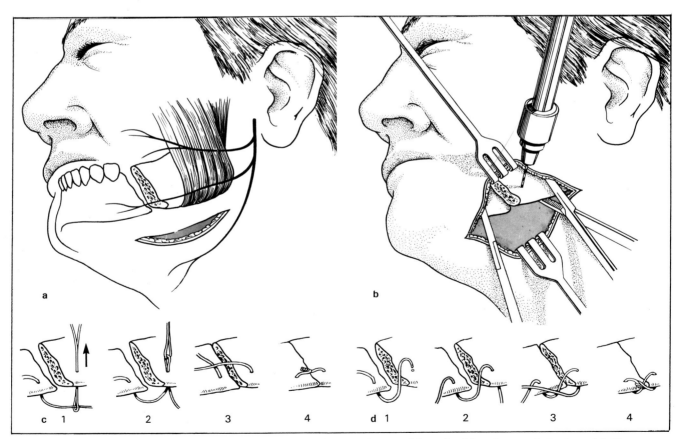

LD-90. *Interosseous wiring. **a**, Submandibular incision placed to avoid cervical branch of facial nerve. **b**, Boring of drill holes. **c**, Simple loop wire. **d**, Figure-of-eight wire*

TEST-YOURSELF QUESTIONS
Part 8 – Trauma

1. In the general examination of a patient with a facial injury the most important points to note and treat are:
a) possible fracture of spine
b) blindness
c) compound limb fracture
d) airway obstruction
e) significant external bleeding
f) facial palsy

2. In severe facial bony trauma requiring immediate surgery, which of the following is the most useful X-ray:
a) postero-anterior of face
b) submento-vertical
c) chest X-ray
d) lateral oblique
e) orthopantomogram

3. Which of the following can obstruct the airway:
a) facial burns
b) dentures
c) blow-out fractures of the orbit
d) mandibular fractures
e) facial muscle weakness

4. In facial and cervical injury is serious haemorrhage:
a) common in the face
b) usually associated with intra-oral lacerations
c) easily controlled by positioning the patient
d) associated with suicide attempts by cutting the neck
e) life threatening especially in the neck

5. What of the following soft tissue facial injuries may require specialist help:
a) laceration of palatal mucosa
b) injury to facial nerve
c) laceration through eyebrow
d) laceration through eyelid
e) laceration of ear
f) skin loss on nose

6. In soft tissue facial lacerations which of the following is true:
a) mucosal wounds are not sutured
b) skin stitches in the face should be left for at least 8 days to ensure sound healing
c) long, thin flaps of skin should be sutured back in place
d) the wound should not be scrubbed vigorously in case this provokes haemorrhage.

7. A 20-year-old man presents with severe full thickness burns of the whole of his face. Which of the following should be carried out:
a) immediate excision and skin grafting of his burns
b) early tarsorraphy or eyelid skin grafting
c) close watch kept on airway

8. Regarding mandibular fracture, which of the following are true:
a) they are usually compound into the mouth
b) they are always unstable
c) they may be difficult to diagnose
d) they need immobilisation for at least 4 weeks

9. A patient has a severe facial bone injury and has the following symptoms and signs: anosmia, rhinnorhea, a long face, trismus, (R) infraorbital anaesthesia. Which of the following fractures may he have:
a) Le Fort I
b) Le Fort II
c) Le Fort III
d) fracture malar complex
e) fracture of the mandible

10. The clinical features of fractures of the malar are:
a) bleeding from nose
b) elongation of the face
c) diplopia
d) infra-orbital anaesthesia
e) malocclusion

The answers to these questions will be found on p. 191.

ANSWERS TO
TEST-YOURSELF QUESTIONS

Part 1 The Ear

1   a, c and d (page 8)
2   b, c and d (pages 8, 22–24)
3   b, c and d (page 28)
4   b and c (page 31)
5   a, b and c (pages 19, 20)
6   b and d (page 21)
7   a and c (page 24)
8   b, c, d and e (pages 25, 26)
9   a and c (page 38)
10 a (pages 31–33)

Part 2 The Nose

1   c and e (page 47)
2   c (page 51)
3   b and d (page 53)
4   c (page 54)
5   e (page 54)
6   b (page 55)
7   d (page 57)
8   a and c (page 57)
9   b (page 59)
10 c (page 59)

Part 3 The Pharynx

1   a – Nasopharynx; b – Oropharynx; c – Hypopharynx (page 72)
2   1 – Is the obstruction unilateral or bilateral?; 2 – Is the obstruction variable?; 3 – Is there associated bleeding?; 4 – Is there an associated nasal secretion? (page 74)
3   a – 2, 3; b – 1, 4; c – 5 (page 78)
4   Compare your list with the list on page 80
5   Your list should include five of the following: nasal infections; oral infections; nasal obstruction; local irritants; general conditions; emotional and psychological problems (page 82)
6   a – Yes; b – Yes; c – Yes; d – No; e – Yes (page 83)
7   a – Yes; b – Yes; c – Yes; d – Yes; e – Yes (page 83)
8   General anaesthesia is used for rigid oesophagoscopy, local anaesthesia if a fibre optic instrument is used (page 86)

Part 4 The Larynx

1   a, c and d (Section I)
2   a and b (Section II)
3   a and c (Section III)
4   a, b, c and d (Section III)
5   d (Section III)
6   a (Section IV)
7   b and c (Section IV)
8   a, b and d (Section III)
9   b (Section V)
10 a, b and d (Section III)

Part 5 The Oral Cavity

1   b, c and e (page 112)
2   a and b (page 121)
3   a, c and e (page 119)
4   c and e (page 113)
5   a and c (page 121)
6   a, b and c (see page 120)
7   a and e (page 114)
8   a and e (page 118)
9   a, c and e (pages 118 and 119)
10 a, b and c (pages 118 and 119)

Part 6 The Salivary Glands

1   a and d (Section II)
2   d (Section I)
3   a and d (Section III)
4   a and b (Section III)
5   b (Section III)
6   a and c (Section IV)
7   a (Section IV)
8   a, b and c (Section IV)
9   a, b and d (Section IV)
10 b and d (Section V)

Part 7 The Neck

1   b and c (page 154)
2   b and d (page 155)
3   a (page 156)
4   a and d (page 158)
5   a, b and c (page 159)
6   a and d (page 160)
7   b, c, d and e (page 161)
8   c (page 162)
9   b and e (page 163)
10 a and c (page 164)
11 d (page 165)
12 a (pages 166 and 167)

Part 8 Trauma

1   d and e (pages 172 and 175)
2   c (page 174)
3   a, b and d (page 175)
4   e (pages 175 and 170)
5   b, d and f (page 176)
6   c (page 177)
7   b and c (page 178)
8   a (page 179)
9   a, b, c, d and e (pages 179, 181 and 182)
10 c and d (page 182)

COLOUR PICTURES

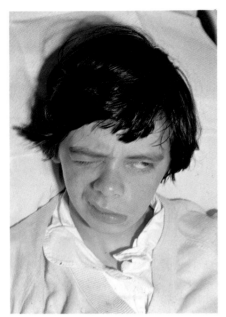

CP-1. *Facial palsy – after skull fracture*

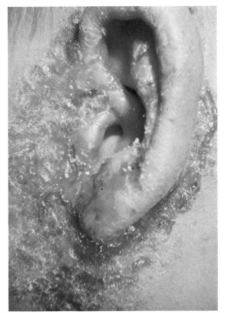

CP-4. *External otitis with excoriation*

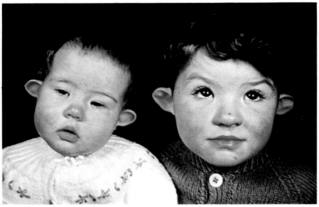

CP-2. *Bat ears*

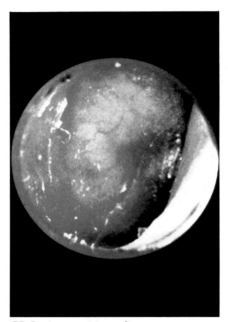

CP-5. *Acute otitis media*

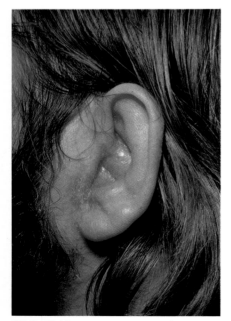

CP-3. *Otitis externa*

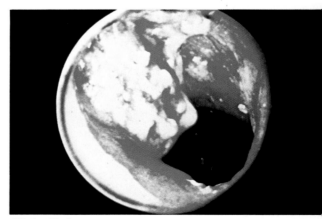

CP-6. *Cholesteatoma*

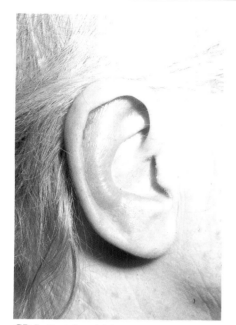

CP-7. *Perichondritis*

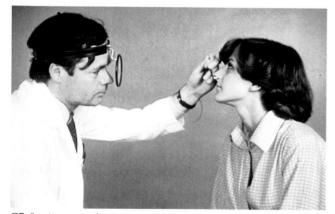

CP-8. *Anterior rhinoscopy*

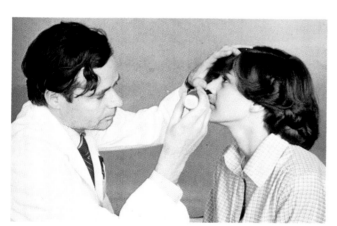

CP-9. *Anterior rhinoscopy with auroscope*

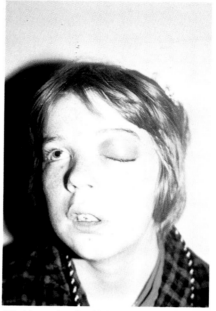

CP-10. *Orbital cellulitis from ethmoidal sinusitis*

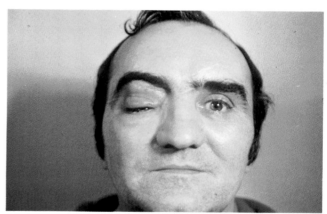

CP-11. *Frontal sinus abscess*

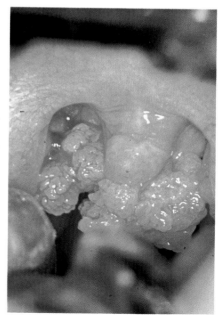

CP-12. *Nasal polyps in choana*

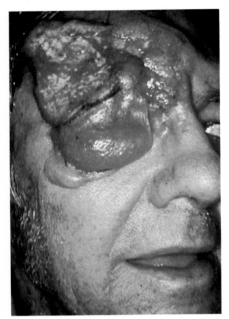

CP-13. Ethmoid carcinoma

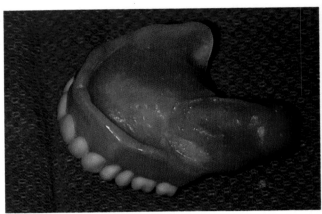

CP-16. Denture with obturator for palate

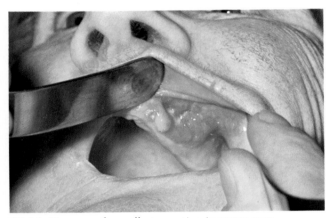

CP-14. Tumour of maxilla presenting in upper gum

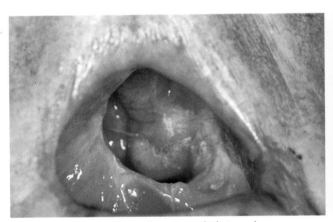

CP-17. Postoperative maxillectomy – hole in palate

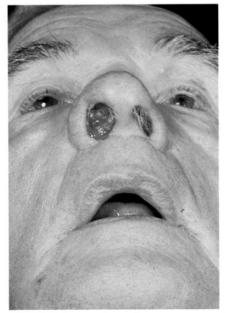

CP-15. Tumour of maxilla presenting in the nose

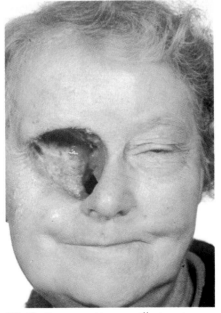

CP-18. Postoperative maxillectomy

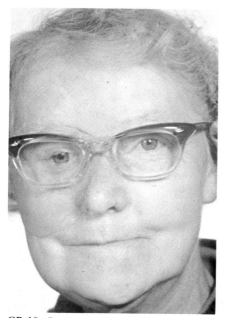

CP-19. *Postoperative maxillectomy with prosthesis*

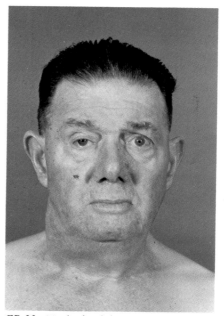

CP-22. *Neck gland from carcinoma of the nasopharynx*

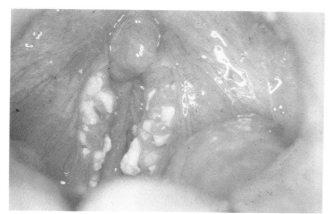

CP-20. *Follicular tonsillitis*

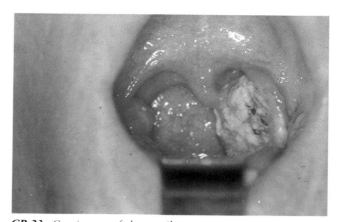

CP-23. *Carcinoma of the tonsil*

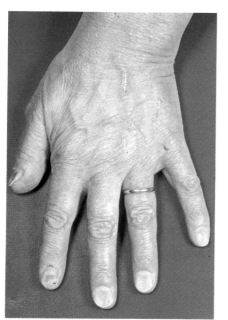

CP-21. *Koilonychia in Plummer–Vinson syndrome*

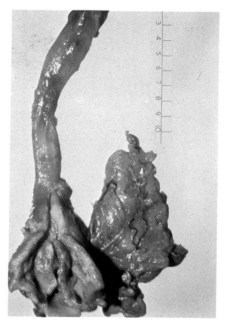

CP-24. *Specimen of postcricoid carcinoma*

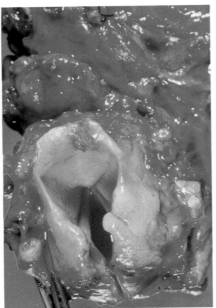

CP-25. *Specimen from laryngectomy and neck dissection for a piriform sinus carcinoma*

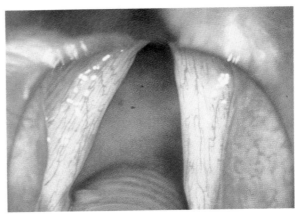

CP-28. *Normal vocal cord*

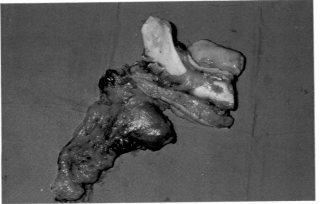

CP-26. *Specimen of carcinoma of the tonsil removed in commando operation*

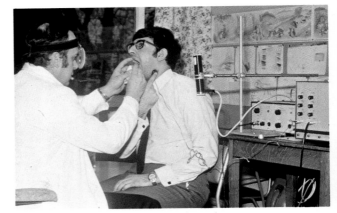

CP-29. *Indirect laryngoscopy with stroboscope*

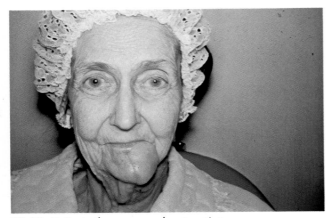

CP-27. *Patient after commando operation*

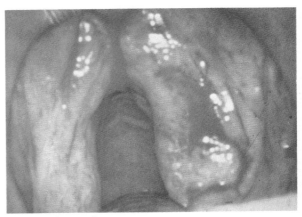

CP-30. *Chronic laryngitis*

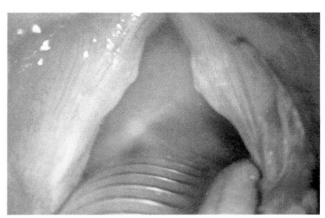

CP-31. Vocal cord nodules

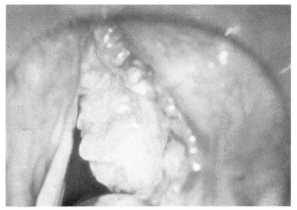

CP-34. Carcinoma of vocal cords

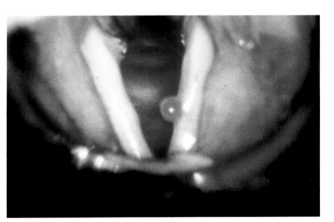

CP-32. Vocal cord polyp

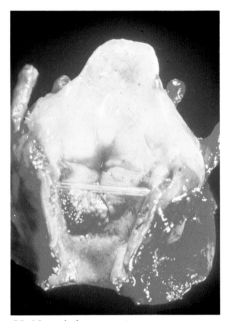

CP-35. Subglottic carcinoma

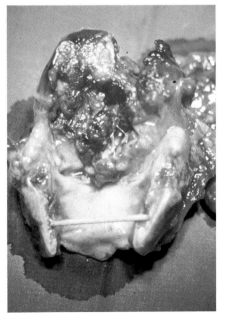

CP-33. Supraglottic carcinoma

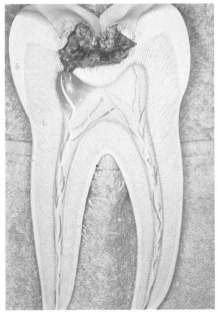

CP-36. Caries

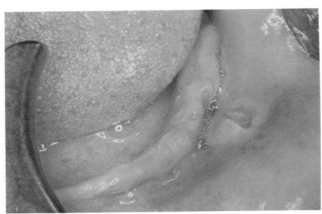

CP-37. *Dental ulcer*

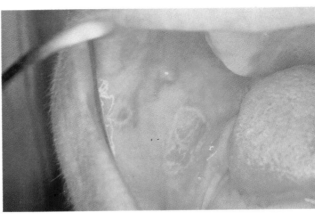

CP-40. *Bullous lichen planus*

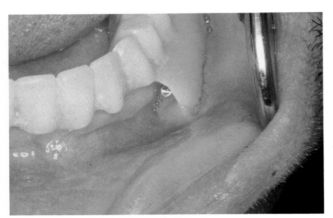

CP-38. *Denture causing dental ulcer*

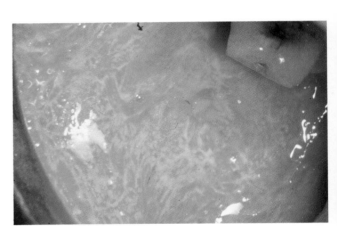

CP-41. *Lichen planus*

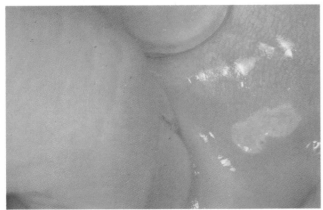

CP-39. *Aphthous ulcer*

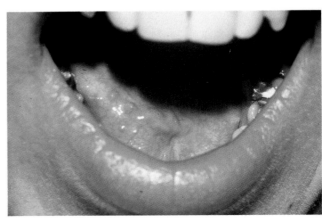

CP-42. *Ranula on floor of mouth*

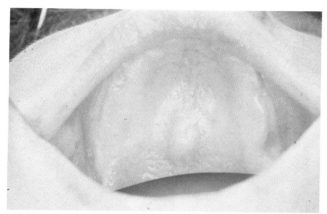

CP-43. Torus palatinus

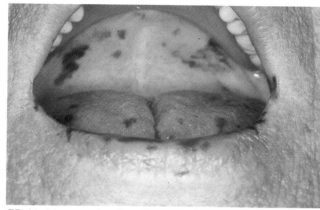

CP-46. Pigmentation from Peutz–Jeghers syndrome

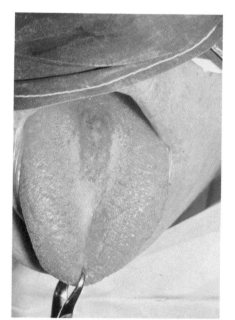

CP-44. Median rhomboid glossitis

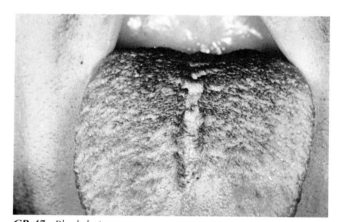

CP-47. Black hairy tongue

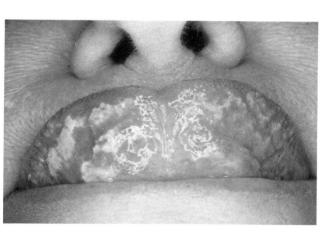

CP-45. Leukoplakia of the tongue

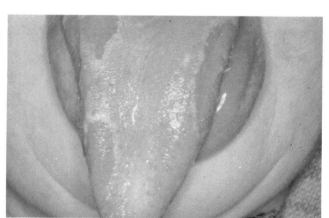

CP-48. A geographic tongue

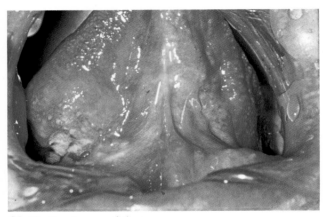

CP-49. *Carcinoma of the tongue*

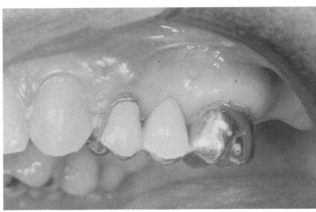

CP-52. *Gum abscess from a root abscess*

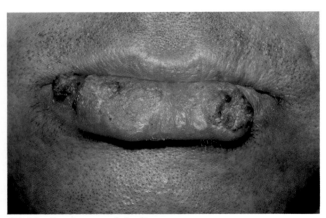

CP-50. *Carcinoma of the lip*

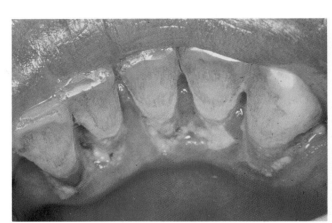

CP 53. *Periodontal disease*

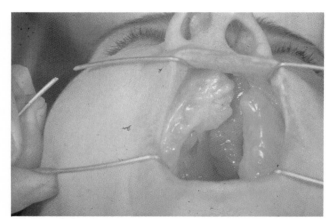

CP-51. *Cleft palate*

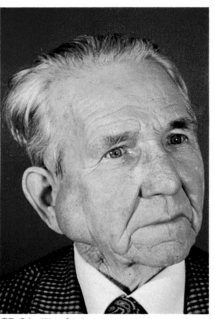

CP-54. *Warthin's tumour*

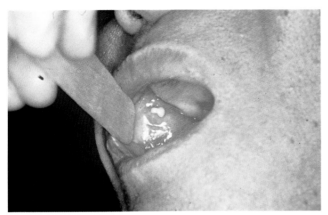

CP-55. Pus in parotid duct

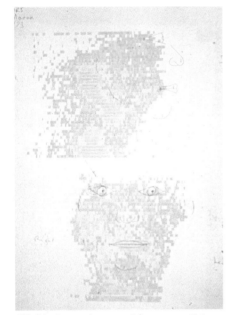

CP-56. Parotid scan with tumour (L)

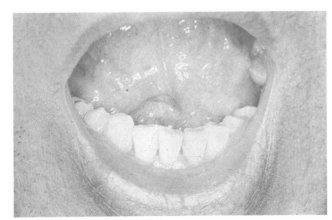

CP-57. Stone in submandibular duct

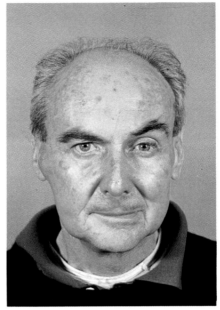

CP-58. Carcinoma of the parotid

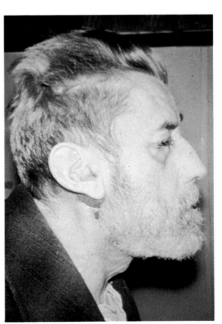

CP-59. Carcinoma of the parotid with
facial nerve paralysis

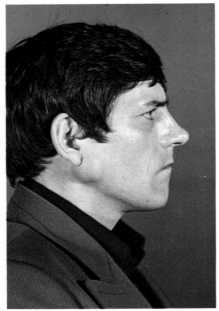

CP-60. *Mixed tumour of the parotid*

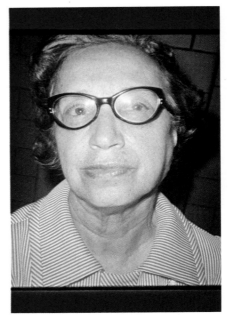

CP-62. *Sjögren's syndrome*

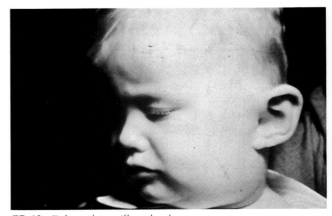

CP-63. *Enlarged tonsillar gland*

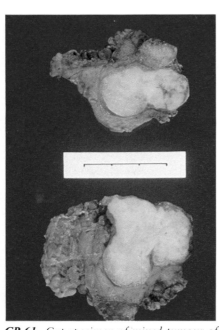

CP-61. *Cut specimen of mixed tumour of the parotid*

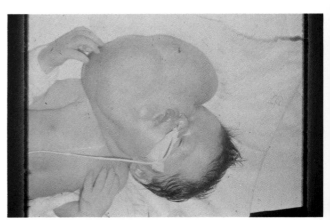

CP-64. *Cystic hygroma*

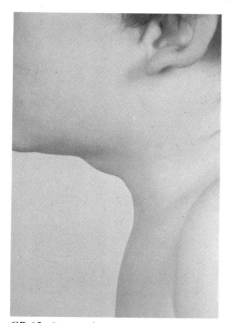

CP-65. *Dermoid cyst*

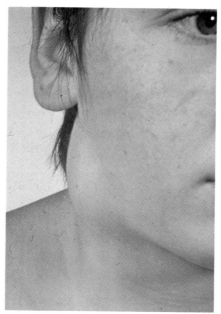

CP-67. *Branchial cyst*

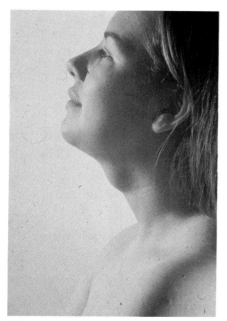

CP-66. *Thyroglossal cyst*

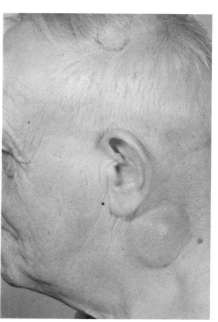

CP-68. *Sebaceous cyst*

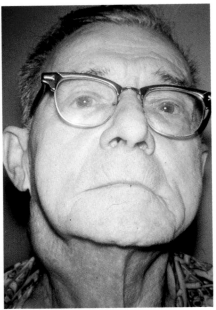

CP-69. *Metastatic neck glands from primary tumour at base of the tongue*

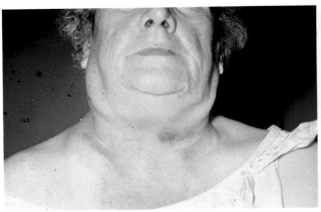

CP-71. *Neck gland enlargement due to lymphoma*

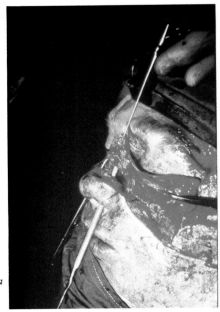

CP-72. *Typical example of a sharp soft tissue facial trauma after a windscreen injury. The edges of the lacerations are cleancut*

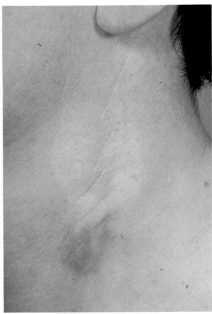

CP-70. *Tuberculous neck glands*

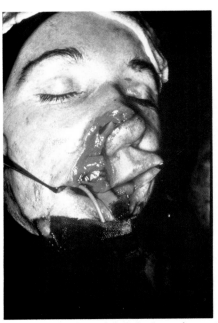

CP-73. *Complicated full thickness laceration of right upper lip and right side of nose*

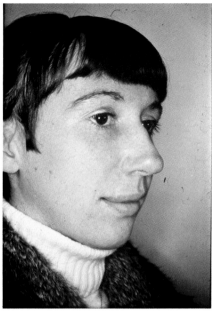

CP-74. *Same patient as in CP-73. Nine months after injury the initial repair has produced an inconspicuous scar*

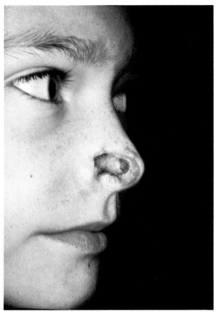

CP-77. *Same patient as CP-75, 76, 4 weeks after the bitten-off piece was sutured back in place.*

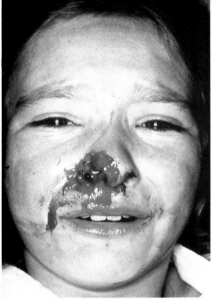

CP-75. *Dog bite of the nose. A full thickness piece of the right side of the tip of this girl's nose was bitten off*

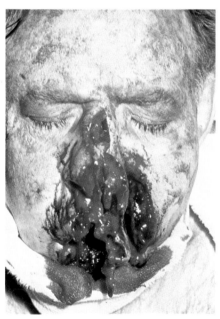

CP-78. *Gunshot wound of the face. This resulted in loss of bone of the mandible, maxilla and nose as well as loss of soft tissues of the mouth*

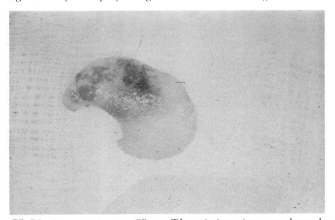

CP-76. *Same patient as CP-75. The missing piece was brought to hospital by the parents and sutured back onto the nose*

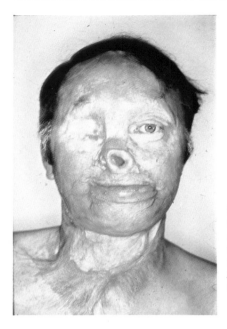

CP-79. Severe facial
injuries after a burn. Loss
of right eye and destruction
of nasal bones and
cartilage. Several skin
grafting procedures have
been performed

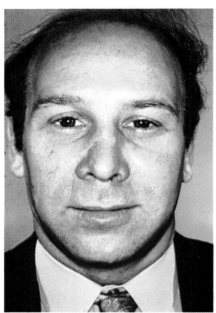

CP-82. Same patient as CP-81, 4 months after injury. The
wounds have healed well and the facial fractures are united

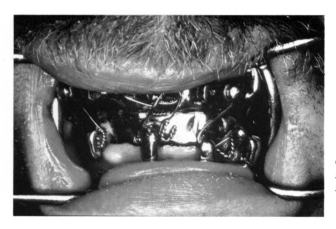

CP-80. Splints on the upper and lower jaws of the patient
seen in CP-81 and CP-82. These are wired together to
stabilize the reduced fracture in occlusion.

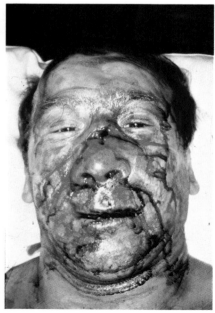

CP-81. Multiple small
bursting facial lacerations
from auto accident. Le Fort
II maxillary fracture,
comminuted fracture of
facial bones and midline
fracture of hard palate

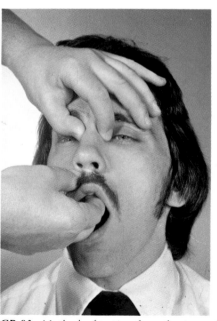

CP-83. Method of testing for a fracture of the maxilla

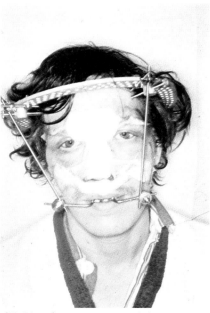

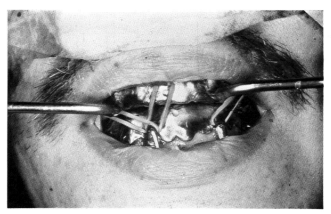

CP-86. Fixation of the rods to splints over the upper alveolus and attachment of the lower dental splint to the upper by elastic bands.

CP-84. This man sustained fractures of his maxilla and nose. A 'halo' has been screwed into the outer table of the skull. From this fixed point bars are suspended which hold the intermaxillary fixation in place and immobilize the reduced maxilla. A nasal plaster keeps the reduced fractured nose in position

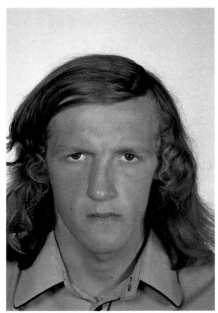

CP-87. A deviated fractured nose

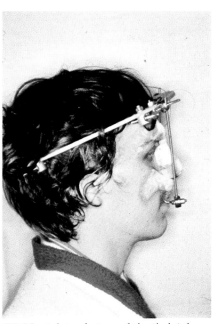

CP-85. A lateral view of the 'halo' frame

X–RAYS

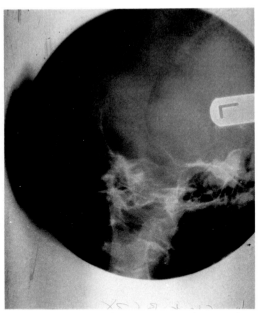

X-1. Stenver's view showing petrous bone and antrum

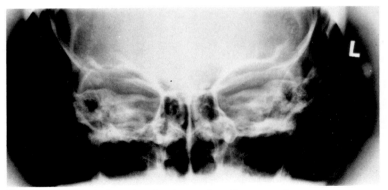

X-3. Transorbital view showing internal auditory canal

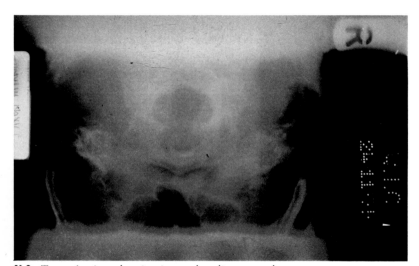

X-2. Towne's view showing internal auditory canal

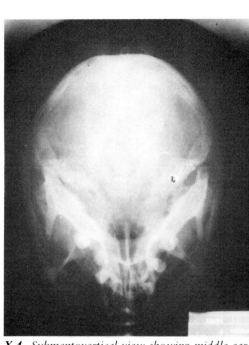

X-4. Submentovertical view showing middle ear, Eustachian tube, petrous apex and antrum

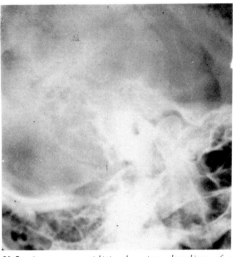

X-5. *Acute mastoiditis showing clouding of cells and destruction of individual cell boundaries*

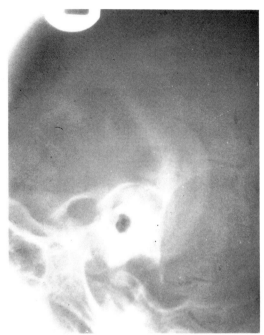

X-7. *Cholesteatoma. There is evidence of bony erosion within the attic and the mastoid*

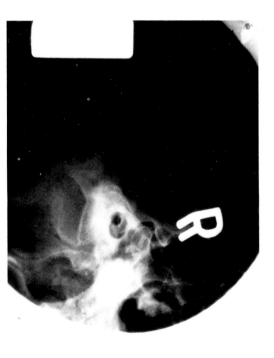

X-6. *Sclerosis of the mastoid following chronic infection*

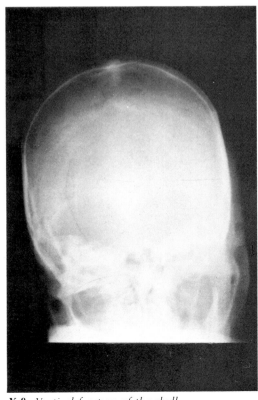

X-8. *Vertical fracture of the skull*

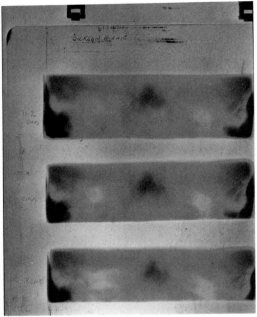

X-9. *Tomography showing expansion of the internal auditory canal from an acoustic neuroma*

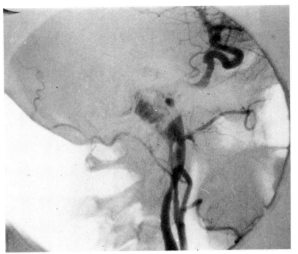

X-11. *Lateral subtraction angiogram*

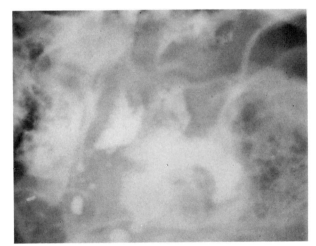

X-12. *Acoustic neuroma demonstrated by pantopaque*

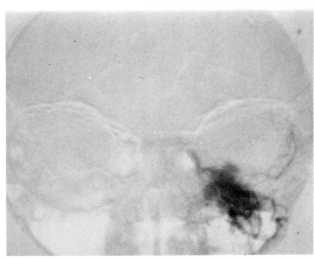

X-10. *Anteroposterior subtraction angiogram*

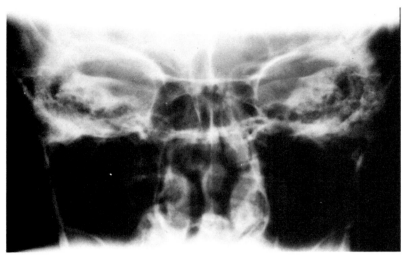

X-13. *Transorbital view – acoustic neuroma*

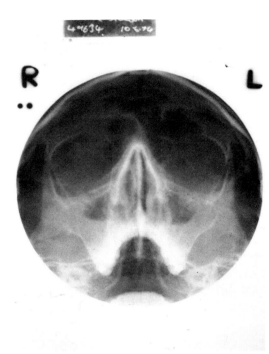

X-15. *Fluid level in sinuses*

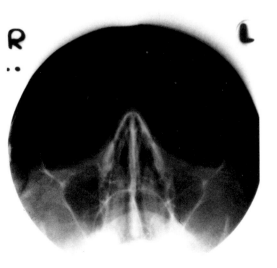

X-14. *Normal sinuses*

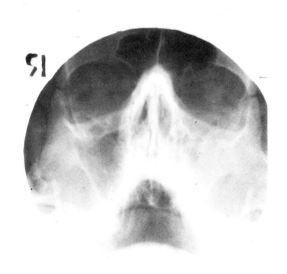

X-16. *Opaque maxillary sinuses*

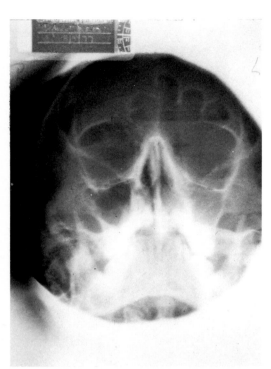

X-17. Thickening of mucous membrane of left antrum

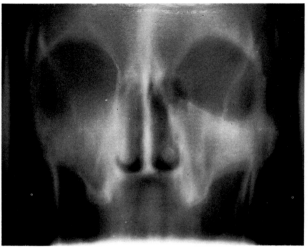

X-19. Erosion of right maxillary sinus wall by tumour (tomography)

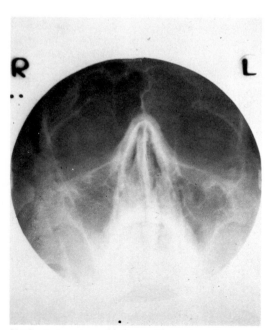

X-18. Expansion of left maxillary sinus by cyst

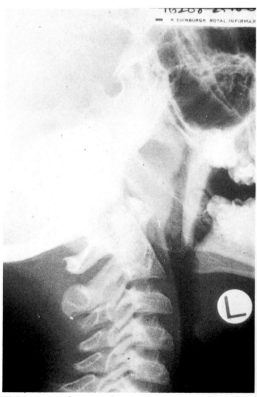

X-20. Lateral view of nasopharynx – enlarged adenoids

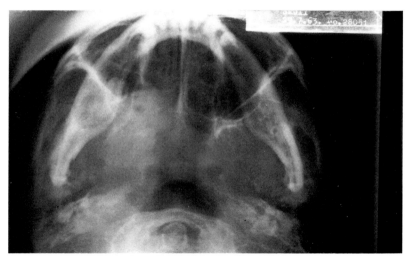

X-21. *Erosion of base of skull – carcinoma of nasopharynx*

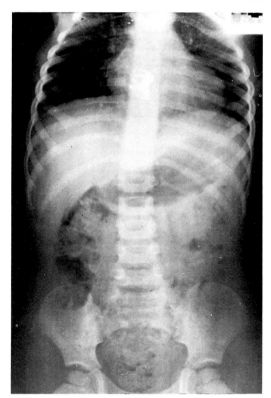

X-23. *White horse in oesophagus*

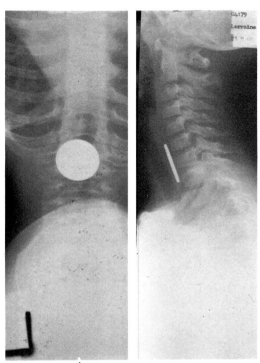

X-22. *Coin in oesophagus*

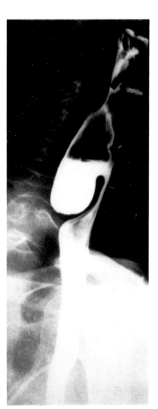

X-24. *Pharyngeal pouch*

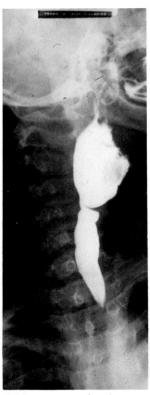

X-25. Postcricoid web

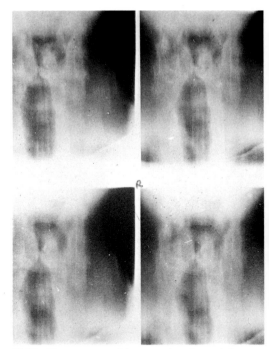

X-27. Tomograms of larynx, showing a left transglottic carcinoma

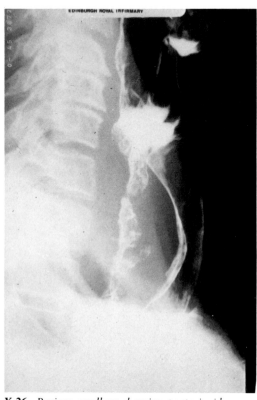

X-26. Barium swallow showing postcricoid carcinoma

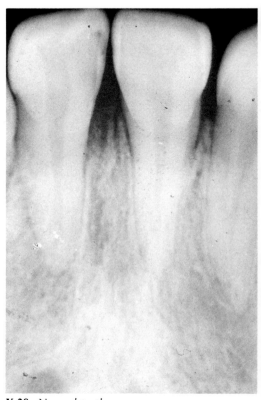

X-28. Normal teeth

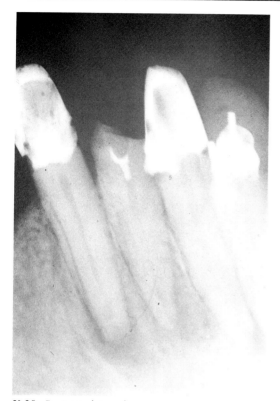

X-29. Periapical translucency

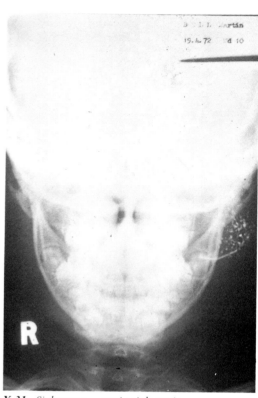

X-31. Sialogram – cystic sialectasis

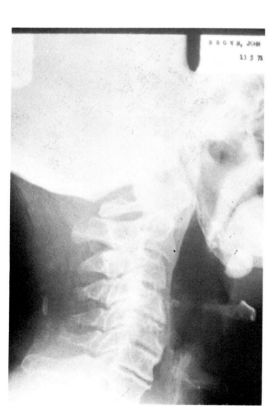

X-30. Stone in submandibular gland

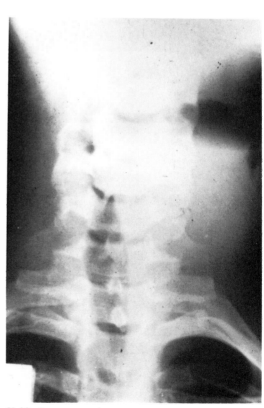

X-32. Laryngocoele

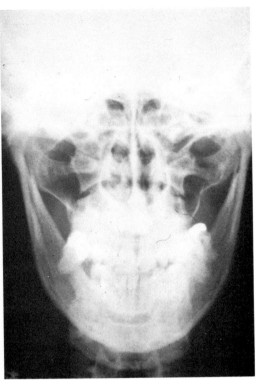

X-33. Posteroanterior X-ray of the unfractured face

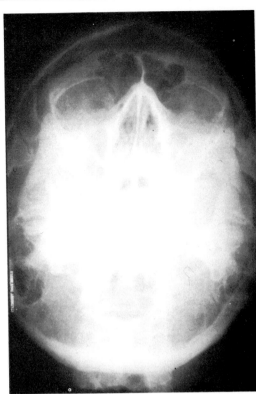

X-35. 30° occipitomental X-ray of unfractured facial bones. This view shows the maxillary antra and the infraorbital margins and is a most informative X-ray

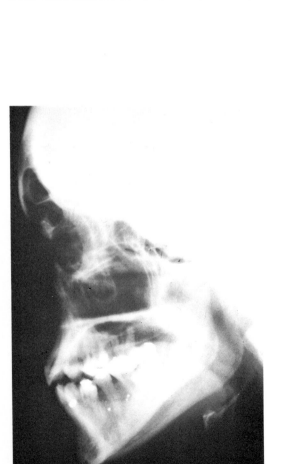

X-34. Lateral X-ray of facial bones. This is difficult to interpret owing to overlapping of bones

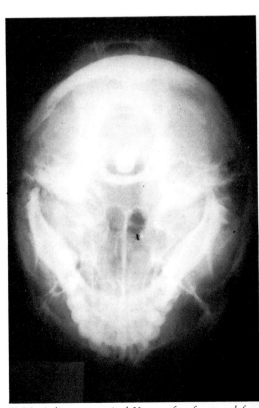

X-36. Submentovertical X-ray of unfractured face

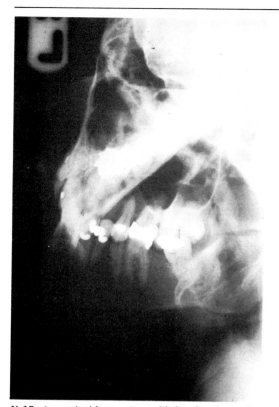

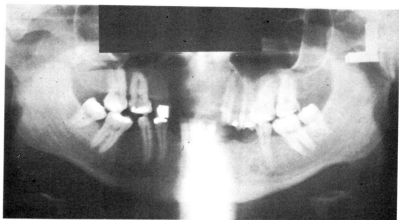

X-40. An orthopantomogram of the mandible that shows bilateral subcondylar fractures. A fracture of the mandibular symphysis is also present

X-37. Lateral oblique view of left side of mandible. This shows the body and ramus of the mandible well

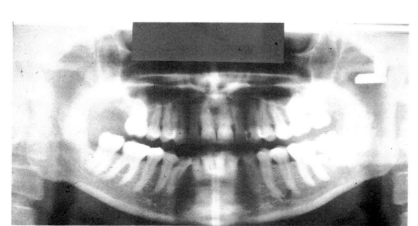

X-38. An orthopantomogram of the mandible 'straightens out' the mandible and makes interpretation of mandible fractures easier

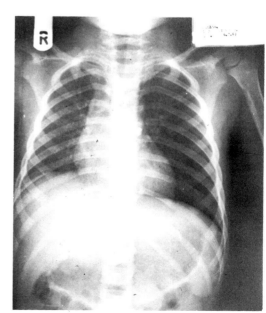

X-39. Chest X-ray showing inhaled tooth and distal changes in the lung

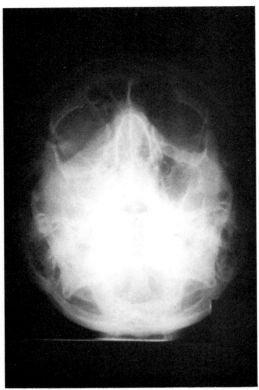

X-41. Fracture of right malar bone on the lateral and infraorbital margins. Observe the break in continuity of the margin of the right orbital rim as compared to the left. The right maxillary antrum is also opaque

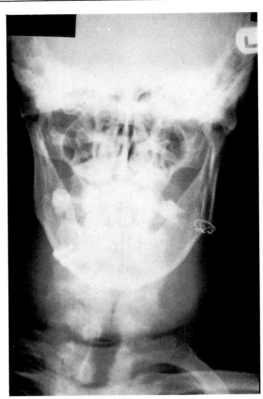

X-43. X-ray of a mandible which has been fractured. The fragments are held together on the left by wiring and on the right by plating

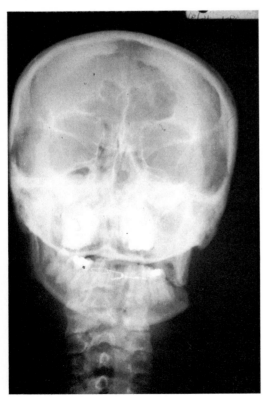

X-42. Fractured maxilla and double fracture of mandible. A temporary wire secures the middle fragment of the fractured mandible

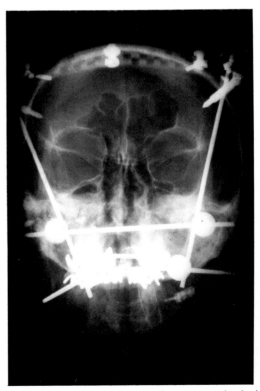

X-44. X-ray of facial bones of a patient who had mandibular and maxillary fractures. A halo is fixed to the skull by four screws. The fracture of the right angle of the mandible has been plated

INDEX

1 ie or ei?

i before *e*, except after *c*.

believe, deceive

Exceptions to the rule

seize   weird   weir   protein   either   neither

ei has an *ee* sound after *c*, but at other times usually has an *ay* sound.

neigh, sleigh, reindeer

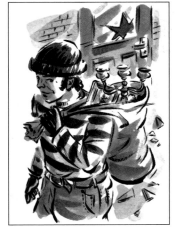

thief

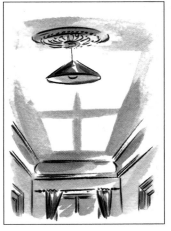

ceiling

Test yourself

1 Complete these words with **ie** or **ei**.

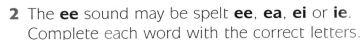

a   sh___ld

b   ch___f

c   rec___ve

d   n___ce

e   s___ze

f   bel___ve

g   c___ling

h   rec___pt

i   f___ld

j   n___ther

2 The **ee** sound may be spelt **ee**, **ea**, **ei** or **ie**. Complete each word with the correct letters.

a   disapp___r

b   ch___se

c   scr___m

d   p___ce (of cake)

e   p___ce (and quiet)

f   dec___ve

g   handkerch___f

h   sw___p

i   pr___st

j   c___ling

k   s___ling

l   w___rd

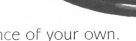

3 Use each word in question **2** in a sentence of your own.

4 Which is correct?

a   greif or grief?

b   diesel or deisel?

c   wieght or weight?

d   neighbour or nieghbour?

e   shreik or shriek?

f   belief or beleif?

g   mischeif or mischief?

h   decieve or deceive?

i   neice or niece?

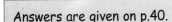

Answers are given on p.40.

3

2 Plurals: -s and -es

Most words add an *s* after the last letter to make the plural form.

book, books; computer, computers

When words end with the letters *s*, *x*, *z*, *sh* or *ch*, add -es to make the plural.

bus, buses; box, boxes; wish, wishes; match, matches

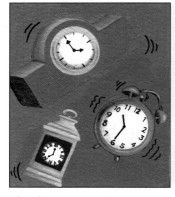
clocks

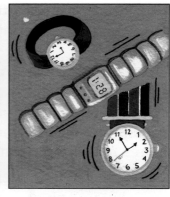
watches

Test yourself

1 Change these singular nouns to plurals by adding **s** or **es**.

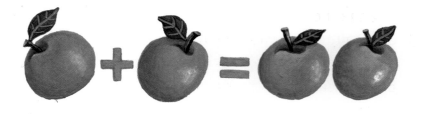

a apple	**g** switch
b peach	**h** fox
c torch	**i** dish
d desk	**j** chair
e kiss	**k** stitch
f road	**l** brush

2 Rewrite these sentences changing the underlined words to plural. Notice that you may also need to change other words too.

  a Is there a <u>witness</u> to the accident?

    <u>Begin</u>: Are there any ...?

  b I went to the <u>church</u>.

  c He hid behind the <u>bush</u>.

  d She bought a <u>clock</u> and a <u>watch</u>.

  e Bring me that <u>box</u> and then wash the <u>dish</u>.

  f The workers dug a <u>trench</u>.

  g The rabbit lives in a <u>hutch</u>.

  h He bought a <u>bunch</u> of flowers.

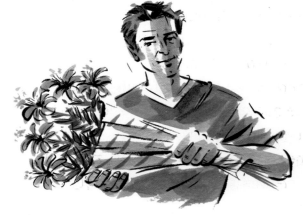

3 Change these words to plurals and use them in sentences of your own.

a lunch	**c** catch	**e** coach	**g** six
b church	**d** ditch	**f** fish	**h** dash

4 Pick out the plurals which are spelt incorrectly and write the correct spelling.

misses foxs crashs wishes crosses lunchs bunchs

Answers are given on p.40.

3 Plurals: words ending in -y

When a singular noun ends in _y_, there are two rules to remember when making the plural:

If there is a vowel before the _y_, then add _s_.

boy, boys; chimney, chimneys

If there is a consonant before the _y_, then change the _y_ to _ies_.

baby, babies; curry, curries

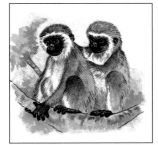
monkeys

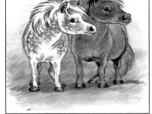
ponies

The **vowels** are a, e, i, o and u.
Consonants are all those letters which are not vowels.

Test yourself

1 Change these singular nouns to plurals. Use the rules above to help you.

   a spray   e journey   i valley

   b lady   f berry   j opportunity

   c sky   g cherry   k body

   d day   h lorry   l ruby

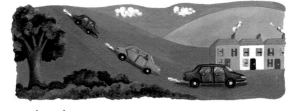

2 Rewrite these sentences changing the underlined words to plural.
Change other words as necessary.

   a The <u>lorry</u> suffered a <u>delay</u>.

   b The <u>boy</u> went under the <u>subway</u>.

   c There was a <u>fly</u> on the <u>cherry</u>.

   d There was a <u>reply</u> to their <u>invitation</u> to the <u>party</u>.

   e She had an <u>inquiry</u> about the silver <u>tray</u> she had for sale.

   f He found a <u>penny</u>, a <u>key</u> and a <u>ruby</u>.

   g The <u>family</u> were looking forward to their <u>holiday</u>.

   h He read a <u>story</u> about a <u>monastery</u>.

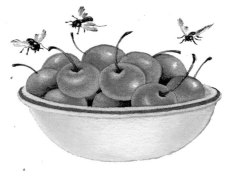

3 Change these words to plurals and use them in sentences of your own.

   a bully   b spy   c donkey   d play   e baby   f enquiry

4 Pick out the spelling mistakes and write each sentence correctly.

   a The house had three stories and had views of two vallies.

   b The lorries made several journies, crossing the channel on ferrys.

   c She worked for government ministerys, inspecting highways.

   d There were bunches of cherrys on the trayies.

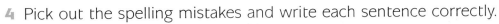

Answers are given on p.40.

When a word ends in *f*, change the *f* to *ve* and then add *s*.

wolf, wolves; wife, wives; life, lives

Exceptions to the rule

Some words ending in *f* just add add *s* when forming their plurals:

chief, chiefs   cliff, cliffs   roof, roofs

staff, staffs   skiff, skiffs

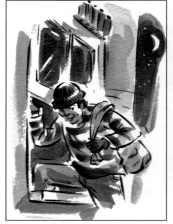
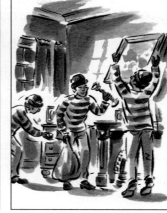

thief   thieves

Test yourself

1 Change these singular nouns to plurals.

a half		**f** roof
b calf		**g** hoof
c self		**h** yourself
d cliff		**i** staff
e wolf		**j** wife

2 Use the plurals you made in question **1** in sentences of your own.

3 Rewrite these sentences changing the underlined words to plurals. Change other words as necessary.

  a The <u>loaf</u> was on the baker's <u>shelf</u>.

  b He cut the <u>leaf</u> with a <u>knife</u>.

  c She bought a <u>handkerchief</u> and a <u>scarf</u>.

  d The <u>wharf</u> was at the foot of the <u>cliff</u>.

  e The <u>thief</u> stole the <u>skiff</u>.

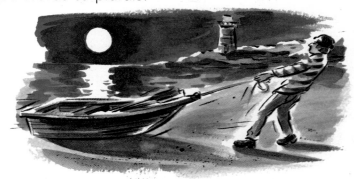

4 Which are the correct plurals?

  a cliff – cliffs or clives?   **e** chief – chiefs or chieves?

  b wife – wifes or wives?   **f** roof – roofs or rooves?

  c elf – elfs or elves?   **g** self – selfs or selves?

  d life – lifes or lives?   **h** staff – staffs or starves?

Answers are given on p.41.

5 Plurals: words ending in -o

When a word ending in *o* has a consonant before the *o*, then add *es* to make the plural.

potato, potatoes; domino, dominoes

> ### Exceptions to the rule
>
> pianos   solos   kilos   zeros   banjos
> photos   memos   dynamos

When a word ending in *o* has a vowel before the *o*, then add *s* to make the plural.

cuckoo, cuckoos; video, videos

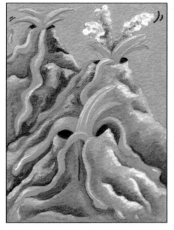
volcanoes

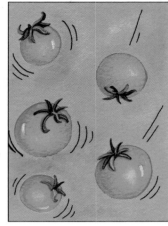
tomatoes

Test yourself

1 Write the plural of these words.

a tomato	**d** mosquito	**g** solo	**j** piano
b radio	**e** photo	**h** kilo	
c hero	**f** zero	**i** memo	

2 Use the plurals you made in question **1** in sentences of your own.

3 Rewrite these sentences changing the underlined words to plurals. Change other words as necessary.

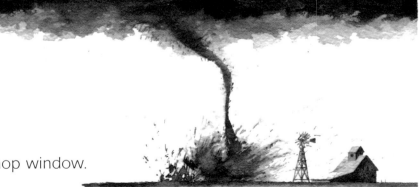

   a She was bitten by a <u>mosquito</u>.
   b The <u>tornado</u> destroyed many houses.
   c She bought a <u>potato</u> and a <u>mango</u>.
   d The <u>radio</u> weighed a <u>kilo</u>.
   e The <u>echo</u> rang round the <u>volcano</u>.
   f He had a <u>piccolo</u> and a <u>banjo</u> for sale.
   g There was a <u>stereo</u> and a <u>video</u> in the shop window.

4 One word in each pair is spelled incorrectly. Write the correct spelling.

   a potatos, tomatoes
   b banjos, pianoes
   c cuckoos, flamingoes
   d cargos, dominoes
   e haloes, heroes
   f sopranos, soloes

Answers are given on p.41.

6 Unusual plurals

A few words make their plurals in unusual ways.

foot, feet; man, men; tooth, teeth;
goose, geese; mouse, mice; child, children

Some words are the same in singular and plural.

sheep   deer   grouse   cod   trout   pike   salmon
aircraft   series   species

Some words are only used in the plural.

cattle   scissors   shears   pliers   pincers   trousers

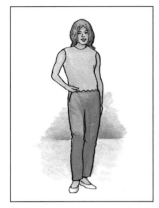
woman

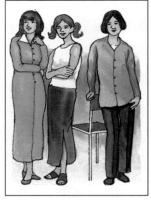
women

Test yourself

1 Write the plurals of these words.

   a man   **d** sheep   **g** goose   **j** deer

   b scissors   **e** child   **h** aircraft

   c foot   **f** salmon   **i** mouse

2 Use the plurals you made in question **1** in sentences of your own.

3 Rewrite these sentences changing the underlined words to plurals, and making any other changes as necessary. Sometimes the word will remain the same.

   a His <u>tooth</u> was aching.

   b The <u>man</u> and <u>woman</u> flew in the <u>aircraft</u>.

   c The <u>fisherman</u> caught a <u>trout</u> and a <u>pike</u>.

   d She cut out a pair of <u>trousers</u> with the <u>scissors</u>.

   e There was a <u>series</u> about <u>salmon</u> on television.

   f The <u>postman</u> was chased by a <u>goose</u>.

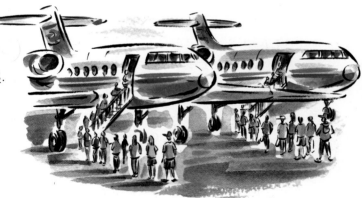

4 One word in each pair is spelled incorrectly. Write the correct spelling.

   a shears, plier   **e** houses, mouses

   b trouser, scissors   **f** geese, grouses

   c childs, women   **g** tooths, feet

   d sharks, salmons

Answers are given on p.41.

7 Adding -ly

For most words, simply add **ly**. You may need to do this to make an adjective into an adverb or a noun into an adjective.

complete, completely; friend, friendly

When a word ends in *le*, remove the *e* and add *y*.

simple, simply; possible, possibly

When a word of two or more syllables ends in *y*, remove the *y* and add *ily*.

busy, busily; merry, merrily

When a word ends in *ll*, simply add *y*.

full, fully; shrill, shrilly

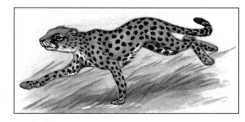

quickly

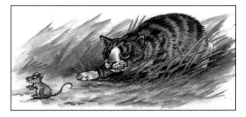

quietly

Test yourself

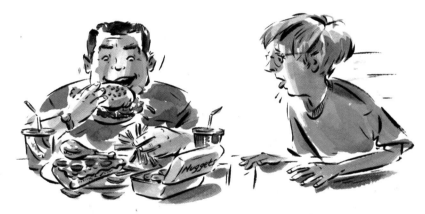

1 Add **ly** to these words.

a lone	**f** crazy
b brave	**g** hungry
c greedy	**h** full
d sensible	**i** tidy
e bubble	**j** beautiful

2 Add **ly** to these words and use each one in a sentence of your own.

a careful	**c** comfortable	**e** shabby	**g** necessary	**i** responsible
b happy	**d** shrill	**f** terrible	**h** steady	**j** desperate

3 Use the clues to find the words. Write it with its correct **ly** ending.

a doing something in a stupid way:

b behaving like a friend:

c done in a dangerous manner:

d a word meaning 'totally': c_____

e done in a way which cannot be seen: inv_____

f in a truthful manner:

g used at the end of a friendly letter: Yours s_____

h likely: pr_____

4 Pick out the words which are spelt incorrectly and write the correct spelling.

busyly   immediately   powerfully   finaly   fortunatly   lonely   wonderfuly   lovly

Answers are given on p.41.

9

8 Adding -ing and -ed

With most verbs, simply add *-ing* or *-ed*.

wash, washing, washed; look, looking, looked;
listen, listening, listened

**When a word ends in e, then drop the e before
adding *-ing* or *-ed*.**

hope, hoping, hoped; stare, staring, stared;
love, loving, loved

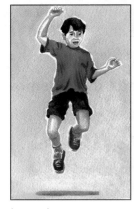 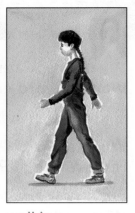

jumping   walking

Test yourself

1 Add **-ing** to these words and use them in sentences of your own.

  a plant   **c** rain   **e** live   **g** tease

  b invite   **d** rest   **f** shine   **h** take

2 Add **-ed** to these words and use them in sentences of your own.

  a measure **c** imagine **e** look   **g** mix

  b snow   **d** scrape   **f** type   **h** mumble

3 Use the clues to find the verb. Write it with its correct **-ing** ending.
The first has been done for you.

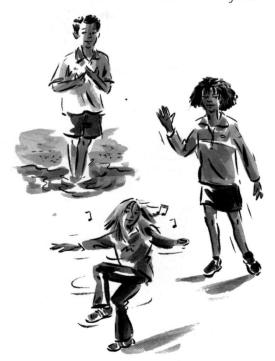

  a opening your eyes after sleeping: waking

  b using the phone:

  c getting into a place where no one can see you:

  d picking the one you want:

  e standing with your feet in shallow water:

  f giving some of what you have to someone else:

  g moving your hand backwards and forwards to say hello
or goodbye:

  h cooking a cake in an oven:

  i complaining and moaning about something:

  j moving about in time to music:

Answers are given on p.41.

10

9 Adding -ing and -ed to verbs ending in y

When the letter before the *y* is a vowel, simply add *ing* or *ed*.

stay, stayed, staying; destroy, destroyed, destroying

When the letter before the *y* is a consonant, change the *y* to *i* before adding *ed*.

fry, fried; carry, carried

When adding *ing*, keep the *y* to avoid having two 'i's together.

carrying – not carriing!

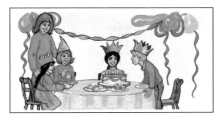

enjoying

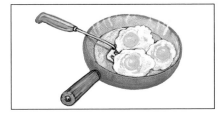

frying

Test yourself

1 Add **ed** to these words. Use them in sentences of your own.

a cry
b marry
c play
d obey
e dry
f employ
g rely
h journey

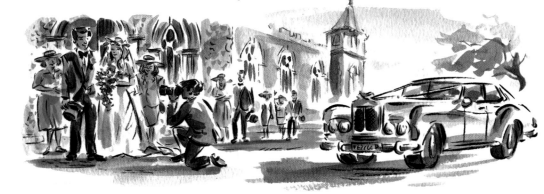

2 Add **ing** to these words. Use them in sentences of your own.

a hurry
b try
c bury
d say
e pay
f worry
g fly
h stray

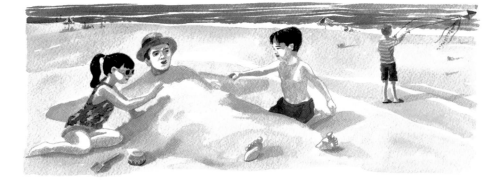

3 Pick out the words which are spelt incorrectly and write the correct spelling.

flying	envyed	carryed	paying	hurriing
tryed	relyed	crying	pitied	buryed

Answers are given on p.42.

10 Doubling letters when adding -ed or -ing

Rule 1

In words of one syllable, with a short vowel, and ending in a consonant, double the consonant when adding *ed* or *ing*.

hop, hopped, hopping; slip, slipped, slipping

Each beat in a word is a syllable. 'Hop' has one beat and 'hopping' has two beats.

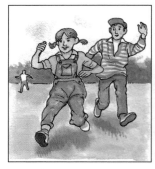 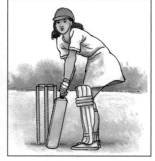

running   batting

Test yourself

1 Add **ing** to these words.

a sit	d skip	g hit
b tug	e lap	h spin
c swim	f rip	

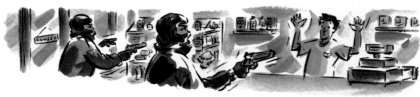

2 Add **ed** to these words.

a knit	d stop	g rob
b bat	e trip	h shop
c sip	f fit	

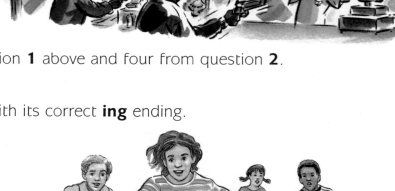

3 Choose four of your answers from question **1** above and four from question **2**.
   Use each one in a sentence of your own.

4 Use the clues to find the verb. Write it with its correct **ing** ending.
   The first one has been done for you.
   a coming first in a race: winning
   b moving away soil to make a hole:
   c fastening things with a pin:
   d letting something fall to the ground:
   e falling in small drops:
   f pulling something along behind you:
   g running gently and slowly for exercise:
   h falling over something:

5 Pick out the words which are spelt incorrectly and write the correct spelling.
   runing   lapped   raining   tiping   flaping   rested   bating   stoping   winning   geting

Rule 2

This applies to words of more than one syllable ending in a consonant. If the last syllable is stressed, then double the final consonant when adding *ed* or *ing*.

admit, admitted, admitting; regret, regretted, regretting

But if the consonant is not stressed, then simply add *ed* or *ing*.

sharpen, sharpened, sharpening; happen, happened, happening

Rule 3

In words of more than one syllable, if the last syllable ends in one vowel plus an *l*, then double the *l* when adding *ed* or *ing*.

cancel, cancelled, cancelling; instil, instilled, instilling

Test yourself

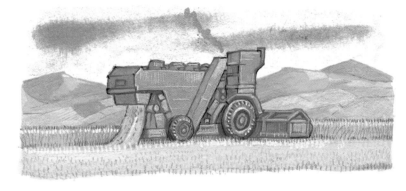

6 Make **ing** words from each of these.

a	propel	f	gallop
b	forget	g	compel
c	harvest	h	fulfil
d	begin	i	chisel
e	quarrel	j	permit

7 Make **ed** and **ing** words from each of these. Use each one in a sentence of your own.

a label

b commit

c target

d travel

e trumpet

f shovel

g gossip

h tunnel

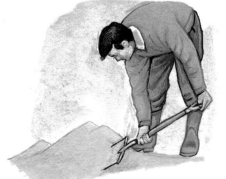

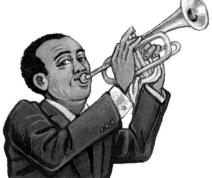

8 Pick out the words below which are spelt incorrectly and write the correct spelling.

installing   channeled   signaled   refered   refitted   profited
canceling   forgetting   begining   permitted   leveled   parcelled

9 Write out from memory all the rules for doubling letters when adding **ed** or **ing**.

Answers are given on p.42.

13

11 Adding -er and -est

When a one-syllable word ends in a consonant, double the consonant before adding *er* or *est*.

big, bigger, biggest;
sad, sadder, saddest

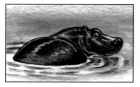 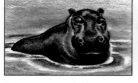 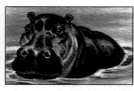

big   bigger   biggest

Exceptions to the rule

● Where the consonant is w, x or y: slow, slower, slowest.
● Where there are two consonants at the end: fast, faster; tall, taller.

When a word of more than two syllables ends in *y*, change the *y* to *i* before adding *er* or *est*.

tidy, tidier, tidiest; happy, happier, happiest

Test yourself

1 Add **er** to these words.

a long	**e** slippy	**i** wet
b fit	**f** small	**j** sweet
c slim	**g** lonely	**k** happy
d warm	**h** proud	**l** smooth

2 Add **est** to these words. Use each one in a sentence of your own.

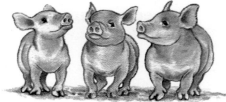

a slow	**d** tasty	**g** fat	**j** red
b thin	**e** busy	**h** hungry	
c flat	**f** narrow	**i** crazy	

3 Use the clues to find the words. Write each adjective with its correct **er** or **est** ending.

a the most shy:	**e** the most flat:	**i** more sad:
b the most unhappy:	**f** more friendly:	**j** the most heavy:
c more thin:	**g** the most mad:	
d more slimy:	**h** more dusty:	

4 Which is correct?

a happyer or happier?	**e** nastyest or nastiest?
b slowwer or slower?	**f** coldest or colddest?
c fastest or fasttest?	**g** fewwer or fewer?
d trimer or trimmer?	**h** merriest or merryest?

Answers are given on p.42.

12 Adding -y and -ful

Many nouns can be made into adjectives by adding **y** or *ful*.

rain, rainy; peace, peaceful

When a word ends in a silent e, drop the e before adding y.

ice, icy; stone, stony

When a single-syllable word with a short vowel ends in a consonant, double the consonant before adding y.

sun, sunny; fog, foggy

Words ending in y change the y to i before adding *ful*.

beauty, beautiful; duty, dutiful

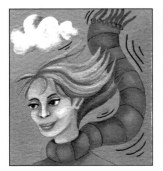
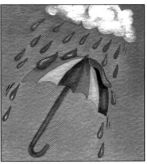

windy   rainy

Test yourself

1 Make adjectives from these words by adding **y** or **ful**.

a	frost	**e**	care	**i**	fun
b	help	**f**	ease	**j**	hope
c	run	**g**	truth	**k**	beauty
d	colour	**h**	use	**l**	plenty

2 Use each of the words you made in question **1** in a sentence of your own.

3 Use the clues to find the adjectives. Write its correct spelling.

   a full of rust: r_____
   b talkative: ch_____
   c turned to mud: m_____
   d causing pain: p_____
   e full of hope: h_____
   f arousing pity: p_____

   g rather cold: n_____
   h showing gratitude: g_____
   i marvellous: w_____
   j filled with noise: n_____
   k covered in spots: s_____
   l terrible: fr_____

4 Which is correct?

   a clouddy or cloudy?
   b choppy or chopy?
   c beautiful or beautyful?
   d nuty or nutty?
   e easy or easey?

   f tastey or tasty?
   g plentyful or plentiful?
   h sogy or soggy?
   i hopeful or hopful?
   j bagy or baggy?

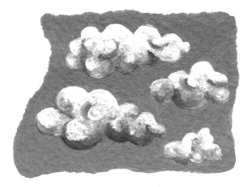

Answers are given on p.42.

13 The apostrophe in shortened forms

When people speak they use shortened forms of some words. The apostrophe shows us where one or more letters have been missed out.

do not, don't; could not, couldn't; I am, I'm

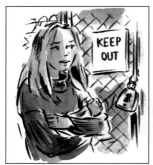
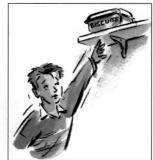

She <u>shouldn't</u> go in.   He <u>can't</u> reach it.

Test yourself

1 Write the shortened form of these:

a did not	**d** you have	**g** you are	**j** would not
b she will	**e** they are	**h** I will	
c I am	**f** he is	**i** we will	

2 Use each of the shortened forms in question **1** in a sentence of your own.

3 Rewrite these sentences using shortened forms for the words underlined.

  a <u>It will</u> start raining as soon as <u>we are</u> ready to go out. <u>That is</u> what happens every time.

  b She <u>did not</u> do the work because she had not got a pen.

  c <u>She is</u> keeping the ring locked up. <u>It is</u> very valuable.

  d <u>You are</u> sure that your sister <u>cannot</u> come to help us? <u>I am</u> disappointed!

  e <u>I have</u> written a letter, <u>he has</u> painted a picture, but <u>you have</u> wasted your time.

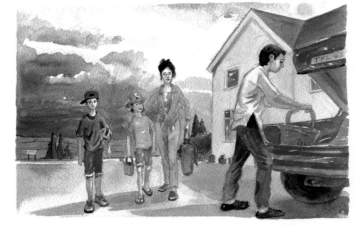

4 Copy and complete these sentences, using apostophes to show that some letters have been missed out.

  a You cant go out now. Its far too late. Youd better go tomorrow instead.

  b Whyre you so slow? I wont let you come again if you dont hurry up.

  c Hes a faster runner than his brothers, but theyre better at football.

  d Im going out at five oclock. Cant I do my homework when I get back?

  e Theyll be very pleased that hes bought them each an ice cream, wont they?

Answers are given on p.42.

14 Homophones

Homophones are words which have the same sound, but are spelt differently.

here, hear; their, there; piece, peace; its, it's

There are no rules to help you get the spellings right, but try inventing your own ways of remembering which word is which. Here are some ideas to start you off.

● **Hear** has the word **ear** in it. **Here** does not.
● **Pie**ce has the word **pie** in it. A piece of pie! **Peace** does not.

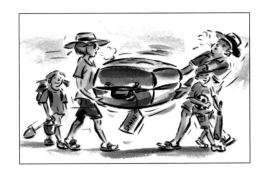

They are going **to** Spain.
The case is **too** heavy.
It needs **two** people to carry it.

Test yourself

1 The words *its* and *it's* are often confused.
When something *belongs to* it we use *its*: The dog buried its bone.
It's is the short form of *it is*: I think it's going to rain.

Write *it's* or *its* in these sentences.

a The cat waited for _____ owner.
b _____ a beautiful picture.
c _____ impossible.
d The dog was in _____ basket.
e _____ time for school.

2 Complete each sentence with the correct homophone.

a I'd love some _____ and quiet. (peace, piece)
b Do you eat _____? (meet, meat)
c The _____ men were _____ tired _____ work any longer. (to, too, two)
d He took a can _____ beans _____ the shelf. (off, of)
e The wind _____ the boat across the _____ sea. (blue, blew)
f Do you _____ with your left hand or your _____ ? (write, right)
g The first _____ past the post _____ the race. (won, one)
h I could do with a _____ after all this work. (brake, break)
i _____ you sell me that plank of _____? (would, wood)
j _____ looking for _____ coats over _____. (there, their, they're)
k I _____ she had bought a _____ pair of shoes. (knew, new)
l He's feeling _____ now but this time next _____ he'll be fit again. (week, weak)

3 Use these words in sentences of your own to show their different meanings.

a here, hear
b there, their
c dear, deer
d hair, hare
e mail, male
f plain, plane

Answers are given on p.43.

17

15 How to begin and end sentences

All sentences begin with a capital letter.

A statement ends with a full stop:

He ran away.

A question ends with a question mark:

Did he run away?

An exclamation ends with an exclamation mark:

Stop, thief!

Proper nouns begin with a capital letter, e.g. London, Ahmed.

Test yourself

1 Rewrite these sentences, adding capital letters, full stops, question marks or exclamation marks where appropriate.

   a the stranger entered town on a black horse
   b how does a question end
   c is roald dahl your favourite author
   d what a fantastic film
   e bill met jake on the way to the library
   f is this the right way to bristol
   g open the door this minute
   h the elephant sensed danger and trumpeted loudly
   i did you see katy when you went to liverpool
   j the aeroplane roared low overhead
   k i don't believe it
   l you did post my letter, didn't you

2 Write four statements about things which interest you.

3 Write four questions you would like to know the answers to.

4 Write three exclamations.

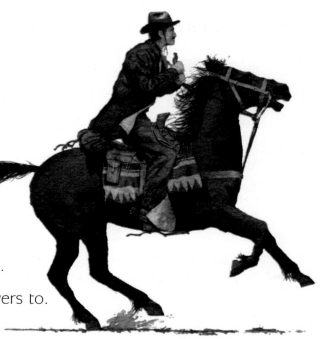

Answers are given on p.43.

18

16 Commas

Commas are used whenever a reader ought to pause in a sentence.

If you aren't sure where to put commas, then read your writing aloud (or inside your head). At each point you pause to make the meaning clear, you need a comma.

Commas are used to separate items in a list:

In the wizard's cave were several wands, a wooden chest, shelves of magic books and bottles of all shapes and colours.

Commas are also used to mark the different sections of complex sentences (see pages 32–33):

After digging all day, Tim was exhausted.

Jamie Baxter, who is our football captain, has been selected to play for the town team.

Note that you don't need a comma before *and*:

He opened the door and let the dog out.

Test yourself

Answers are given on p.43.

1 Rewrite these sentences putting in commas where necessary.
   a Don't forget to bring boots an anorak sandwiches and a drink.
   b Looking very pleased with himself Ben stepped up to collect the prize.
   c Although he was very busy he found time to help Mrs Dunn.
   d There were coats scarves and gloves scattered all over the room.
   e Before you go clean all this mess up!
   f Daffodils tulips crocuses and hyacinths are all spring flowers.

2 Complete each list sentence with at least four items, adding commas where necessary.
   a My favourite books are ...
   b At the market Mr Walsh bought ...
   c The school subjects I like best are ...
   d To play cricket you need ...
   e In my room I have ...
   f ... are all animals found in Africa.

3 Rewrite this passage, putting in capital letters, full stops, question marks, exclamation marks and commas as necessary. There are eight sentences.

without waiting for the others sam entered the dark room until his eyes adjusted to the dark he couldn't make anything out then he saw the room was filled with piles of old magazines, newspapers and books what was that a slithering sound came from the corner sam froze then he saw the snake sliding towards him what a fright that gave him

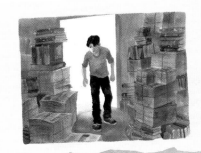

17 Other punctuation in sentences

The comma is the most common punctuation mark used in sentences, but the colon, semi-colon, dashes and brackets have their uses too.

The colon (:)

The colon is usually used to show that some kind of explanation or a list is to follow:

There was a terrible crash: John had fallen through the ceiling.

We travelled through several countries: France, Belgium, Germany, Switzerland and Italy.

Dashes (–)

Dashes are used to show a sudden change of thought:

We'll go to Australia – no, let's go to New Zealand.

A dash is also used to show a strong idea added to a sentence:

Leanne thinks – but I'm not at all sure – that we'll be given a holiday next Monday.

Brackets ( )

Brackets are used around words in a sentence to explain something:

My watch has an LCD (liquid crystal display).

Or they may show an afterthought:

All this mess was made by Tom (a usually well-behaved boy).

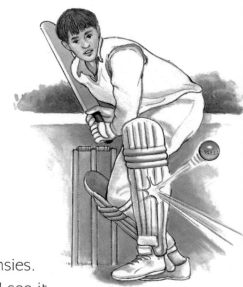

Test yourself

1 Rewrite these sentences with appropriate punctuation.
   a He was out LBW leg before wicket.
   b I'll have a hamburger no make that a hot dog.
   c He ran all the way to school he was late.
   d Matt says but I don't believe him that he's got full marks.
   e We bought several plants petunias marigolds geraniums and pansies.
   f The forecast is for a sunny bank holiday which I'll believe when I see it.
   g Breakfast consisted of coffee boiled eggs toast and marmalade.
   h The computer has a very large VDU visual dsplay unit.

Answers are given on p.43.

20

18 The apostrophe to show possession

In Chapter 12 you learned how to use an apostrophe to show missing letters.

The apostrophe is also used to show that something belongs to someone.

the painter's brushes (the brushes belonging to the painter)

Jenny's father (the father of Jenny)

the firefighters' ladders (the ladders of the firefighters)

Placing the apostrophe correctly is not difficult. First ask yourself who the owner is. Then put the apostrophe immediately after the owner or owners:

the bike of the boy – the boy's bike   the shoes of the boys – the boys' shoes

Test yourself

1 Write each of these using an apostophe. The first one has been done for you.

  a the mother of Pat: *Pat's mother*

  b the desk of the teacher:

  c the dress of the lady:

  d the cars of the ladies:

  e the helmets of the policemen:

  f the helmet of the policeman:

  g the collar of my dog:

  h the cover of the book:

  i the shirts of the boy:

  j the house of Mr Green:

  k the wings of the bee:

  l the nest of the wasps:

2 Add apostrophes where required in these sentences.

  a Kates bag is bigger than Yasmins.

  b The postmans van stopped outside Mr Smiths shop.

  c On the table were: a referees whistle, a gardeners trowel and a ladys brooch.

  d The teacher confiscated Ravis comic, the twins sweets and Gerrys crisps.

  e He delivered leaflets to the Browns house and the Jones flat.

3 Match up these people to their belongings. Write a sentence of your own about each one.

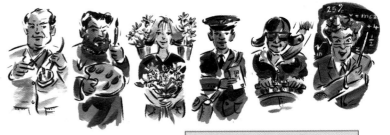

the electrician	books
the artists	flowers
the postman	paints
the pilots	screwdrivers
the teachers	letters
the florist	aeroplanes

Answers are given on p.44.

21

19 Punctuating speech

Speech marks

When we write the actual words spoken, we put them inside speech marks.

Think of speech marks as ^{66} and ^{99}.

" goes before the first word spoken;

" goes after the last word spoken.

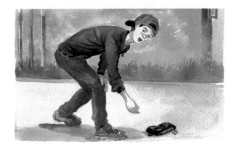

"This is my lucky day," said Lee.

"What is yellow and highly dangerous?" asked Carla.

"I don't know," replied Zena.

"Shark infested custard," said Carla.

The passage above has examples of four rules for using speech marks:

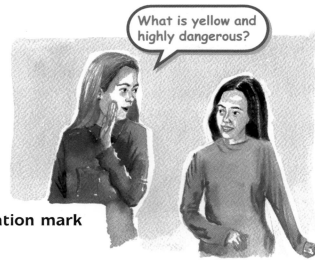

* **Put "** before the first spoken word.
* **Begin the first spoken word with a capital letter.**
* **Put a comma, full stop, question mark or exclamation mark after the last spoken word.**
* **Put " to show the spoken words have ended.**

Test yourself

1 Complete these sentences with words from the speech bubbles.

    a "_____," said Dad.

    b Tim said, "_____."

    c Mum said, "_____."

    d "_____," said Laura.

2 Copy these sentences. Put speech marks round the spoken words.

    a I'll tidy my room when I get back, he promised.

    b Mark said, It's time we took a break.

    c Are you going to the shops? he asked.

    d That's a job well done, said Dad.

    e What time is it? asked Charlie.

    f Watch out! yelled Craig.

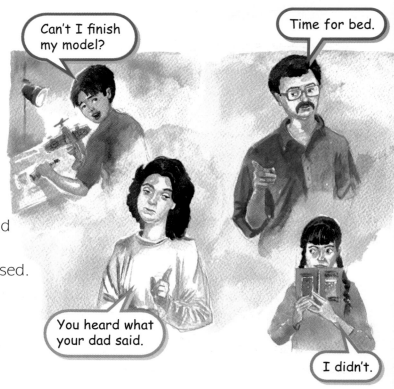

3 Write five sentences of your own using speech sparks.

Other punctuation in speech

Words such as "she said" may come before, after, or in the middle of the spoken words. Use commas to separate the spoken words from the rest of the sentence.

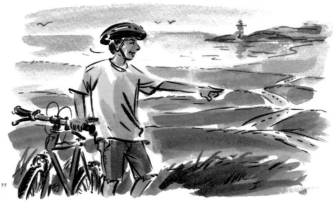

a "If it's fine, I'll cycle to the beach," said Richard.

b Richard said, "If it's fine, I'll cycle to the beach."

c "If it's fine," said Richard, "I'll cycle to the beach."

Notice that in sentences **b** and **c** the spoken words end in a full stop because they come at the end of the sentence. The speech marks come after the full stop.

Beginning speech on new lines

When writing a conversation begin a new line for each speaker.

"What are you looking for?" asked Amrik.
"My keys," replied Ben.
"Where did you lose them?"
"Over there," answered Ben.
"If you lost them over there," said Amrik,
"why are you looking for them over here?"
"Because there's more light over here," said Ben.

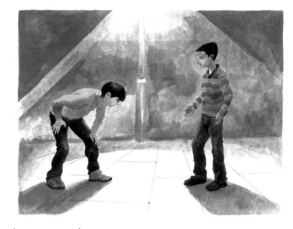

Test yourself

4 Copy these sentences. Put speech marks round the spoken words. Add any other punctuation necessary.

   a Stop cried Jamie.

   b Aunty Lisa said what would you like for your birthday?

   c Unless we set off right away said Nicola we won't get there in time.

   d Oh no cried Jonathan I've forgotten my money.

   e The teacher said we're going to the museum tomorrow.

   f If I'm not mistaken said the man we met last year at Brighton.

5 Write three sentences of your own with the spoken words at the end of the sentence.

6 Write three sentences of your own, placing the words which tell who is speaking in the middle of the spoken words.

7 Write a short conversation (about ten lines) between a parent and a child. Use appropriate punctuation, and don't forget to begin a new line for each speaker.

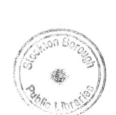

Answers are given on p.44.

20 Using paragraphs

A paragraph is a group of sentences about a single topic.

Begin a new paragraph when:

- **the topic changes**
- **a character begins speaking**
- **the speaker changes.**

Look at how the passage below has been organised into paragraphs.

Opening paragraph: the topic is Number 21 Lincoln Street

New paragraph: character begins speaking

New paragraph: the speaker changes

New paragraph: topic change (the young woman)

Number 21 Lincoln Street was an old Victorian house in a poor state of repair. The garden gate had dropped on its hinges and the postman had difficulty pushing it open. The path up to the house was overgrown with weeds, and paint was peeling from the front door.

"What do you want?" said a voice from above, as he was about to ring the bell.

"I've got a package for you," replied the postman, looking up.

A young woman was looking down from an open window. She was fashionably dressed and looked slightly out of place in the old house.

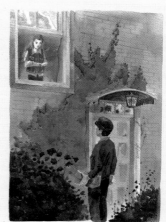

In your own writing, start each paragraph on a new line, and about 5 cm in from the left-hand side.

Test yourself

1 Read this passage carefully. Pick out the topics. Then rewrite the passage with a separate paragraph for each topic.

The boys were sitting at the top of a hill. On one side was a village, while on the other were open fields and a lonely cottage. They began to eat their packed lunches. Suddenly Mick tugged at Carl's sleeve. "Look," he whispered. Down below, half hidden in bushes, was a man. He was facing away from them, looking through binoculars at the cottage. "What do you think he's up to?" asked Mick. "Nothing good I expect," replied Carl. At that moment a young man and a woman came out of the cottage and set off walking to the village. The man with binoculars watched until they were out of sight, and then set off towards the cottage. "They're definitely up to no good," said Mick.

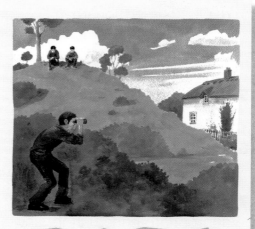

Answers are given on p.44.

21 Checking your work

Checking your work for mistakes is very important. Punctuation and spelling errors can spoil an otherwise good piece of writing. This is particularly important in your National Test Writing paper, where you will lose marks if you are careless with spelling or punctuation.

The activities below give you practice in spotting and correcting errors.

Test yourself

1 Pick out the spelling errors in this passage. Write the correct spellings.

Yesterday we went on a nature walk. The whether was suny and the veiw across the vallies was beautyful. We were hopeing to see deers, but they were not to be scene. We walked across some feilds and busyly picked some blackberrys. They were very tastey. Ms Jones took some photoes of us.

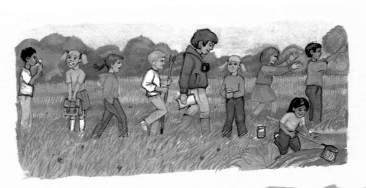

2 Rewrite this passage in paragraphs, putting in the missing or incorrect punctuation.

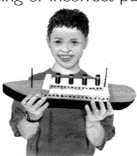

My names daniel hargreaves. I live at 15 belgrave terrace newtown. I have two sister's joanne and louise. My favourite hobbies are swimming football and building models yesterday i went to my friends house. Jake and I are building a model of the titanic. That's a great job youre doing there said Jakes dad but whos going to keep the model when its finished. Well take turns I said.

3 Rewrite this passage correcting both spelling and punctuation errors. Don't forget to use paragraphs.

Help. The cry came from behind a wall Simon and I tryed to clime the wall but it was to high. Dont worry I shouted were coming. In no time at all we were runing round the corner and racing for a gate we new was their. We ran threw it without stoping. The crys were comeing from a big pile of junk. Someone had tunneled there way in and it had collapsed. Are you hurt I shouted no replyed the voice Im all write but im traped. Simon then went for help while I stayed five minutes later too men pulled a girl out safly.

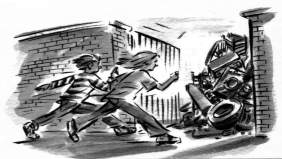

Answers are given on p.44.

25

22 Verbs

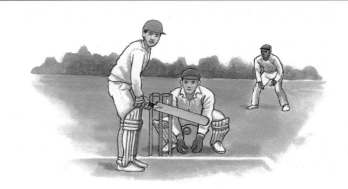

Subject–verb agreement

A verb must always agree with its subject.

This can best be explained by looking at a sentence where the verbs do not agree with their subjects:

We plays cricket when the weather are fine.

The correct way of writing the above sentence is:

<u>We play</u> cricket when <u>the weather is fine</u>.

Tense

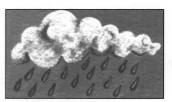

It rained.

The tense of a verb tells us when the action takes place.

Present tense: It <u>rains</u> without stopping. It <u>is raining</u> hard today.

Past tense: Yesterday it <u>rained</u>. Last Saturday it <u>was raining</u>.

Future tense: It <u>will rain</u> again this afternoon. It <u>will be raining</u> again tomorrow.

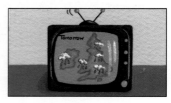

It will rain.

When we say "it rained", we are using the **simple past** form of the verb, where the action was completed.

When we say "it was raining", we are using the **past continuous** form, where the action was still going on. The continuous form of the verb always ends in **ing**.

The present and future tenses also have simple and continuous forms.

Test yourself

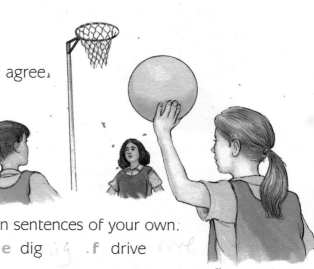

1 Rewrite these sentences so that the subjects and verbs agree.
   a The girls is playing netball.
   b Help your mother when you gets home.
   c They was running as fast as they could.
   d The dog were barking all night.
   e Jo and I is going to the park.

2 Change these verbs into the **simple past** and use them in sentences of your own.
   a paint   b walk   c swim   d win   e dig   f drive

3 Change these verbs into the **past continuous** (with **ing**) and use them in sentences of your own. Use the spelling rules for adding **ing**.
   a watch   b run   c quarrel   d carry   e take

4 Change these verbs into the **future tense**. Use them in sentences of your own.
   a come   b listen   c fasten   d pretend   e dust   f arrive

Keeping the tense consistent

In your writing always keep the tense consistent.

This can best be explained by looking at sentences where the writer has not been consistent:

Jack <u>moved</u> cautiously to the edge of the cliff and looks over. He <u>sees</u> two men on the beach below. They <u>were looking</u> out to sea.

The writer has begun in the past tense, lapsed into the present and then gone back into the past.

When to use other tenses

Although you will mainly use the simple past when you write a story, at times you will need to use other tenses.

You may find the **past continuous** useful when describing a setting:

The moon was rising over the hill.

When you write speech you may need the **past**, **present** or **future** tense:

"I left my bag on the bus," said Yasmin. (past)

"What will you do?" asked Nadine. (future)

"There is nothing I can do at the moment." (present)

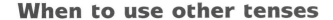

Test yourself

5 Rewrite this passage, correcting any mistakes in tense consistency and verb-subject agreement.

> We set off jogging down the road. After half an hour we was exhausted and sit down for a short rest. It was then we hear the strange noise. It were like a cry. I thought it was a bird, but Liam thinks it is some animal. We sets off to look for it. It seemed to came from behind a clump of bushes. When we got there we was disappointed. It were only a long strip of plastic, wrap fast round a twig. It were the wind that make it produced that strange sound.

6 Change this passage into the past tense. Correct any mistakes in verb-subject agreement as you do so. Make sure you keep the tense consistent.

> Lee packs his bag and hurries to the station, but when he gets there he finds the train is already pulling out of the station. His watch is slow. There are an hour to the next train. He buys a sports magazine, and sit down. He reads it and find it so interesting he forgets what time it is and only just catch his train.

Answers are given on p.45.

23 Making simple sentences more interesting

A simple sentence has a subject and a verb, and sometimes an object.

| *subject* | *verb* | | *subject* | *verb* | *object* |
| The dog | barked. | | The dog | ate | the meat. |

Using adjectives and adverbs

Simple sentences may be made more interesting by adding adjectives or adverbs.

An **adjective** describes a noun: The <u>fierce</u> dog barked.

An **adverb** tells us more about a verb: The dog ate the meat <u>greedily</u>.

Most adverbs end in **-ly**. Look back at page 9 to make sure you remember the spelling rules for adding **-ly**.

Test yourself

1 Make these simple sentences more interesting by adding suitable adjectives to the nouns underlined.

   a A <u>van</u> stopped outside the <u>house</u>.

   b He found a <u>key</u> under a <u>stone</u>.

   c The <u>lady</u> wore a <u>dress</u> and a <u>necklace</u>.

   d The <u>man</u> bought a <u>television</u> and a <u>kettle</u>.

   e The <u>boy</u> ate a <u>cake</u> and two <u>ice creams</u>.

   f In the <u>box</u> was a <u>ring</u>, a <u>chain</u> and <u>ear-rings</u>.

2 Make these sentences more interesting by adding a suitable adverb to each underlined verb.

   a He <u>crept</u> up to the door.

   b She <u>writes</u> and <u>sings</u>.

   c When he <u>fell</u> he <u>hurt</u> himself.

   d He <u>woke up</u> when the phone <u>rang</u>.

   e He <u>tied</u> the knot so that he could <u>climb</u> down the rope.

   f She <u>swam</u> and <u>won</u> the race.

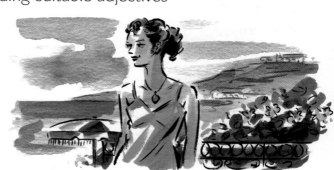

3 Make these simple sentences more interesting by adding adjectives and adverbs.

   a The girl spoke to the boy.   **d** The boy played the piano.

   b A woman walked up the hill.   **e** The sun shone on the lake.

   c The cat watched the bird.   **f** The girl climbed the tree.

Using phrases

Simple sentences may be made more interesting by adding phrases.

A phrase is a group of words which does not make complete sense on its own. It has no verb.

An **adjective phrase** tells us more about a noun.

A man <u>with red hair</u> delivered a parcel.

A man delivered a parcel <u>tied up with string</u>.

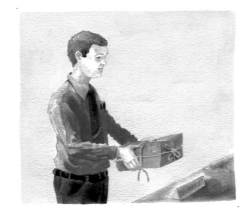

An **adverb phrase** tells us more about a verb.

He won the race <u>earlier today</u>. (tells us when)

He won the race <u>up the hill</u>. (tells us where)

He won the race <u>with ease</u>. (tells us how)

Test yourself

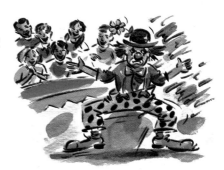

4 Make each of these sentences more interesting by adding a suitable adjective phrase. Do it like this: He met a man <u>with a beard</u>.

  a He drove a car.   **e** He lives in a house.

  b The clown made us laugh.   **f** Those flowers are roses.

  c The box was too heavy to lift.   **g** The boy is my cousin.

  d A dog kept us awake.

5 Make each of these sentences more interesting by adding a suitable adverb phrase. Do it like this: She finished her work in <u>double quick time</u>.

  a They fell.

  b He crossed the road.

  c She tidied the room.

  d He finished the job.

  e She hit the ball.

  f He left the building.

  g He walked home.

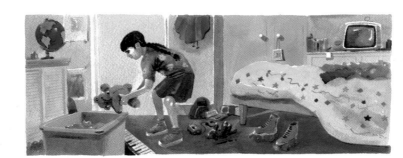

6 Make these simple sentences more interesting by adding an adjective phrase and an adverb phrase. Do it like this: The boy <u>with the blue shirt</u> played football <u>all afternoon</u>.

  a The boy fell into the river.   **e** She chose a book.

  b The man dived in to save him.   **f** There was a girl.

  c The squirrel ran up the tree.   **g** The workers stopped work.

  d The man climbed the hill.

Answers are given on p.45.

24 Joining sentences

Two simple sentences can be joined to make a compound sentence. To do this we use a linking word, or conjunction:

It was a glorious day. We decided to have a picnic.

It was a glorious day <u>and</u> we decided to have a picnic.

We decided to have a picnic <u>because</u> it was a glorious day.

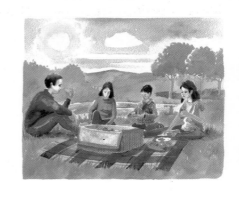

Common conjunctions

and   but   yet   although   because   therefore . so   while   or

But, **yet** and **although** are used to join one idea with an unexpected or contrasting idea:

I had a sore leg <u>but</u> I played football.

I had a sore leg, <u>yet</u> I played football.

I played football, <u>although</u> I had a sore leg.

Because, **therefore** and **so** are used to join one idea with another which explains it:

I got high marks <u>because</u> my work was good.

His work was excellent, <u>therefore</u> he got high marks.

His work was excellent, <u>so</u> he got high marks.

While is used to join two actions which are going on at the same time:

<u>While</u> you were watching television, I was doing my homework.

Or is used to show two alternative courses of action, one of which might be a consequence of the first:

Take care <u>or</u> you will get into trouble.

Test yourself

1 Join these sentences with a suitable conjunction. Try to use a different conjunction for each sentence.

  a She went to buy some sugar. There was none in the shop.

  b I painted the door. My brother painted the window frame.

  c Mr Green's car broke down. He never serviced it.

  d I stayed in. It was a sunny day.

  e I washed up. My sister dusted.

  f The streets were like a maze. Joanne found her way to the hotel.

  g Smeeta arrived home early. She had time to walk the dog.

  h Hurry up. You will be late.

Varying your sentences

Most conjunctions are placed in the middle of a compound sentence:

He decided to go hiking <u>although</u> the weather looked threatening.

With conjunctions such as **because**, **although**, **while** and **so**, you may sometimes choose to put the conjunction at the beginning. This will add interest and variety to your writing.

<u>Because</u> the clock needed repairing, I decided to buy a new one.

<u>Although</u> the weather seemed threatening, he went hiking.

<u>While</u> I was still thinking about it, Jo had the car fixed and running.

<u>So</u> we could set off early, I set the alarm for half past six.

To make your writing interesting, you need to use a mix of simple and compound sentences.

A passage of entirely simple or compound sentences can be very boring. The passage on the right uses a good mix. Here the writer uses simple sentences to build excitement. See if you can pick them out.

Andy slowed down and looked over his shoulder. The men were gaining on him. He tried to run faster, but he could now feel a pain in his side. He had to find a hiding place. At the top of the hill he would be out of sight for a few moments and might be able to find somewhere to hide. The top of the hill came nearer. The pain in his side grew worse. Then Andy was over the top and out of sight. But there was absolutely nowhere to hide!

Test yourself

2 Rewrite this passage joining some, but not all, of the simple sentences. Use an interesting mix of simple and compound sentences.

Mrs King was walking home. She was very tired. She had spent all morning shopping. She stopped. She put her heavy bags down. She waited to get her breath back. She saw a man was hurrying towards her. There was a shout from up the road. A policeman was chasing after the man. Mrs King was old. She decided to stop the man. She blocked the pavement with her bags. She stood facing him. He shouted for her to get out of the way. She did not move. He swerved round her into the road. At that moment Mrs King put out her foot. The man tripped up. He fell headlong into the road.

He was then arrested by the policeman.

"That was a brave thing to do. It was dangerous too," the policeman told her. "You could have been hurt."

"But I wasn't," smiled Mrs King. She was still smiling when she arrived home.

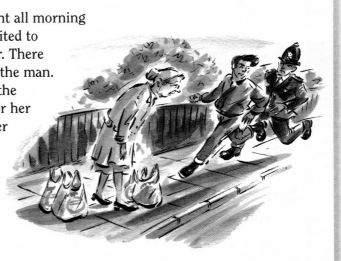

Answers are given on p.46.

25 Complex sentences

A <u>complex sentence</u> is made by adding a clause to a simple sentence.

A <u>clause</u> is a group of words which contains a <u>verb</u>.

Simple sentence: The man decorated the room.

Complex sentence: The man decorated the room <u>before he went on holiday</u>.

Clauses may be adjectival or adverbial.

Adjectival clauses often begin with *who*, *which*, *that*, *whose* or *whom*, and add information about nouns.

Tom read a book, <u>which he bought for 5p</u>.

He knows Mrs Healey, <u>who is our teacher</u>.

The lady, <u>whose dog is missing</u>, has offered a reward.

Notice the use of commas in the above sentences to separate the added clause from the rest of the sentence.

Adverbial clauses answer the questions *how? when? where?* or *why?* about the verb.

The children played <u>where there was no traffic</u>. (tells us where)

He went to meet her <u>after she phoned him</u>. (tells us when)

Test yourself

1 Make these simple sentences into complex sentences by adding a clause of your own. Begin each clause with one of the words from the word bank. Try to use each word only once.

   a They hid the money.

   b She was looking out of the window.

   c He had a coffee.

   d He took the dog for a walk.

   e She bought a book.

   f You won't get good marks.

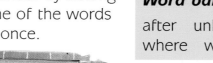

Word bank:

after   unless   before   as
where   which   when

2 Make these simple sentences into complex sentences by adding an adjectival clause of your own.

   a Pat bought a new suit.   c The artist painted a picture.

   b Ben met a man.   d The people built the house.

3 Make these simple sentences into complex sentences by adding an adverbial clause of your own.

   a He did not look.   c Sam brought an umbrella.

   b She went for a walk.   d A girl opened the door.

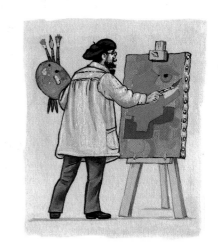

Varying complex sentences

You can add a clause <u>at the beginning</u> of a simple sentence. Remember that when you do this, you need to use a comma to separate the two parts of the sentence:

<u>While he was on the phone</u>, I went out for a walk.

<u>As it was raining</u>, he stayed in and read a book.

<u>After I hurt my hand</u>, I stopped work.

You can also add a clause <u>in the middle</u> of a simple sentence. Remember to use commas to separate the added clause from the main sentence:

Tammy, <u>who is my cousin</u>, is coming to stay with us.

The boy, <u>charging madly down the street</u>, bumped into a lady.

The gold watch, <u>which used to belong to his grandfather</u>, was stolen.

Test yourself

4 Make these simple sentences into complex sentences by adding a clause of your own <u>at the beginning</u>. Begin each clause with one of the words from the word bank. Try to use each word only once. Don't forget to use a comma to separate the two parts.

> **Word bank:**
>
> if unless as since until although because when

a You will not be picked for the team.

b She went out without a coat.

c I went to see my friend.

d We will go for a walk.

e You may go out.

f I can't buy you an ice cream.

g You have grown quite tall.

h I'm going to keep on trying.

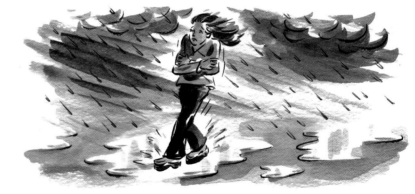

5 Change each of these simple sentences into three different complex sentences by adding a different clause at the end, at the beginning and in the middle. The first one has been done for you.

a The girl played football.

The girl played football <u>when she had finished her work</u>.
<u>Whenever she got the chance</u>, the girl played football.
The girl, <u>who was wearing Manchester United kit</u>, played fotball.

b The cyclist locked up his bike.

c The firefighters put out the fire.

d A man knocked at the door.

e The cat chased the dog.

f A box was left on the doorstep.

g The wind uprooted the tree.

Answers are given on p.46.

Camping

The Richards family had chosen a perfect spot for their campsite. It was near to a clear stream, but raised well above it to avoid flooding, and protected from the prevailing wind by a hill.

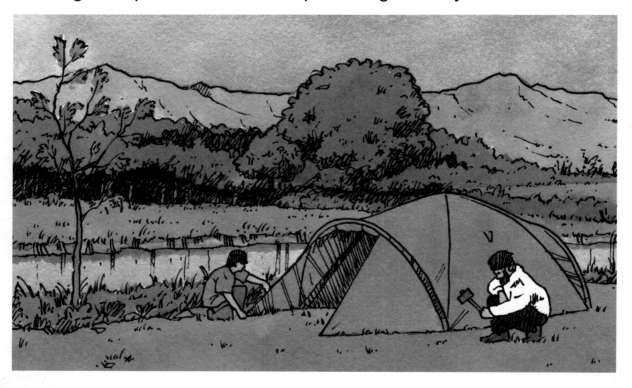

They had almost finished _____ up the tent. The ground was firm, and Dad was sure the tent pegs _____ hold well. As he was _____ hammering in the last of the tent pegs, Sam's _____ was unpacking their first meal. The forecast said there _____ be rain, but the weather was _____ and all Sam's worries _____.

Spelling Test 1

They sat _____, listening to the sound of the birds and

the babble of the stream. A few _____ flew around them

and Dad decided to _____ a fire to keep them away.

He _____ some wood and fire-lighters from the car.

Soon a fire was blazing. Sam helped Mum wash the

_____. Then they put some _____ in foil to

cook in the fire. Sam _____ into the fire,

_____ a world of magic in the flames. He was

_____ that tomorrow they could go _____

in a nearby pool. He could not _____ that it was only

three hours since they left home. Now here they were in the

_____ of the countryside. He smiled. This is a great

place, he _____ to himself.

Stockton Borough Public Libraries

The Sea Chest

The children never tired of watching the sea. That day the waves rolled onto the beach, breaking up into plumes of spray as they smashed onto the rocks around the sandy bay.

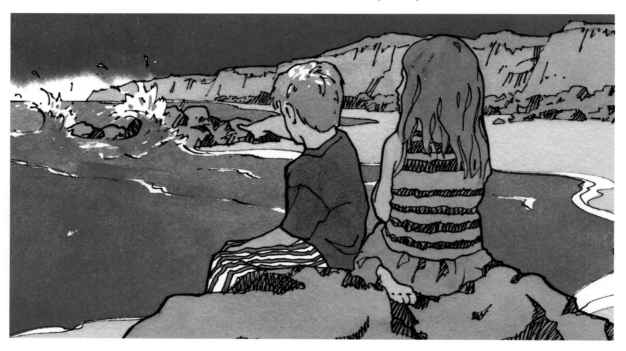

Dark clouds _____ across the sky. Suddenly the sun

broke _____, casting a shaft of sunlight which struck the

_____ waves. In its light a strange object could be seen:

a chest _____ on the waves. _____ that the

sea was dangerous on such days, Rob _____ down the

beach. In no time he was _____ towards the chest.

Lucy called to him but her _____ were lost in the

Spelling Test 2

_____ of the surf and the sea. The chest was being

carried _____ towards Rob. Then as the waves lifted it

as if offering it to him, Rob grabbed one of its _____.

The sea still supported its _____ and Rob was able to

pull it towards the beach. But as the sea got _____

the chest got _____. Lucy came to help him.

_____ they were far from any of the _____

rocks. They _____ the chest onto the beach. The box

was shut _____, but not locked. Rob and Lucy forced

open the lid. To their bitter _____ the chest was

_____ empty.

The UFO

Nadia did not believe in UFOs, or unidentified flying objects to give them their proper name. Some people will believe anything, won't they? Little green men in alien spacecraft with flashing lights – what a lot of nonsense! But something was about to happen to change her mind.

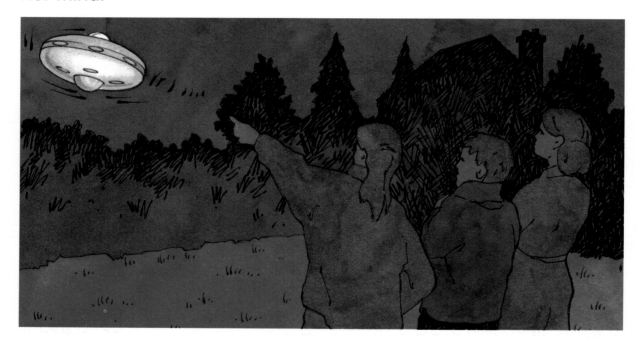

Nadia _____ had a party on her _____.

The house was full of her _____, and so was the

_____. It was a starry night, filled with the sound of the

children's _____. Suddenly someone noticed a green

light low over the _____ opposite. Then the light grew

Spelling Test 3

_____. There was a strange _____ sound as it

came over the _____.

"It's a _____ saucer!" someone cried excitedly.

"There's no _____ thing," replied Nadia, but she

_____ sound sure. In fact she was _____ to

feel afraid.

"Did you send them an _____?" someone said. No one

_____ thought it funny. The children were standing close

_____ watching the flying saucer hovering above them.

The light was _____ now, changing colour from green to

red. Then suddenly the object shot across the sky, _____

to some unknown destination. Nadia began to wonder if there might

be _____ from other worlds. Was it _____?

At least it was exciting to think so.

Answers and Guidance

Here is a chance for you to check your answers to the questions. Examples are given of possible ways of answering the questions and you should compare your answer with those given.

1 ie or ei?

1
a shield   d niece   g ceiling   j neither
b chief   e seize   h receipt
c receive   f believe   i field

2
a disappear   g handkerchief
b cheese   h sweep
c scream   i priest
d piece (of cake)   j ceiling
e peace (and quiet)   k sealing
f deceive   l weird

3 Check your spellings with **2** above.

4
a grief   d neighbour   g mischief
b diesel   e shriek   h deceive
c weight   f belief   i niece

2 Plurals: –s and –es

Most people have difficulty with English spelling, even if only with a few words. But there are several things we can do to help us, and one of these is to learn spelling rules. As you work through this book <u>make sure you learn each spelling rule</u>.

Now check your own work:

1
a apples   d desks   g switches   j chairs
b peaches   e kisses   h foxes   k stitches
c torches   f roads   i dishes   l brushes

2
a Are there any <u>witnesses</u> to the accident?
b I went to the <u>churches</u>.
c He hid behind the <u>bushes</u>.
d She bought some <u>clocks</u> and <u>watches</u>.
e Bring me those <u>boxes</u> and then wash the <u>dishes</u>.
f The men dug some <u>trenches</u>.
g The rabbits live in <u>hutches</u>.
h He bought some <u>bunches</u> of flowers.

3 These are the correct spellings of the words you should have used in your own sentences:
a lunches   c catches   e coaches   g sixes
b churches   d ditches   f fishes   h dashes

4 foxes, crashes, lunches, bunches

3 Plurals: words ending in -y

Check your own work:

1
a sprays   e journeys   i valleys
b ladies   f berries   j opportunities
c skies   g cherries   k bodies
d days   h lorries   l rubies

2
a The <u>lorries</u> suffered <u>delays</u>.
b The <u>boys</u> went under the <u>subway</u>.
c There were <u>flies</u> on the <u>cherries</u>.
d There were <u>replies</u> to their <u>invitations</u> to the <u>parties</u>.
e She had <u>some inquiries</u> about the silver <u>trays</u> she had for sale.
f He found <u>pennies</u>, <u>keys</u> and <u>some rubies</u>.
g The <u>families</u> were looking forward to their <u>holidays</u>.
h He read some <u>stories</u> about <u>monasteries</u>.

3 These are the correct spellings of the words you should have used in sentences of your own:
a bullies   c donkeys   e babies
b spies   d plays   f enquiries

4
a The house had three <u>storeys</u> and had views of two <u>valleys</u>.
b The lorries made several <u>journeys</u>, crossing the channel on <u>ferries</u>.
c She worked for government <u>ministeries</u>, inspecting highways.
d There were bunches of <u>cherries</u> on the <u>trays</u>.

If after learning the spelling rules you still find some words difficult, then try the **Look, Say, Cover, Write, Check** method. This can be used with any word, especially the ones you find most difficult to spell.

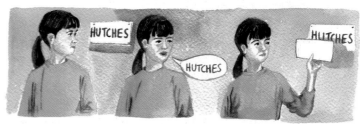

Look   Say   Cover

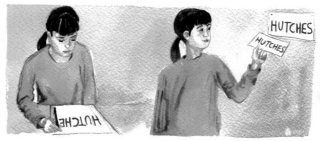

Write   Check

Answers and Guidance

4 Plurals: words ending in –f

1 Note that in **g** the plural of hoof has two acceptable plural endings.
- **a** halves
- **b** calves
- **c** selves
- **d** cliffs
- **e** wolves
- **f** roofs
- **g** hoofs or hooves
- **h** yourselves
- **i** staffs
- **j** wives

2 Check your spellings with the list above.

3
- **a** The <u>loaves</u> were on the baker's <u>shelves</u>.
- **b** He cut the <u>leaves</u> with <u>knives</u>.
- **c** She bought <u>some handkerchiefs</u> and <u>scarves</u>.
- **d** The <u>wharves</u> were at the foot of the <u>cliffs</u>.
- **e** The <u>thieves</u> stole the <u>skiffs</u>.

Note that the following plurals may have either an *s* or a *ves* ending:
handkerchief – handkerchiefs or handkerchieves
scarf – scarfs or scarves
wharf – wharfs or wharves

4
- **a** cliffs
- **b** wives
- **c** elves
- **d** lives
- **e** chiefs
- **f** roofs
- **g** selves
- **h** staffs

5 Plurals: words ending in –o

1
- **a** tomatoes
- **b** radios
- **c** heroes
- **d** mosquitoes
- **e** photos
- **f** zeros
- **g** solos
- **h** kilos
- **i** memos
- **j** pianos

2 Check your spellings with the list above.

3
- **a** She was bitten by <u>mosquitoes</u>.
- **b** The <u>tornadoes</u> destroyed many houses.
- **c** She bought some <u>potatoes</u> and some <u>mangos</u>.
- **d** The <u>radios</u> weighed two <u>kilos</u>.
- **e** The <u>echoes</u> rang round the <u>volcanoes</u>.
- **f** He had <u>piccolos</u> and <u>banjos</u> for sale.
- **g** There were <u>stereos</u> and <u>videos</u> in the shop window.

Note that in **c** mangos or mangoes are acceptable.

4
- **a** potatoes
- **b** pianos
- **c** flamingos
- **d** cargoes
- **e** halos
- **f** solos

6 Unusual plurals

1
- **a** men
- **b** scissors
- **c** feet
- **d** sheep
- **e** children
- **f** salmon
- **g** geese
- **h** aircraft
- **i** mice
- **j** deer

2 Check your spellings with the list above.

3
- **a** His <u>teeth were</u> aching.
- **b** The <u>men</u> and <u>women</u> flew in the <u>aircraft</u>.
- **c** The <u>fishermen</u> caught <u>some trout</u> and <u>pike</u>.
- **d** She cut out <u>some pairs of trousers</u> with the <u>scissors</u>.
- **e** There were <u>two series</u> about <u>salmon</u> on television.
- **f** The <u>postmen were</u> chased by <u>some geese</u>.

4
- **a** pliers
- **b** trousers
- **c** children
- **d** salmon
- **e** mice
- **f** grouse
- **g** teeth

If you have trouble spelling any of these unusual plurals, use one of these tried and tested ways of remembering:
- Look, Say, Cover, Write, Check
- Split up words for easier spelling: child-ren; trous-ers
- Say silent letters out loud: salmon
- Imagine silent letters as coloured and moving: scissors
- Mark the parts you have trouble with: scissors

7 Adding –ly

1
- **a** lonely
- **b** bravely
- **c** greedily
- **d** sensibly
- **e** bubbly
- **f** crazily
- **g** hungrily
- **h** fully
- **i** tidily
- **j** beautifully

2
- **a** carefully
- **b** happily
- **c** comfortably
- **d** shrilly
- **e** shabbily
- **f** terribly
- **g** necessarily
- **h** steadily
- **i** responsibly
- **j** desperately

3
- **a** stupidly
- **b** friendly
- **c** dangerously
- **d** completely
- **e** invisibly
- **f** truthfully
- **g** sincerely
- **h** probably

4 busily, finally, fortunately, wonderfully, lovely

8 Adding –ing and –ed

1
- **a** planting
- **b** inviting
- **c** raining
- **d** resting
- **e** living
- **f** shining
- **g** teasing
- **h** taking

2
- **a** measured
- **b** snowed
- **c** imagined
- **d** scraped
- **e** looked
- **f** typed
- **g** mixed
- **h** mumbled

3
- **a** waking
- **b** phoning
- **c** hiding
- **d** choosing
- **e** paddling
- **f** sharing
- **g** waving
- **h** baking
- **i** grumbling
- **j** dancing

Answers and Guidance

9 Adding -ing and -ed to verbs ending in y

1
a cried   c played   e dried   g relied
b married   d obeyed   f employed   h journeyed

2
a hurrying   d saying   g flying
b trying   e paying   h straying
c burying   f worrying

3 envied, carried, hurrying, tried, relied, buried

10 Doubling letters when adding -ed or ing

1
a sitting   d skipping   g hitting
b tugging   e lapping   h spinning
c swimming   f ripping

2
a knitted   c sipped   e tripped   g robbed
b batted   d stopped   f fitted   h shopped

3 Check your spellings with **1** and **2** above.

4
a winning   d dropping   g jogging
b digging   e dripping   h tripping
c pinning   f dragging

5 running, tipping, flapping, batting, stopping, getting

6
a propelling   e quarrelling   h fulfilling
b forgetting   f galloping   i chiselling
c harvesting   g compelling   j permitting
d beginning

7
a labelled, labelling
b committed, committing
c targeted, targeting
d travelled, travelling
e trumpeted, trumpeting
f shovelled, shovelling
g gossiped, gossiping
h tunnelled, tunnelling

8 channelled, signalled, referred, cancelling, beginning, levelled

9 Check your writing with the rules on pages 12–13.

11 Adding -er and -est

1
a longer   d warmer   g lonelier   j sweeter
b fitter   e slippier   h prouder   k happier
c slimmer   f smaller   i wetter   l smoother

2
a slowest   d tastiest   g fattest   j reddest
b thinnest   e busiest   h hungriest
c flattest   f narrowest   i craziest

3
a shyest   e flattest   h dustier
b unhappiest   f friendlier   i sadder
c thinner   g maddest   j heaviest
d slimier

4
a happier   c fastest   e nastiest   g fewer
b slower   d trimmer   f coldest   h merriest

12 Adding -y and -ful

1
a frosty   d colourful   g truthful   j hopeful
b helpful   e careful   h useful   k beautiful
c runny   f easy   i funny   l plentiful

2 Check your spellings with **1** above.

3
a rusty   d painful   g nippy   j noisy
b chatty   e hopeful   h grateful   k spotty
c muddy   f pitiful   i wonderful   l frightful

4
a cloudy   d nutty   g plentiful   j baggy
b choppy   e easy   h soggy
c beautiful   f tasty   i hopeful

13 The apostrophe in shortened forms

1
a didn't   d you've   g you're   j wouldn't
b she'll   e they're   h I'll
c I'm   f he's   i we'll

2 Check your spellings with those in **1** above.

3
a It'll start raining as soon as we're ready to go out. That's what happens every time.
b She didn't do the work because she hadn't got a pen.
c She's keeping the ring locked up. It's very valuable.
d You're sure that your sister can't come to help us? I'm disappointed!
e I've written a letter, he's painted a picture, but you've wasted your time.

4
a You can't go out now. It's far too late. You'd better go tomorrow instead.
b Why're you so slow? I won't let you come again if you don't hurry up.
c He's a faster runner than his brothers, but they're better at football.

Answers and Guidance

d I'm going out at five o'clock. Can't I do my homework when I get back?

e They'll be very pleased that he's bought them each an ice cream, won't they?

14 Homophones

1 a The cat waited for its owner.
   b It's a beautiful picture.
   c It's impossible.
   d The dog was in its basket.
   e It's time for school.

2 a I'd love some peace and quiet.
   b Do you eat meat?
   c The two men were too tired to work any longer.
   d He took a can of beans off the shelf.
   e The wind blew the boat across the blue sea.
   f Do you write with your left hand or your right?
   g The first one past the post won the race.
   h I could do with a break after all this work.
   i Would you sell me that plank of wood?
   j They're looking for their coats over there.
   k I knew she had bought a new pair of shoes.
   l He's feeling weak now but this time next week he'll be fit again.

3 These are examples of sentences to show the difference in meaning between the homophones.
   a Here is the pen I lost. Did you hear that shout?
   b I left it over there by the fire. Their parents came to see me this afternoon.
   c These shoes are far too dear! The deer is a graceful animal.
   d Comb your hair! A hare has long ears.
   e An important letter arrived in the mail. A lion is male and a lioness is female.
   f Have you got this material in a plain colour? The plane roared overhead.

15 How to begin and end sentences

1 a The stranger entered town on a black horse.
   b How does a question end?
   c Is Roald Dahl your favourite author?
   d What a fantastic film!
   e Bill met Jake on the way to the library.
   f Is this the right way to Bristol?
   g Open the door this minute!
   h The elephant sensed danger and trumpeted loudly.
   i Did you see Katy when you went to Liverpool?
   j The aeroplane roared low overhead.

k I don't believe it!
l You did post my letter, didn't you?

2 Make sure your statements begin with a capital letter and end with a full stop. Have you used capital letters for proper nouns?

3 Make sure your questions begin with a capital letter and end with a question mark.

4 Make sure your exclamations begin with a capital letter and end with an exclamation mark.

16 Commas

1 a Don't forget to bring boots, an anorak, sandwiches and a drink.
   b Looking very pleased with himself, Ben stepped up to collect the prize.
   c Although he was very busy, he found time to help Mrs Dunn.
   d There were coats, scarves and gloves scattered all over the room.
   e Before you go, clean all this mess up!
   f Daffodils, tulips, crocuses and hyacinths are all spring flowers.

2 Make sure you have a comma after each item in your list, but remember you don't need a comma before *and*.

3 Without waiting for the others, Sam entered the dark room. Until his eyes adjusted to the dark, he couldn't make anything out. Then he saw the room was filled with piles of old magazines, newspapers and books. What was that? A slithering sound came from the corner. Sam froze. Then he saw the snake sliding towards him. What a fright that gave him!

17 Other punctuation in sentences

1 a He was out LBW (leg before wicket).
   b I'll have a hamburger – no, make that a hot dog.
   c He ran all the way to school: he was late.
   d Matt says – but I don't believe him – that he's got full marks.
   e We bought several plants: petunias, marigolds, geraniums and pansies.
   f The forecast is for a sunny bank holiday (which I'll believe when I see it).
   g Breakfast consisted of: coffee, boiled eggs, toast and marmalade.
   h The computer has a very large VDU (visual display unit).

Answers and Guidance

18 The apostrophe to show possession

1 b the teacher's desk
 c the lady's dress
 d the ladies' cars
 e the policemen's helmets
 f the policeman's helmet
 g my dog's collar
 h the book's cover
 i the boy's shirts
 j Mr Green's house
 k the bee's wings
 l the wasps' nest

2 a <u>Kate's</u> bag is bigger than <u>Yasmin's</u>.
 b The <u>postman's</u> van stopped outside Mr <u>Smith's</u> shop.
 c On the table were: a <u>referee's</u> whistle, a <u>gardener's</u> trowel and a <u>lady's</u> brooch.
 d The teacher confiscated <u>Ravi's</u> comic, the <u>twins'</u> sweets and <u>Gerry's</u> crisps.
 e He delivered leaflets to the <u>Brown's</u> house and the <u>Jones'</u> flat.

3 the electrician's screwdrivers; the artists' paints; the postman's letters; the pilots' aeroplanes; the teachers' books; the florist's flowers

19 Punctuating speech

1 a "Time for bed," said Dad.
 b Tim said, "Can't I finish my model?"
 c Mum said, "You heard what your dad said."
 d "I didn't," said Laura.

2 a "I'll tidy my room when I get back," he promised.
 b Mark said, "It's time we took a break."
 c "Are you going to the shops?" he asked.
 d "That's a job well done," said Dad.
 e "What time is it?" asked Charlie.
 f "Watch out!" yelled Craig.

3 Check that you have used the four rules for using speech marks.

4 a "Stop!" cried Jamie.
 b Aunty Lisa said, "What would you like for your birthday?"
 c "Unless we set off right away," said Nicola, "we won't get there in time."
 d "Oh, no!" cried Jonathan, "I've forgotten my money."
 e The teacher said, "We're going to the museum tomorrow."

 f "If I'm not mistaken," said the man, "we met last year at Brighton."

5 and 6 Check that you have used correct punctuation.

7 Check that you have used correct punctuation, and begun a new line for each speaker.

20 Using paragraphs

1 The boys were sitting at the top of a hill. On one side was a village, while on the other were open fields and a lonely cottage. They began to eat their packed lunches. Suddenly Mick tugged at Carl's sleeve.
 "Look," he whispered. Down below, half hidden in bushes, was a man. He was facing away from them, looking through binoculars at the cottage.
 "What do you think he's up to?" asked Mick.
 "Nothing good I expect," replied Carl.
 At that moment a young man and a woman came out of the cottage and set off walking to the village. The man with binoculars watched until they were out of sight, and then set off towards the cottage.
 "They're definitely up to no good," said Mick.

21 Checking your work

1 Yesterday we went on a nature walk. The weather was sunny and the view across the valleys was beautiful. We were hoping to see deer, but they were not to be seen. We walked across some fields and busily picked some blackberries. They were very tasty. Ms Jones took some photos of us.

2 My name's Daniel Hargreaves. I live at 15, Belgrave Terrace, Newtown. I have two sisters, Joanne and Louise. My favourite hobbies are: swimming, football and building models.
 Yesterday I went to my friend's house. Jake and I are building a model of the Titanic.
 "That's a great job you're doing there," said Jake's dad, "but who's going to keep the model when it's finished?"
 "We'll take turns," I said.

3 "Help!" The cry came from behind a wall. Simon and I tried to climb the wall, but it was too high.
 "Don't worry," I shouted. "We're coming!"
 In no time at all we were running round the corner and racing for a gate we knew was there. We ran through it without stopping. The cries were coming from a big pile of junk. Someone had tunnelled their way in and it had collapsed.
 "Are you hurt?" I shouted.

Answers and Guidance

"No," replied the voice, "I'm all right, but I'm trapped."

Simon then went for help, while I stayed. Five minutes later two men pulled a girl out safely.

22 Verbs

1 a The <u>girls are</u> playing netball.
   b Help your mother when <u>you get</u> home.
   c <u>They were</u> running as fast as they could.
   d The <u>dog was</u> barking all night.
   e <u>Jo and I are</u> going to the park.

2 These are the correct forms of verbs you should have used in your sentences:
   a painted   c swam   e dug
   b walked   d won   f drove

3 Notice the use of the spelling rules from pages 12–13 in questions **b-d**. If you got the spelling wrong learn the rules again.
   a was (or were) watching   d was carrying
   b was running   e was taking
   c were quarrelling

4 a will come   c will fasten   e will dust
   b will listen   d will pretend   f will arrive

5 We set off jogging down the road. After half an hour we <u>were</u> exhausted and sat down for a short rest. It was then we <u>heard</u> the strange noise. It was like a cry. I thought it was a bird, but Liam <u>thought</u> it was some animal. We <u>set</u> off to look for it. It seemed to <u>come</u> from behind a clump of bushes. When we got there we <u>were</u> disappointed. It <u>was</u> only a long strip of plastic, <u>wrapped</u> fast round a twig. It <u>was</u> the wind that made it produce that strange sound.

6 Lee <u>packed</u> his bag and <u>hurried</u> to the station, but when he <u>got</u> there he <u>found</u> the train <u>was</u> pulling out of the station. His watch <u>was</u> slow. There <u>was</u> an hour to the next train. He <u>bought</u> a sports magazine, and <u>sat</u> down. He <u>read</u> it and <u>found</u> it so interesting he forgot what time it <u>was</u> and only just <u>caught</u> his train.

23 Making simple sentences more interesting

These are just some of the ways in which the simple sentences can be made more interesting:

1 a A <u>white</u> van stopped outside the <u>semi-detached</u> house.
   b He found a <u>rusty</u> key under a <u>large</u> stone.
   c The <u>beautiful</u> lady wore a <u>velvet</u> dress and a <u>gold</u> necklace.
   d The <u>young</u> man bought a <u>wide-screen</u> television and an <u>electric</u> kettle.
   e The <u>greedy</u> boy ate a <u>delicious</u> cake and two <u>chocolate</u> ice creams.
   f In the <u>wooden</u> box was a <u>diamond</u> ring, a <u>silver</u> chain and <u>emerald</u> ear-rings.

2 a He crept <u>silently</u> up to the door.
   b She writes <u>neatly</u> and sings <u>sweetly</u>.
   c When he fell <u>awkwardly</u> he hurt himself <u>badly</u>.
   d He woke up <u>suddenly</u> when the phone rang <u>unexpectedly</u>.
   e He tied the knot <u>tightly</u> so that he could climb <u>safely</u> down the rope.
   f She swam <u>strongly</u> and won the race <u>easily</u>.

3 a The <u>angry</u> girl spoke <u>sharply</u> to the <u>naughty</u> boy.
   b A <u>tired</u> woman walked <u>slowly</u> up the <u>steep</u> hill.
   c The <u>crouching</u> cat watched the <u>unsuspecting</u> bird <u>intently</u>.
   d The <u>clever</u> boy played the <u>old</u> piano <u>beautifully</u>.
   e The <u>fierce</u> sun shone <u>brightly</u> on the <u>sparkling</u> lake.
   f The <u>agile</u> girl <u>swiftly</u> climbed the <u>tall</u> tree.

4 These are just some of the ways in which the simple sentences can be made more interesting by adding phrases:
   a He drove a car <u>with a broken headlamp</u>.
   b The clown <u>in baggy trousers</u> made us laugh.
   c The box <u>of iron</u> was too heavy to lift.
   d A dog <u>with a loud bark</u> kept us awake.
   e He lives in a house <u>by the river</u>.
   f Those flowers <u>on the table</u> are roses.
   g The boy <u>with the charming smile</u> is my cousin.

5 a They fell <u>in a heap</u>.
   b He crossed the road <u>without looking</u>.
   c She tidied the room <u>before dinner</u>.
   d He finished the job <u>with time to spare</u>.
   e She hit the ball <u>high in the air</u>.
   f He left the building <u>in a great hurry</u>.
   g <u>After school</u> he walked home.

Note that you can often put an adverb phrase at the beginning of a sentence, as in **5g** above. Doing this occasionally will make your sentences more varied and interesting.

Answers and Guidance

6 a The boy <u>on the bank</u> fell into the river <u>with a great splash</u>.
  b <u>Without hesitation</u> the man <u>on the bridge</u> dived in to save him.
  c <u>In a flash</u> the squirrel ran up the tree <u>by the gate</u>.
  d The man <u>with a limp</u> climbed the hill <u>with great difficulty</u>.
  e <u>After a great deal of thought</u> she chose a book <u>about the Ancient Egyptians</u>.
  f <u>At the top of the path</u> there was a girl <u>with a backpack</u>.
  g <u>At half past two</u> the workers <u>on the bypass</u> stopped work.

24 Joining sentences

1 a She went to buy some sugar <u>but</u> there was none in the shop.
  b I painted the door <u>while</u> my brother painted the window frame.
  c Mr Green's car broke down <u>because</u> he never serviced it.
  d I stayed in <u>although</u> it was a sunny day.
  e I washed up <u>while</u> my sister dusted.
  f The streets were like a maze <u>yet</u> Joanne found her way to the hotel.
  g Smeeta arrived home early <u>so</u> she had time to walk the dog.
  h Hurry up <u>or</u> you will be late.

It is often acceptable to change the order of simple sentences when joining them with a conjunction. For example **1d** above might be written: <u>Although</u> it was a sunny day, I stayed in.

2 Mrs King was walking home. She was very tired <u>because</u> she had spent all morning shopping. She stopped <u>and</u> put her heavy bags down. <u>While</u> she waited to get her breath back, she saw a man was hurrying towards her. There was a shout from up the road. A policeman was chasing after the man. <u>Although</u> Mrs King was old, she decided to stop the man. She blocked the pavement with her bags <u>and</u> stood facing him. He shouted for her to get out of the way <u>but</u> she did not move. He swerved round her into the road <u>and</u> at that moment Mrs King put out her foot. The man tripped <u>and</u> fell headlong into the road. He was then arrested by the policeman.

    "That was a brave thing to do, yet dangerous too," the policeman told her. "You could have been hurt."

    "But I wasn't," smiled Mrs King. She was still smiling when she arrived home.

25 Complex sentences

1 These are examples of good complex sentences:
  a They hid the money where no one would find it.
  b She was looking out of the window when the taxi arrived.
  c He had a coffee after he had finished mowing the lawn.
  d He took the dog for a walk before he had his tea.
  e She bought a book which was full of interesting facts about animals.
  f You won't get good marks unless you work hard.

2 a Pat bought a new suit, which made (him/her) look smart.
  b Ben met a man who knew my father.
  c The artist painted a picture which he sold for £300.
  d The people built the house on land owned by my uncle.

3 a He did not look where he was going.
  b She went for a walk before she had her dinner.
  c Sam brought an umbrella even though it was sunny.
  d A girl, who had her arm in a sling, opened the door.

4 These are good examples. Notice the comma which separates the two parts of the sentence.
  a Unless you practise, you will not be picked for the team.
  b Although it looked stormy, she went out without a coat.
  c When I got back from Egypt, I went to see my friend.
  d As it is fine, we will go for a walk.
  e If you do all your homework, you may go out.
  f Because I have spent all my money, I can't buy you an ice cream.
  g Since I saw you last, you have grown quite tall.
  h Until I can play the piano perfectly, I'm going to keep on trying.

5 This is a good example of **b**. Notice the use of commas. Make sure you have made appropriate use of commas in all your own sentences.
  b The cyclist locked up his bike, because there had been several thefts in the area.
    When he arrived home, the cyclist locked up his bike.
    The cyclist, who was worried about theft, locked up his bike.

How to use the Spelling Tests

Your child's Spelling Tests are on pages 34–39. Printed below are the full versions of the Tests which you will read out, with the words printed in **bold** that your child has to spell. You may want to cut these pages out of the book so that your child does not have a chance to see the words.

Carrying out each Test

- Each Test should take about 15 minutes.
- Ask your child to turn to their version of the Spelling Test.
- Read the Test out aloud without stopping. Make sure your child doesn't write anything at this time, but simply follows his/her version of the passage as you read it.
- Read the passage a second time. Every time you come to a word in bold, read it and then pause to allow time for your child to fill in the missing words in the Test paper.
- Encourage your child to attempt each word, even if he/she is not sure. A good guess may be right but blank spaces cannot gain marks.

Correcting mistakes

Mark the Test with your child. If there are mistakes, revise the appropriate spelling rules from Chapters 1–14 of this book. Where the words do not follow any of the rules, your child should use the Look, Say, Cover, Write strategy to learn them.

Spelling Test 1

Camping

The Richards family had chosen a perfect spot for their campsite. It was near to a clear stream, but raised well above it to avoid flooding, and protected from the prevailing wind by a hill.

They had almost finished **putting** up the tent. The ground was firm, and Dad was sure the tent pegs **would** hold well. As he was **busily** hammering in the last of the tent pegs, Sam's **mother** was unpacking their first meal. The forecast said there **might** be rain, but the weather was **sunny** and all Sam's worries **disappeared**. They sat **quietly**, listening to the sound of the birds and the babble of the stream. A few **flies** flew around them and Dad decided to **build** a fire to keep them away.

He **brought** some wood and fire-lighters from the car. Soon a fire was blazing. Sam helped Mum wash the **dishes**. Then they put some **potatoes** in foil to cook in the fire. Sam **stared** into the fire, **imagining** a world of magic in the flames. He was **hoping** that tomorrow they could go **swimming** in a nearby pool. He could not **believe** that it was only three hours since they left home. Now here they were in the **peace** of the countryside. He smiled. This is a great place, he **thought** to himself.

cut here

Spelling Test 2

The Sea Chest

The children never tired of watching the sea. That day the waves rolled onto the beach, breaking up into plumes of spray as they smashed onto the rocks around the sandy bay.

Dark clouds **raced** across the sky. Suddenly the sun broke **through**, casting a shaft of sunlight which struck the **white** waves. In its light a strange object could be seen: a chest **tossed** on the waves. **Forgetting** that the sea was dangerous on such days, Rob **hurried** down the beach. In no time he was **wading** towards the chest. Lucy called to him but her **cries** were lost in the **sound** of the surf and the sea. The chest was being carried **steadily** towards Rob. Then as the waves lifted it as if offering it to him, Rob grabbed one of its **handles**. The sea still supported its **weight** and Rob was able to pull it towards the beach. But as the sea got **shallower** the chest got **heavier**. Lucy came to help him. **Fortunately** they were far from any of the **dangerous** rocks. They **dragged** the chest onto the beach. The box was shut **tight**, but not locked. Rob and Lucy forced open the lid. To their bitter **disappointment** the chest was **completely** empty.

Spelling Test 3

The UFO

Nadia did not believe in UFOs, or unidentified flying objects to give them their proper name. Some people will believe anything, won't they? Little green men in alien spacecraft with flashing lights – what a lot of nonsense! But something was about to happen to change her mind.

Nadia **always** had a party on her **birthday**. The house was full of her **friends**, and so was the **garden**. It was a starry night, filled with the sound of the children's **laughter**. Suddenly someone noticed a green light low over the **houses** opposite. Then the light grew **brighter**. There was a strange **humming** sound as it came over the **roofs**.

"It's a **flying** saucer!" someone cried excitedly.

"There's no **such** thing," replied Nadia, but she **didn't** sound sure. In fact she was **beginning** to feel afraid.

"Did you send them an **invitation**?" someone said. No one **else** thought it funny. The children were standing close **together** watching the flying saucer hovering above them. The light was **different** now, changing colour from green to red. Then suddenly the object shot across the sky, **travelling** to some unknown destination. Nadia began to wonder if there might be **visitors** from other worlds. Was it **likely**? At least it was exciting to think so.

cut here